Cardiovascular MRI in Practice

Cardiovascular MRI in Practice

Edited by Zachary Garcia

AMERICAN
MEDICAL PUBLISHERS
www.americanmedicalpublishers.com

American Medical Publishers,
41 Flatbush Avenue,
1st Floor, New York,
NY 11217, USA

Visit us on the World Wide Web at:
www.americanmedicalpublishers.com

ISBN: 978-1-63927-021-7

Cataloging-in-Publication Data

Cardiovascular MRI in practice / edited by Zachary Garcia.
p. cm.
Includes bibliographical references and index.
ISBN 978-1-63927-021-7
1. Heart--Magnetic resonance imaging. 2. Cardiovascular system--Diseases--Diagnosis.
3. Heart--Imaging. I. Garcia, Zachary.
RC683.5.M35 C373 2022
616.120 754 8--dc23

Table of Contents

Preface IX

Chapter 1 **Quantitative three-dimensional cardiovascular magnetic resonance myocardial perfusion imaging in systole and diastole** 1
Manish Motwani, Ananth Kidambi, Steven Sourbron, Timothy A Fairbairn, Akhlaque Uddin, Sebastian Kozerke, John P Greenwood and Sven Plein

Chapter 2 **Targeted endomyocardial biopsy guided by real-time cardiovascular magnetic resonance** 12
Christina Unterberg-Buchwald, Christian Oliver Ritter, Verena Reupke, Robin Niklas Wilke, Christine Stadelmann, Michael Steinmetz, Andreas Schuster, Gerd Hasenfuß, Joachim Lotz and Martin Uecker

Chapter 3 **Hemorrhage promotes inflammation and myocardial damage following acute myocardial infarction: insights from a novel preclinical model and cardiovascular magnetic resonance** 22
Nilesh R. Ghugre, Mihaela Pop, Reuben Thomas, Susan Newbigging, Xiuling Qi, Jennifer Barry, Bradley H. Strauss and Graham A. Wright

Chapter 4 **Myocardial perfusion is impaired in asymptomatic renal and liver transplant recipients: a cardiovascular magnetic resonance study** 35
Susie Parnham, Jonathan M. Gleadle, Darryl Leong, Suchi Grover, Craig Bradbrook, Richard J. Woodman, Carmine G. De Pasquale and Joseph B. Selvanayagam

Chapter 5 **Unrecognized myocardial infarctions assessed by cardiovascular magnetic resonance are associated with the severity of the stenosis in the supplying coronary artery** 44
Per Hammar, Anna M. Nordenskjöld, Bertil Lindahl, Olov Duvernoy, Håkan Ahlström, Lars Johansson, Nermin Hadziosmanovic and Tomas Bjerner

Chapter 6 **Role of cardiovascular magnetic resonance in the guidelines of the European Society of Cardiology** 53
Florian von Knobelsdorff-Brenkenhoff and Jeanette Schulz-Menger

Chapter 7 **Blood correction reduces variability and gender differences in native myocardial T1 values at 1.5 T cardiovascular magnetic resonance – a derivation/validation approach** 71
Jannike Nickander, Magnus Lundin, Goran Abdula, Peder Sörensson, Stefania Rosmini, James C. Moon, Peter Kellman, Andreas Sigfridsson and Martin Ugander

Chapter 8 **Myocardial perfusion cardiovascular magnetic resonance: optimized dual sequence and reconstruction for quantification** 82
Peter Kellman, Michael S. Hansen, Sonia Nielles-Vallespin, Jannike Nickander, Raquel Themudo, Martin Ugander and Hui Xue

Chapter 9 **Longitudinal assessment of right ventricular structure and function by cardiovascular magnetic resonance in breast cancer patients treated with trastuzumab** 96
Ashita Barthur, Christine Brezden-Masley, Kim A. Connelly, Vinita Dhir, Kelvin K. W. Chan, Rashida Haq, Anish Kirpalani, Joseph J. Barfett, Laura Jimenez-Juan, Gauri R. Karur, Djeven P. Deva and Andrew T. Yan

Chapter 10 **Impaired right ventricular contractile function in childhood obesity and its association with right and left ventricular changes: a cine DENSE cardiac magnetic resonance study** 105
Linyuan Jing, Arichanah Pulenthiran, Christopher D. Nevius, Abba Mejia-Spiegeler, Jonathan D. Suever, Gregory J. Wehner, H. Lester Kirchner, Christopher M. Haggerty and Brandon K. Fornwalt

Chapter 11 **Hyperpolarized ^{13}C urea myocardial first-pass perfusion imaging using velocity-selective excitation** 115
Maximilian Fuetterer, Julia Busch, Sophie M. Peereboom, Constantin von Deuster, Lukas Wissmann, Miriam Lipiski, Thea Fleischmann, Nikola Cesarovic, Christian T. Stoeck and Sebastian Kozerke

Chapter 12 **Cardiovascular magnetic resonance in an adult human population: serial observations from the multi-ethnic study of atherosclerosis** 127
Kihei Yoneyama, Bharath A. Venkatesh, David A. Bluemke, Robyn L. McClelland and João A. C. Lima

Chapter 13 **Fully quantitative cardiovascular magnetic resonance myocardial perfusion ready for clinical use: a comparison between cardiovascular magnetic resonance imaging and positron emission tomography** 138
Henrik Engblom, Hui Xue, Shahnaz Akil, Marcus Carlsson, Cecilia Hindorf, Jenny Oddstig, Fredrik Hedeer, Michael S. Hansen, Anthony H. Aletras, Peter Kellman and Håkan Arheden

Chapter 14 **CMR fluoroscopy right heart catheterization for cardiac output and pulmonary vascular resistance: results in 102 patients** 147
Toby Rogers, Kanishka Ratnayaka, Jaffar M. Khan, Annette Stine, William H. Schenke, Laurie P. Grant, Jonathan R. Mazal, Elena K. Grant, Adrienne Campbell-Washburn, Michael S. Hansen, Rajiv Ramasawmy, Daniel A. Herzka, Hui Xue, Peter Kellman, Anthony Z. Faranesh and Robert J. Lederman

Chapter 15 **Quantitative cardiovascular magnetic resonance perfusion imaging identifies reduced flow reserve in microvascular coronary artery disease** 159
Benjamin Zorach, Peter W. Shaw, Jamieson Bourque, Sujith Kuruvilla, Pelbreton C. Balfour Jr, Yang Yang, Roshin Mathew, Jonathan Pan, Jorge A. Gonzalez, Angela M. Taylor, Craig H. Meyer, Frederick H. Epstein, Christopher M. Kramer and Michael Salerno

Chapter 16 **Adenosine stress CMR T1-mapping detects early microvascular dysfunction in patients with type 2 diabetes mellitus without obstructive coronary artery disease** 167
Eylem Levelt, Stefan K. Piechnik, Alexander Liu, Rohan S. Wijesurendra, Masliza Mahmod, Rina Ariga, Jane M. Francis, Andreas Greiser, Kieran Clarke, Stefan Neubauer, Vanessa M. Ferreira and Theodoros D. Karamitsos

Chapter 17 **Site-specific association between distal aortic pulse wave velocity and peripheral arterial stenosis severity: a prospective cardiovascular magnetic resonance study** 177
Harrie C M van den Bosch, Jos J M Westenberg, Wikke Setz-Pels, John Wondergem, Ron Wolterbeek, Lucien E M Duijm, Joep A W Teijink and Albert de Roos

Chapter 18 **Use of a 1.0 Tesla open scanner for evaluation of pediatric and congenital heart disease** 186
Jimmy C Lu, James C Nielsen, Layne Morowitz, Muzammil Musani, Maryam Ghadimi Mahani, Prachi P. Agarwal, El-Sayed H. Ibrahim and Adam L. Dorfman

Chapter 19 **Measurement of myocardial blood flow by cardiovascular magnetic resonance perfusion: comparison of distributed parameter and Fermi models with single and dual bolus** 194
Giorgos Papanastasiou, Michelle C Williams, Lucy E Kershaw, Marc R Dweck, Shirjel Alam, Saeed Mirsadraee, Martin Connell, Calum Gray, Tom MacGillivray, David E Newby and Scott IK Semple

Chapter 20 **The distribution and prognosis of anomalous coronary arteries identified by cardiovascular magnetic resonance: 15 year experience from two tertiary centres** 204
David P Ripley, Ansuman Saha, Albert Teis, Akhlaque Uddin, Petra Bijsterveld, Ananth Kidambi, Adam K McDiarmid, Mohan Sivananthan, Sven Plein, Dudley J Pennell and John P Greenwood

Permissions

List of Contributors

Index

Preface

This book has been an outcome of determined endeavour from a group of educationists in the field. The primary objective was to involve a broad spectrum of professionals from diverse cultural background involved in the field for developing new researches. The book not only targets students but also scholars pursuing higher research for further enhancement of the theoretical and practical applications of the subject.

The medical imaging technology used for the non-invasive assessment of the function and structure of the cardiovascular system is termed as cardiovascular magnetic resonance imaging. It corresponds to other imaging techniques such as cardiac CT, echocardiography and nuclear medicine. It plays an important role in evidence-based diagnostic and therapeutic pathways in cardiovascular diseases. It helps in the assessment of cardiomyopathies, vascular diseases, myocarditis, congenital heart disease, and myocardial ischemia and other cardiac diseases. It also plays a crucial role in surgical planning in complex congenital heart disease. Cardiovascular magnetic resonance imaging utilizes the basic principles of image reconstruction and acquisition like other MRI techniques. The various advancements in cardiovascular magnetic resonance imaging are glanced at and their applications as well as ramifications are looked at in detail in this book. It elucidates new techniques and their applications in a multidisciplinary manner. This book will serve as a reference to a broad spectrum of readers.

It was an honour to edit such a profound book and also a challenging task to compile and examine all the relevant data for accuracy and originality. I wish to acknowledge the efforts of the contributors for submitting such brilliant and diverse chapters in the field and for endlessly working for the completion of the book. Last, but not the least; I thank my family for being a constant source of support in all my research endeavours.

Editor

1

Quantitative three-dimensional cardiovascular magnetic resonance myocardial perfusion imaging in systole and diastole

Manish Motwani[1], Ananth Kidambi[1], Steven Sourbron[2], Timothy A Fairbairn[1], Akhlaque Uddin[1], Sebastian Kozerke[3], John P Greenwood[1] and Sven Plein[1*]

Abstract

Background: Two-dimensional (2D) perfusion cardiovascular magnetic resonance (CMR) remains limited by a lack of complete myocardial coverage. Three-dimensional (3D) perfusion CMR addresses this limitation and has recently been shown to be clinically feasible. However, the feasibility and potential clinical utility of *quantitative* 3D perfusion measurements, as already shown with 2D-perfusion CMR and positron emission tomography, has yet to be evaluated. The influence of systolic or diastolic acquisition on myocardial blood flow (MBF) estimates, diagnostic accuracy and image quality is also unknown for 3D-perfusion CMR. The purpose of this study was to establish the feasibility of quantitative 3D-perfusion CMR for the detection of coronary artery disease (CAD) and to compare systolic and diastolic estimates of MBF.

Methods: Thirty-five patients underwent 3D-perfusion CMR with data acquired at both end-systole and mid-diastole. MBF and myocardial perfusion reserve (MPR) were estimated on a per patient and per territory basis by Fermi-constrained deconvolution. Significant CAD was defined as stenosis ≥70% on quantitative coronary angiography.

Results: Twenty patients had significant CAD (involving 38 out of 105 territories). Stress MBF and MPR had a high diagnostic accuracy for the detection of CAD in both systole (area under curve [AUC]: 0.95 and 0.92, respectively) and diastole (AUC: 0.95 and 0.94). There were no significant differences in the AUCs between systole and diastole (p values >0.05). At stress, diastolic MBF estimates were significantly greater than systolic estimates (no CAD: 3.21 ± 0.50 vs. 2.75 ± 0.42 ml/g/min, $p < 0.0001$; CAD: 2.13 ± 0.45 vs. 1.98 ± 0.41 ml/g/min, $p < 0.0001$); but at rest, there were no significant differences (p values >0.05). Image quality was higher in systole than diastole (median score 3 vs. 2, $p = 0.002$).

Conclusions: Quantitative 3D-perfusion CMR is feasible. Estimates of MBF are significantly different for systole and diastole at stress but diagnostic accuracy to detect CAD is high for both cardiac phases. Better image quality suggests that systolic data acquisition may be preferable.

Keywords: Cardiovascular magnetic resonance, Perfusion, 3-dimensional, Myocardial perfusion imaging, Ischemic heart disease, Myocardial blood flow

* Correspondence: s.plein@leeds.ac.uk
[1]Multidisciplinary Cardiovascular Research Centre & The Division of Cardiovascular and Diabetes Research, Leeds Institute of Genetics, Health & Therapeutics, University of Leeds, Leeds, UK
Full list of author information is available at the end of the article

Background

Myocardial perfusion imaging with cardiovascular magnetic resonance (CMR) is a highly accurate technique for the detection of coronary artery disease (CAD) [1]. However, conventional acquisition with two-dimensional (2D) methods can only acquire a small number of non-contiguous slices of the left ventricle (LV) at each R-R interval, and therefore incomplete myocardial coverage remains a significant limitation.

Recent technological advances have allowed unprecedented acceleration of dynamic CMR and have led to the development of three-dimensional (3D) myocardial perfusion CMR methods providing full LV coverage with preserved temporal and spatial resolution [2-4]. Three recent studies have shown 3D-perfusion CMR to be clinically feasible and highly accurate for the detection of CAD with visual perfusion assessment [5-7]. However, the feasibility and potential clinical application of deriving quantitative estimates of myocardial blood flow (MBF) from 3D-perfusion CMR has not yet been studied.

A further limitation of conventional 2D-perfusion CMR is that each slice is acquired in a different period of the cardiac cycle. Two recent quantitative studies have shown a significant difference in MBF estimates derived from the same mid-ventricular slice acquired in systole and diastole with 2D-perfusion CMR [8,9]. As well as limiting quantitative comparisons between slices, these significant phasic differences impact on inter-study and longitudinal comparisons of MBF. Unlike 2D-perfusion CMR, 3D imaging allows acquisition of data from the entire myocardium in the same, optimised period of the cardiac cycle. Most previous 3D-perfusion CMR studies have acquired data in systole but to date it is unknown whether systolic or diastolic acquisition leads to better image quality and diagnostic yield. Furthermore, it is unknown whether quantitative estimates of MBF from 3D data demonstrate the same phasic differences previously reported for 2D techniques [8,9].

The purpose of this study was therefore to establish the feasibility of quantitative 3D-perfusion CMR for the detection of coronary artery disease (CAD) and to compare systolic and diastolic estimates of MBF. Defining the optimal cardiac phase for acquisition may be more relevant for 3D than 2D-perfusion CMR because it allows the acquisition of all slices in a particular cardiac phase.

Methods

Population

Forty consecutive patients with known or suspected CAD were recruited. All patients were imaged within 30 days of clinically scheduled diagnostic coronary angiography. No revascularization or clinical events occurred between angiography and CMR. Exclusion criteria were contraindications to CMR, adenosine, or gadolinium contrast agents, recent myocardial infarction (MI) or unstable angina (within 6 months), or poorly controlled arrhythmias. Patients were instructed to refrain from caffeine for 24 hours before their CMR study but continue cardiac medications as normal. The study was approved by the regional ethics committee and all patients gave written consent.

CMR protocol

All studies were performed on a 3.0 T scanner (Achieva TX, Philips Healthcare, Best, The Netherlands) equipped with dual-source parallel radiofrequency transmission technology and a 32-channel cardiac coil. For perfusion imaging, a 3D spoiled turbo gradient-echo sequence was used (TR/TE/flip angle 1.8 ms/0.7 ms/15°; saturation prepulse delay 150 ms; linear *k*-space encoding; 70% partial Fourier acquisition in two dimensions; typical field of view 350 × 350 mm; 10 fold *k-t* acceleration and 11 training profiles leading to a net acceleration of 7.0; typical acquisition duration 192 ms, *k-t* principal component analysis (PCA) reconstruction; reconstructed to 12 contiguous slices with voxel size 2.3×2.3×5 mm^3) [2,7].

Two *k-t* undersampled 3D data sets were acquired in each R-R interval, each preceded by a non-selective saturation prepulse. Vertical and horizontal long-axis cine images were used to identify appropriate trigger delays for systolic and diastolic acquisition [8-10]. Additionally, because of the longitudinal lengthening of the heart from systole to diastole, the position of the end-systolic and mid-diastolic perfusion stacks (12 slices each) were individually planned from the chosen systolic and diastolic cine frames (Figure 1) [8,9]. The same trigger delays were used for stress and rest acquisitions.

Stress perfusion images were acquired during intravenous adenosine-induced hyperemia administered for 4 min at 140mcg/kg/min. Consistent with previous 3D-perfusion CMR studies, an intravenous bolus of 0.075 mmol/kg of gadobutrol (Gadovist, Bayer Schering Pharma, Berlin, Germany) was administered at a rate of 4.0 ml/s followed by a 20 ml saline flush. Stress perfusion CMR was followed by cine imaging covering the left ventricle in 10-12 short-axis sections. Rest perfusion CMR was performed 15 min after stress, using identical imaging parameters. Late gadolinium enhancement (LGE) imaging was acquired in the same short-axis geometry as perfusion imaging after an additional 10-15 min using conventional 2D methods (T1 weighted segmented inversion recovery gradient echo; TR/TE/flip angle 4.9 ms/1.9 ms/15°; inversion time individually adjusted according to Look-Locker scan; spatial resolution 1.35 × 1.35 × 10 mm).

Image quality

Systolic and diastolic perfusion images were analyzed in separate reporting sessions in random order (MM, 2 years

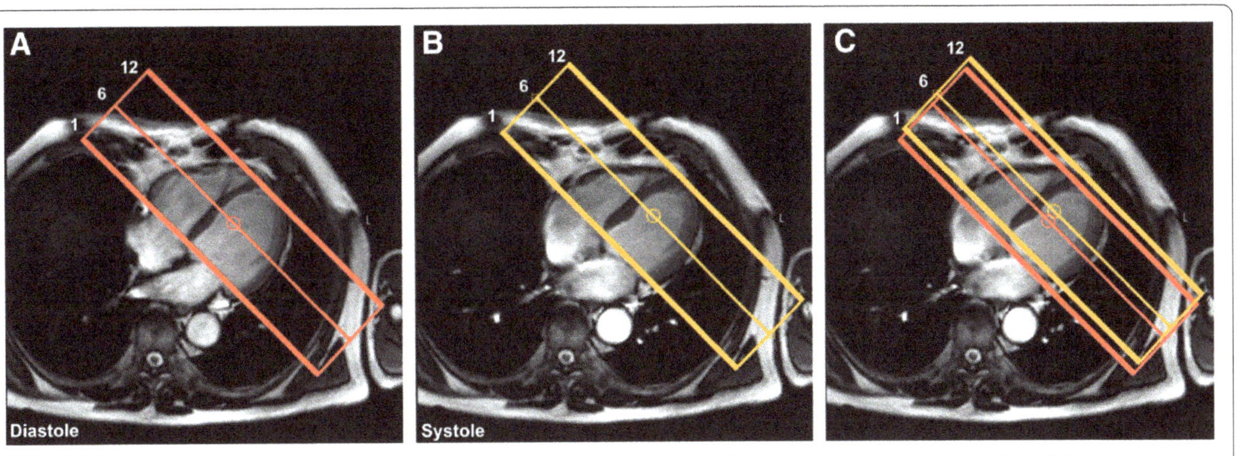

Figure 1 Acquisition planning. Because of the longitudinal lengthening of the heart from systole to diastole, the position of the mid-diastolic (red) and end-systolic perfusion stacks (yellow) (12 slices each) were individually planned from the chosen diastolic (Panel **A**) and systolic (Panel **B**) 4-chamber cine frames. Panel **C** shows both stacks superimposed on the chosen end-systolic frame.

experience of perfusion CMR). Overall image quality was scored as follows: 0 = non-diagnostic, 1 = poor, 2 = adequate and 3 = excellent. The occurrence of artifact related to respiratory-motion, *k-t* reconstruction or dark-rim artifact was scored as follows: 0 = none, 1 = mild, 2 = moderate and 3 = severe.

Myocardial blood flow estimation

Perfusion images were processed offline using previously validated in-house software (PMI 0.4; written in IDL 6.4 (ITT Visual Information Systems, Boulder, CO) [11]. All short-axis slices with clearly identifiable LV cavity enhancement during first-pass perfusion and with >75% circumferential LV myocardium were included in the analysis [5,6].

Per patient analysis

Following manual rigid motion-correction, a circular region of interest (ROI) was drawn in the basal LV cavity in diastole, to derive the arterial input function (AIF). The same (diastolic) AIF was used for both systolic and diastolic estimates of MBF in order to avoid potential variations in the AIF between phases with subsequent effects on MBF estimation [8].

A whole-heart myocardial region of interest (ROI) excluding any dark-rim artifact was drawn for both systolic and diastolic perfusion images (covering all slices containing myocardium). Signal intensity–time data were converted to concentration-time data by subtracting the baseline signal, and global MBF was estimated at stress and rest using constrained deconvolution with a delayed Fermi-model applied to the first pass [9,12,13]. MPR was calculated as stress MBF divided by rest MBF.

Per territory analysis

The above analysis was repeated on a per territory basis using the 17-segment AHA model adjusted for coronary dominance [14]. For this, all slices from an individual patient were first visually allocated to basal, mid or apical sections of the model. For each perfusion territory, a myocardial ROI was then outlined including all segments pertaining to that territory across all slices according to the 17-segment AHA model. MBF and MPR estimates were obtained using the same algorithm as for the whole-heart ROI.

Intra-observer and inter-observer variability

Thirty random territories were re-analyzed 1 month later by the same observer (M.M.) and by a second observer A.K. (2 yrs and 1 yr experience respectively). A.K. was blinded to the results of all previous analyses.

Quantitative coronary angiography

Quantitative coronary angiography was performed (QCA-Plus, Sanders Data Systems, Palo Alto, CA, USA) on anonymised X-ray angiography images (M.M. 6 years experience in coronary angiography). Significant CAD was defined as luminal stenosis ≥70% diameter in any of the main epicardial coronary arteries or their branches with a diameter of ≥2 mm.

Statistical analysis

Analysis was performed using SPSS 17.0 (SPSS, Chicago, IL). Data are presented as mean ± SD. Group means were compared using paired or unpaired Student t-tests; or within-subjects analysis of variance with Greenhouse-Geisser correction for multi-sample sphericity, as appropriate. Ordinal data were compared using the Wilcoxon signed-rank test. Receiver-operating characteristic (ROC) analysis was performed on a per territory basis, to determine the diagnostic accuracy of MPR to detect significant CAD. Diagnostic accuracies are presented as area under the ROC curve (AUC); and were compared between systole and diastole using methods described by Delong and Delong. Optimal MPR cut-off values, for both cardiac phases, were defined as values that maximised the sum of sensitivity and specificity. A secondary ROC analysis was performed to evaluate the diagnostic accuracy of stress MBF diastolic/systolic ratio. To assess reproducibility, the coefficients of variation (CoV) for intra- and inter-observer measurements were calculated. Because three coronary territories were examined per patient, the intra-cluster correlation coefficient (ICC) was calculated for MPR estimates to determine the design effect and the need to adjust data for clustering. All statistical tests were 2-tailed and a p value <0.05 was considered significant.

Results

Study population

Five of the 40 recruited patients were excluded: 3 because of claustrophobia and 2 owing to technical problems (1 mistimed contrast injection; 1 significantly altered patient position between stress and rest scans). A total of 35 patients (105 coronary territories) were therefore available for analysis. Table 1 shows the baseline patient characteristics. QCA confirmed significant CAD in 20 patients (57%) and 38 coronary territories (36%). Only 3 patients had evidence of MI on LGE imaging (the same 3 patients with a clinical history of MI), and this involved only 3 of the 105 territories analysed. Figure 2 shows an example of the stress perfusion images acquired in a patient with significant CAD.

Table 1 Patient characteristics

Parameter	*Data (n = 35)*
Age (yrs ± SD)	62 ± 8
Sex, n (%)	
Male	26 (74)
Female	9 (26)
Risk factors, n (%)	
Hypertension	18 (51)
Hypercholesterolemia	19 (54)
Diabetes Mellitus	6 (17)
Smoking	14 (40)
Previous MI	3 (9)
Previous PCI	3 (9)
Angiography findings, n (%) *	
No significant disease	15 (43)
One-vessel disease	6 (17)
Two-vessel disease	10 (29)
Three -vessel disease	4 (11)
LAD disease	17 (49)
LCX disease	10 (29)
RCA disease	11 (31)

*Significant disease defined as coronary stenosis ≥70% on quantitative coronary analysis.
MI = myocardial infarction; *PCI* = percutaneous coronary intervention; *LAD* = left anterior descending coronary artery; *LCX* = left circumflex coronary artery; *RCA* = right coronary artery.

Image quality

Overall image quality was better in systole than in diastole (median image quality score: 3 vs. 2 respectively; p = 0.002). In diastole, there was a greater frequency of dark-rim artifact (19 patients [54%] vs. 9 patients [26%] and a higher overall artifact score compared to systole (median scores: 1 vs. 0 respectively; p < 0.0001).

In 5 patients (14%), perfusion images (both cardiac phases) were affected by *k-t* reconstruction artifacts at stress and/or rest due to respiratory motion, but all of these artifacts occurred at the end of the breath-hold and did not affect analysis of the first-pass perfusion images.

Myocardial blood flow estimation

Estimates of MBF and MPR for both cardiac phases are seen in Tables 2, 3 and 4. On per patient (n = 35) and per territory analysis (n = 105), mean resting MBF was similar in both cardiac phases (all p values > 0.05); but mean stress MBF and MPR were significantly greater in diastole than systole (all p values <0.001). These relationships existed in normal and CAD subgroups, as well as overall (all p values <0.01) (Tables 2, 3, 4). In both cardiac phases, stress MBF and MPR were significantly lower in the presence of CAD than in normal patients (all p values < 0.01) or normal territories (all p values < 0.0001) (Tables 2, 3, 4).

Analysis of the normal patient group (n = 15) found no significant regional differences in stress MBF, rest MBF or MPR between the LAD, LCX or RCA perfusion territories in both phases (all p values <0.05) (Table 5).

Based on MPR estimates, the ICC for this study was low (r1 =0.09 [95% CI: -0.25 to 0.41]) with a design effect of 1.18 where cluster size = 3. This shows that the study design of using 3 'related' coronary territories per patient (n = 35) to derive a sample size of 105 coronary territories does not significantly diminish statistical power.

Diagnostic performance

Stress MBF

On a per territory analysis (n = 105), the use of stress MBF alone had a high overall diagnostic accuracy for the detection of CAD - which was similar in both cardiac phases (AUC = 0.95 for both; p = 0.70). The optimal stress MBF cut-off value was 2.31 ml/min/g for systole and 2.60 ml/min/g for diastole. At these thresholds, the sensitivity and specificity were 92% and 93% respectively for systole; and 95% and 96% for diastole. There was no significant difference between the diagnostic accuracy of

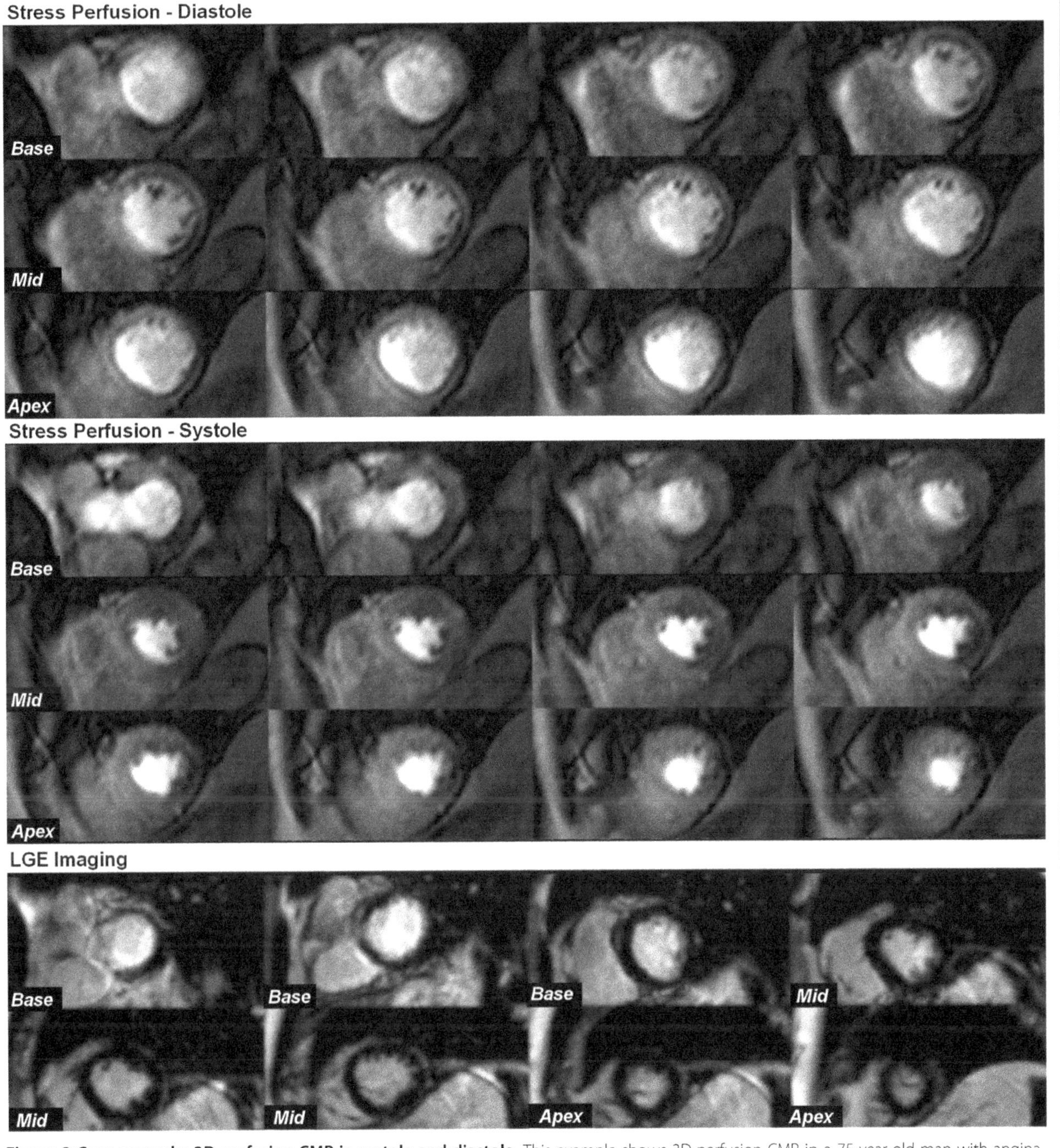

Figure 2 Case example: 3D-perfusion CMR in systole and diastole. This example shows 3D-perfusion CMR in a 75-year-old man with angina. Stress-induced perfusion defects are seen infero-laterally from base to apex and antero-laterally from mid-ventricle to apex in both diastole and systole. However, perfusion defects are difficult to discern from dark-rim artifact in diastole and are more clearly delineated with systolic acquisition. Late-gadolinium enhancement imaging did not reveal any myocardial infarction. X-ray coronary angiography revealed 80% stenosis of a large diagonal branch and significant proximal disease in a large dominant left circumflex artery.

MPR or stress MBF alone for either cardiac phase (both p values >0.05) (Figure 3).

MPR

On per territory analysis ($n = 105$), MPR also had a high overall diagnostic accuracy for the detection of significant CAD, and this was similar in both cardiac phases (AUC, systole: 0.92 vs. diastole: 0.94; $p = 0.41$) (Figure 3). The optimal MPR cut-off value was 1.75 for systole and 2.02 for diastole (Figure 4). At these thresholds, the sensitivity and specificity were 82% and 93% respectively for systole; and 87% and 94% for diastole. The diagnostic accuracy of

Table 2 Estimates of MBF and MPR from 3D perfusion CMR - per patient analysis

	Stress MBF (ml/min/g)			Rest MBF (ml/min/g)			MPR		
	Systole	*Diastole*	*p*	*Systole*	*Diastole*	*p*	*Systole*	*Diastole*	*p*
Normal (n = 15)	2.88 ± 0.32	3.47 ± 0.41	p < 0.0001	1.28 ± 0.17	1.26 ± 0.15	p = 0.45	2.27 ± 0.37	2.78 ± 0.40	p < 0.0001
CAD (n = 20)	2.32 ± 0.42	2.53 ± 0.47	p < 0.0001	1.32 ± 0.19	1.28 ± 0.21	p = 0.06	1.82 ± 0.54	2.08 ± 0.74	p < 0.001
Overall (n = 35)	2.56 ± 0.47	2.93 ± 0.65	p < 0.0001	1.30 ± 0.18	1.27 ± 0.19	p = 0.06	2.01 ± 0.08	2.38 ± 0.05	p < 0.0001

All values expressed as mean ± SD. Coronary artery disease (*CAD*) defined as stenosis ≥70%. *CMR* = cardiovascular magnetic resonance; *MBF* = myocardial blood flow; *MPR* = myocardial perfusion reserve.

MPR to detect CAD in each of the 3 coronary territories is shown in Table 6 and no significant differences were seen between cardiac phases.

Diastolic/systolic stress MBF ratio

The diastolic/systolic stress MBF ratio was significantly lower for territories with CAD than in normal territories (1.07 ± 0.06 vs. 1.17 ± 0.11; p < 0.0001). On ROC analysis, the diagnostic accuracy (AUC) of this ratio to detect significant CAD was 0.79. The optimal cut-off value for the ratio was 1.10 which gave a sensitivity of 82% and specificity of 76% (Figure 5).

Reproducibility

Stress MBF

The mean absolute difference between intra-observer measurements of stress MBF was similar in systole and diastole (0.33 ± 0.14 vs. 0.35 ± 0.16; p = 0.18); and the corresponding CoVs were 16% and 17% respectively. The mean absolute difference between inter-observer measurements of stress MBF was also similar in systole and diastole (0.41 ± 0.22 vs. 0.45 ± 0.20; p = 0.11) with corresponding CoVs of 18% for both.

MPR

The mean absolute difference between intra-observer measurements of MPR was similar in systole and diastole (0.30 ± 0.15 vs. 0.36 ± 0.13; p = 0.09); and the corresponding CoVs were both 18%. The mean absolute difference between inter-observer measurements of MPR was also similar in systole and diastole (0.35 ± 0.17 vs. 0.41 ± 0.15; p = 0.07) with corresponding CoVs of 20% and 21% respectively.

Discussion

The main findings of this study are 1) quantitative 3D-perfusion CMR is feasible and has a high diagnostic accuracy for the detection of CAD; 2) similar to 2D studies, estimates of stress MBF and MPR from 3D data are significantly greater in diastole than systole; and 3) the diastolic dominance of stress MBF estimates is reduced in ischemia.

One of the limitations of myocardial perfusion imaging and standard visual interpretation is the dependence on a reference area of normal perfusion. This is a particular impediment in diffuse or balanced multi-vessel disease. This limitation can be avoided by using absolute quantification of MBF [15]. At present, the most robust technique to quantify MBF noninvasively is positron emission tomography (PET) - but its wide-spread clinical application has been slowed by limited access [16]. PET imaging also involves exposure to ionizing radiation, and its spatial resolution limits evaluation of transmural flow differences in normal thickness myocardium.

Over the last decade, several animal, normal volunteer and patient studies have validated the use of CMR for absolute MBF quantification against microsphere and invasive coronary flow reserve measurements [17-19]. Furthermore, several clinical studies have demonstrated high diagnostic accuracy of CMR derived estimates of absolute MBF and MPR against both QCA and fractional flow reserve [9,13,15,20,21]. Nonetheless, the lack of complete myocardial coverage has been a significant limitation of conventional 2D-perfusion CMR for this purpose.

This study has for the first time demonstrated the feasibility of quantitative whole-heart 3D-perfusion CMR. Shin *et al* have previously reported semi-quantitative measures (time-intensity curve indices) of resting

Table 3 Estimates of MBF and MPR from 3D-perfusion CMR - per territory analysis

	Stress MBF (ml/min/g)			Rest MBF (ml/min/g)			MPR		
	Systole	*Diastole*	*p*	*Systole*	*Diastole*	*p*	*Systole*	*Diastole*	*p*
Normal (n=67)	2.75 ± 0.42	3.21 ± 0.50	p < 0.0001	1.24 ± 0.15	1.25 ± 0.15	p = 0.27	2.26 ± 0.43	2.59 ± 0.44	p < 0.0001
CAD (n=38)	1.98 ± 0.41	2.13 ± 0.55	p < 0.0001	1.24 ± 0.15	1.26 ± 0.14	p = 0.20	1.63 ± 0.14	1.72 ± 0.19	p < 0.01
Overall (n=105)	2.47 ± 0.55	2.82 ± 0.71	p < 0.0001	1.24 ± 0.15	1.25 ± 0.15	p = 0.10	2.03 ± 0.52	2.27 ± 0.61	p < 0.0001

All values expressed as mean ± SD. Coronary artery disease (*CAD*) defined as stenosis ≥70%. *CMR* = cardiovascular magnetic resonance; *MBF* = myocardial blood flow; *MPR* = myocardial perfusion reserve.

Table 4 Regional estimates of MBF and MPR - per territory (n=105)

	Normal			CAD		
	Systole	*Diastole*	*p*	*Systole*	*Diastole*	*p*
Stress MBF (ml/min/g)						
LAD	2.91 ± 0.35	3.43 ± 0.46	p<0.0001	2.11 ± 0.46	2.28 ± 0.52	p<0.001
LCX	2.63 ± 0.33	3.10 ± 0.44	p<0.0001	1.90 ± 0.28	2.04 ± 0.28	p<0.01
RCA	2.77 ± 0.51	3.16 ± 0.55	p<0.0001	1.85 ± 0.39	1.97 ± 0.40	p<0.0001
Rest MBF (ml/min/g)						
LAD	1.26 ± 0.17	1.30 ± 0.17	p=0.10	1.21 ± 0.12	1.23 ± 0.12	p=0.52
LCX	1.26 ± 0.17	1.24 ± 0.13	p=0.56	1.22 ± 0.14	1.20 ± 0.10	p=0.27
RCA	1.20 ± 0.13	1.23 ± 0.15	p=0.28	1.28 ± 0.13	1.24 ± 0.16	p=0.26
MPR						
LAD	2.35 ± 0.42	2.68 ± 0.48	p<0.0001	1.75 ± 0.37	1.87 ± 0.51	p=0.02
LCX	2.12 ± 0.35	2.52 ± 0.38	p<0.0001	1.58 ± 0.32	1.72 ± 0.29	p<0.01
RCA	2.33 ± 0.51	2.59 ± 0.48	p<0.001	1.46 ± 0.34	1.60 ± 0.34	p<0.01

All values expressed as mean ± SD. Coronary artery disease (*CAD*) defined as stenosis ≥70%. *MBF* = myocardial blood flow; *MPR* = myocardial perfusion reserve; *LAD* = left anterior descending coronary artery; *LCX* = left circumflex coronary artery; *RCA*= right coronary artery.

myocardial perfusion from a 3D acquisition in 3 healthy volunteers - but no stress acquisition or absolute MBF quantification was performed [10]. The MBF values derived with 3D-perfusion CMR in normal patients in the present study are comparable to values from PET studies and the previous CMR literature [22,23]. For example, in a large study of 160 healthy men and women with PET, the mean resting MBF was 0.98 ± 0.23 ml/min/g (range 0.59-2.05 ml/min/g) and the mean stress MBF was 3.77 ± 0.85 ml/min/g (range 1.85-5.99 ml/min/g) [23]. Intra- and inter-observer reproducibility for stress MBF and MPR in our study was also similar to that seen in 2D-perfusion CMR and PET studies [24,25].

The finding of lower estimates of stress MBF in systole compared to diastole is consistent with the expected physiology and a number of previous studies. Physiologically, one explanation is that during systole, the effect of adenosine-mediated vasodilatation is diminished by the compression of intramyocardial vessels [26]. Two previous 2D-perfusion CMR studies have shown the same phasic differences with higher stress MBF estimates in diastole, but no difference between the phases at rest [8,9]. One previous 3D-perfusion CMR study confirmed similar semi-quantitative measures of resting myocardial perfusion between systole and diastole - but no stress perfusion was performed [10]. Our study has now demonstrated that these phasic differences are also seen with 3D-perfusion CMR quantification and underline the importance of stating the phase of acquisition in future studies to allow comparison in the literature.

Table 5 Comparison of regional MBF and MPR estimates – in normal patients (n=15)

	Perfusion territory			
	LAD	*LCX*	*RCA*	*p*
Stress MBF (ml/min/g)				
Systole	2.95 ± 0.36	2.66 ± 0.29	2.88 ± 0.46	P=0.11
Diastole	3.51 ± 0.46	3.19 ± 0.27	3.27 ± 0.47	P=0.10
Rest MBF (ml/min/g)				
Systole	1.27 ± 0.17	1.29 ± 0.19	1.20 ± 0.13	p=0.25
Diastole	1.29 ± 0.17	1.27 ± 0.14	1.22 ± 0.15	p=0.47
MPR				
Systole	2.36 ± 0.42	2.10 ± 0.32	2.45 ± 0.53	P=0.06
Diastole	2.76 ± 0.45	2.54 ± 0.33	2.71 ± 0.48	P=0.27

All values expressed as mean ± SD. *MBF* = myocardial blood flow; *MPR* = myocardial perfusion reserve; *LAD* = left anterior descending coronary artery; *LCX* = left circumflex coronary artery; *RCA*= right coronary artery.

Quantitative analysis with MPR yielded high diagnostic accuracies in both systole and diastole (AUC: 0.92 and 0.94 respectively). The optimal MPR cut-off values for detecting significant CAD (1.75 for systole and 2.02 for diastole) were within the range of 1.50–2.06 reported in previous 2D-perfusion CMR studies [9,13,20,21,27]. Recently, in 2D-perfusion CMR, Huber *et al* (n = 31) showed that the use of stress MBF alone had a similar diagnostic accuracy as MPR (AUC 0.92 vs. 0.84 respectively; $p < 0.18$) [11]. Our study has shown a similar finding in 3D-perfusion CMR and the implication is that a rest perfusion sequence could potentially be omitted in quantitative studies, thus reducing both scanning and post-processing times without a loss in diagnostic yield (Figure 3).

The noted reduction in diastolic/systolic stress MBF ratio in territories with CAD is consistent with previous invasive studies measuring coronary flow velocity throughout the cardiac cycle [28]. The loss of diastolic dominance has been explained by the increased influence of a significant stenosis on flow during periods of low vascular resistance

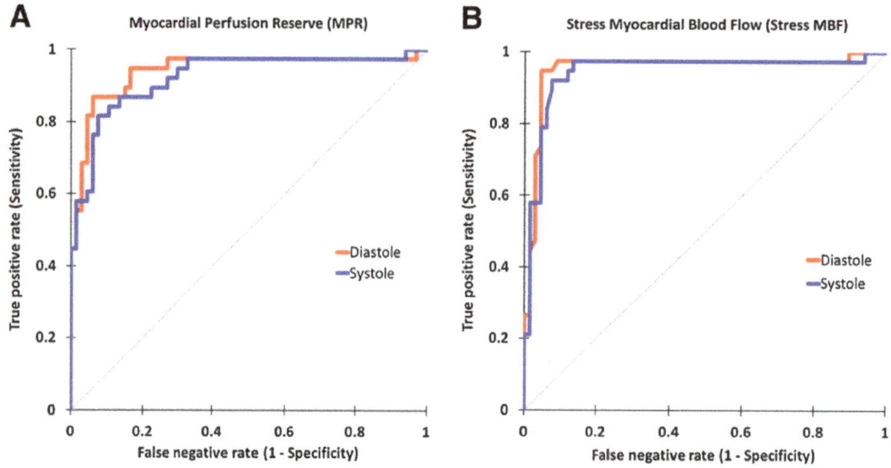

Figure 3 Diagnostic accuracy of quantitative 3D-perfusion CMR. (A) Receiver-operator characteristic curves shows a high diagnostic accuracy in both systole and diastole for MPR (area under curve [AUC]: 0.92 vs. 0.94 respectively; p = 0.41). **(B)** Use of stress MBF alone also had a high diagnostic accuracy in both cardiac phases (AUC: 0.95 for both; p = 0.70) and in fact there was no significant difference compared to MPR (p > 0.05 for both cardiac phases).

and low intramyocardial tension (diastole); as compared with that during periods of high vascular resistance and high intramyocardial tension (systole) [29]. As such, the diastolic/systolic stress MBF ratio is a novel diagnostic index with moderate diagnostic accuracy (AUC = 0.79) – and this may warrant further evaluation in future studies.

In our quantitative study, both phases had similar diagnostic performance and reproducibility. However, similar to previous 2D studies, diastole was more prone to dark-rim artifact with an adverse effect on image quality; and this is thought to relate to the thinner myocardium, making it more prone to partial volume effects at a given spatial resolution [9]. For this reason, as well as the fact that contour delineation is easier in systole because of the thicker myocardium, we would suggest systole as the preferred phase for 3D-perfusion CMR acquisition - particularly for quantitative studies. Although analysis time was not specifically measured, each 3D perfusion dataset took approximately 20 min to analyse on a per patient basis (including stress and rest analyses for either the systolic or diastolic cardiac phase). Quantifying 3D-perfusion CMR can be simpler than quantifying conventional 2D datasets, because as in our study, fewer dynamic images are often acquired and there is a degree

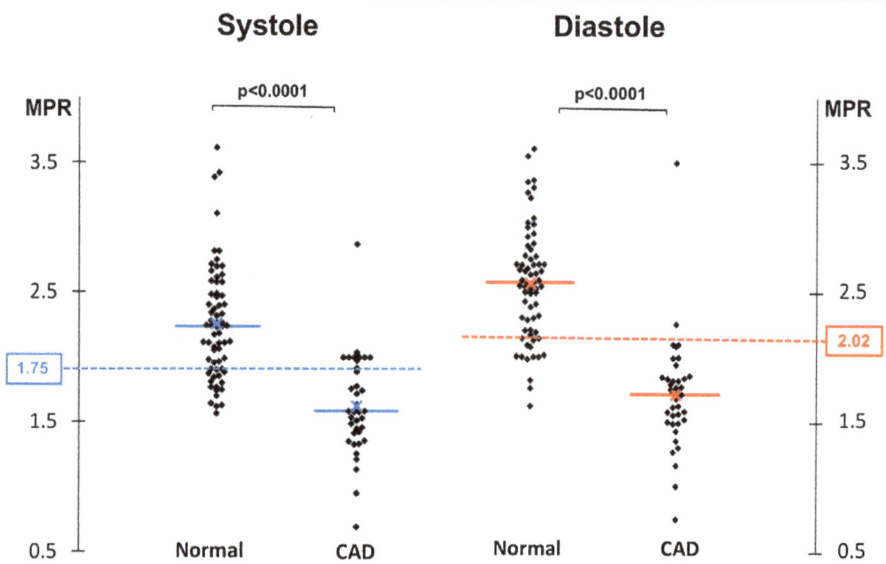

Figure 4 Myocardial perfusion reserve threshold. The scatter-plots show myocardial perfusion reserve (MPR) values from normal and significantly diseased perfusion territories with both systolic and diastolic 3D-perfusion CMR (x = mean value, solid line = median value). The optimal MPR cut-off values determined by receiver-operating characteristic analysis are also plotted (dashed lines, 1.75 for systole and 2.02 for diastole).

Table 6 Diagnostic accuracy of quantitative 3D-perfusion CMR–per territory (n=105)

	AUC for MPR		
	Systole	*Diastole*	*P*
All territories	0.92 (0.87-0.98)	0.94 (0.88-0.99)	p=0.41
LAD	0.89 (0.78-0.99)	0.90 (0.79-1.00)	p=0.76
LCX	0.88 (0.77-0.99)	0.98 (0.93-1.00)	p=0.34
RCA	0.92 (0.86-0.99)	0.98 (0.93-1.00)	p=0.50

Values are area under the curve (*AUC*) and (95% confidence interval). *LAD* = left anterior descending coronary artery; *LCX* = left circumflex coronary artery; *RCA*= right coronary artery.

of temporal filtering due to the undersampling in the temporal domain which reduces the amount of time-consuming manual motion correction required.

Finally, there is considerable scope for quantitative perfusion CMR in clinical practice and therefore demonstrating the feasibility of 3D whole-heart coverage and quantification is important. Nonetheless, there still remain a number of other limitations that hold back the wider clinical adoption of quantitative perfusion CMR. The current lack of standardisation in image acquisition, contrast dosing protocols, post-processing, mathematical modelling and interpretation is addressed by an international standardisation task force [30,31]. There is also no widely available and validated analysis software for quantitative analysis of perfusion CMR data and research groups generally use in-house solutions. Analysis can be time-consuming, precluding routine clinical application. Finally, the incremental value of quantitative analysis of myocardial perfusion CMR analysis needs to be shown in large clinical studies.

Study limitations

The spatio-temporal undersampling methods required for 3D data acquisition are sensitive to respiratory motion, cardiac arrhythmia and low-pass temporal filtering - all of which pose additional challenges to quantitative assessment. Low-pass temporal filtering in particular may lead to underestimation of MBF. We reduced these limitations by use of the constrained *k-t* PCA framework for image reconstruction, which has been shown to improve temporal fidelity, permitting robust measurements of MBF at very high acceleration factors [32]. The latter is also less prone to respiratory artifact as temporal basis functions are derived based on the low-resolution training data acquired in every heartbeat [2].

Although MPR performed well in our study, perfusion imaging is a measurement of the hemodynamic consequences of a stenosis rather than its anatomy, and therefore our use of QCA is an imperfect reference standard. Following this initial feasibility study, future validation against fractional flow reserve is planned in a larger clinical population. Another limitation, common to many previous studies, is the potential effect of data clustering as three perfusion territories are examined per patient [20,27]. However, the design effect of this was low (1.18) owing to a small ICC and cluster size.

Finally, the model used for estimating MBF assumes a linear relation between signal and contrast agent concentration i.e. ignoring saturation effects in the LV blood pool which can lead to underestimation of MBF [33]. This is particularly relevant as we used a relatively high contrast agent dose of 0.075 mmol/kg bodyweight to be consistent with previous 3D-perfusion CMR studies. Proposed solutions include the use of a non-linear signal model combined with precontrast T1-mapping and/or the use of a small pre-bolus to measure the AIF. There is currently no evidence that either of these potential solutions actually leads to improved diagnostic accuracy for the detection of CAD in the clinical setting. In fact

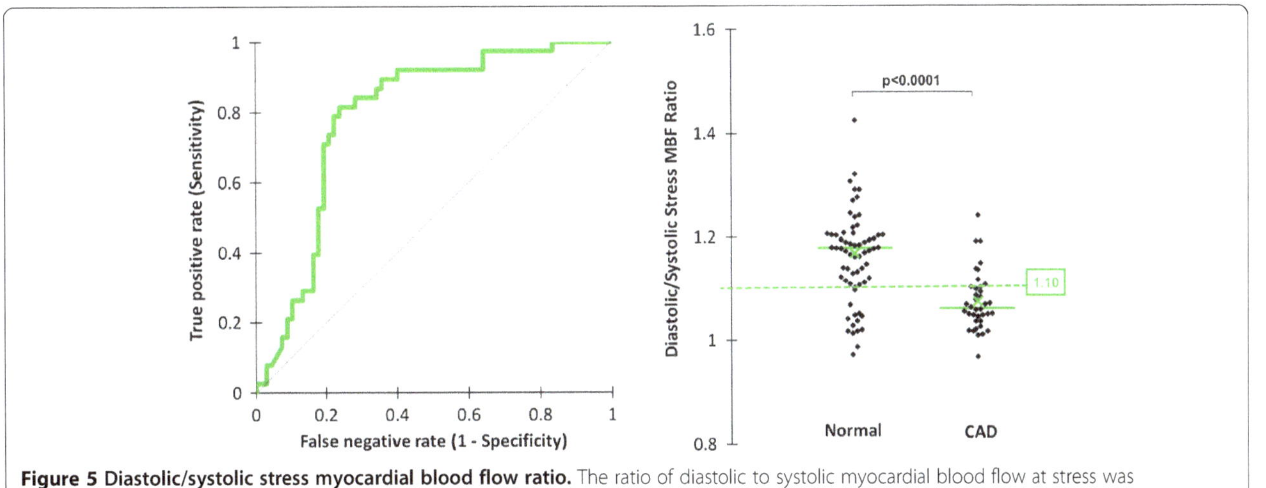

Figure 5 Diastolic/systolic stress myocardial blood flow ratio. The ratio of diastolic to systolic myocardial blood flow at stress was significantly lower for territories with coronary artery disease (CAD) than in normal territories (1.07 ± 0.06 vs. 1.17 ± 0.11; p < 0.0001). On receiver-operator characteristic analysis, the diagnostic accuracy (area under the curve) of this ratio to detect significant CAD was 0.79. The optimal cut-off value for the ratio was 1.10, which gave a sensitivity of 82% and specificity of 76%.

the only study directly addressing this question came to the opposite conclusion i.e. the use of a pre-bolus AIF was found to reduce diagnostic accuracy compared to a single-bolus approach [34].

Conclusions

We have shown that quantitative 3D-perfusion CMR is feasible and can be used to detect CAD with high diagnostic accuracy. In addition, we have found that there are significant differences in systolic and diastolic MBF estimates. Both cardiac phases provide comparable diagnostic yield, albeit at different thresholds. Because systolic images had fewer artifacts and higher image quality, systole may be the preferred phase for acquisition of 3D perfusion data.

Abbreviations

CAD: Coronary artery disease; CMR: Cardiovascular magnetic resonance; MBF: Myocardial blood flow; MPR: Myocardial perfusion reserve; *k-t*: *k*-space and time; PCA: Principal component analysis; ROI: Region of interest; AIF: Arterial input function; AUC: Area-under-the-curve; ROC: Receiver-operator characteristic.

Competing interests

The authors declare that they have no competing interests. SP and AK are funded by a British Heart Foundation Senior Clinical Research Fellowship (FS/1062/28409). SP and JPG receive an educational research grant from Philips Healthcare.

Authors' contributions

MM: conception and design, acquisition, analysis and interpretation of data, drafting of manuscript; AK: acquisition, analysis and interpretation of data, critical and intellectual revision of manuscript; SS: analysis and interpretation of data, critical and intellectual revision of manuscript; TAF: critical and intellectual revision of manuscript; AU: acquisition of data, critical and intellectual revision of manuscript; SK: critical and intellectual revision of manuscript; JPG: interpretation of data, critical and intellectual revision of manuscript; SP: conception and design, interpretation of data, critical and intellectual revision of manuscript. All authors read and approved the final manuscript.

Acknowledgements

We thank Gavin Bainbridge, Margaret Saysell and Caroline Richmond (radiographers) for their technical assistance; and Petra Bijsterveld and Fiona Richards (research nurses) for their assistance with patient recruitment.

Author details

[1]Multidisciplinary Cardiovascular Research Centre & The Division of Cardiovascular and Diabetes Research, Leeds Institute of Genetics, Health & Therapeutics, University of Leeds, Leeds, UK. [2]Division of Medical Physics, University of Leeds, Leeds, UK. [3]Institute for Biomedical Engineering, University and ETH Zurich, Zurich, Switzerland.

References

1. Greenwood JP, Maredia N, Younger JF, Brown JM, Nixon J, Everett CC, Bijsterveld P, Ridgway JP, Radjenovic A, Dickinson CJ, Ball SG, Plein S. **Cardiovascular magnetic resonance and single-photon emission computed tomography for diagnosis of coronary heart disease (CE-MARC): a prospective trial.** *Lancet.* 2012; **379:**453–460.
2. Vitanis V, Manka R, Giese D, Pedersen H, Plein S, Boesiger P, Kozerke S. **High resolution three-dimensional cardiac perfusion imaging using compartment-based k-t principal component analysis.** *Magn Reson Med.* 2011; **65:**575–587.
3. Shin T, Nayak KS, Santos JM, Nishimura DG, Hu BS, McConnell MV. **Three-dimensional first-pass myocardial perfusion MRI using a stack-of-spirals acquisition.** *Magn Reson Med.* 2013; **69:**839–844.
4. Chen L, Adluru G, Schabel MC, McGann CJ, Dibella EV. **Myocardial perfusion MRI with an undersampled 3D stack-of-stars sequence.** *Med Phys.* 2012; **39:**5204–5211.
5. Manka R, Jahnke C, Kozerke S, Vitanis V, Crelier G, Gebker R, Schnackenburg B, Boesiger P, Fleck E, Paetsch I. **Dynamic 3-dimensional stress cardiac magnetic resonance perfusion imaging: detection of coronary artery disease and volumetry of myocardial hypoenhancement before and after coronary stenting.** *J Am Coll Cardiol.* 2011; **57:**437–444.
6. Manka R, Paetsch I, Kozerke S, Moccetti M, Hoffmann R, Schroeder J, Reith S, Schnackenburg B, Gaemperli O, Wissmann L, Wyss CA, Kaufmann PA, Corti R, Boesiger P, Marx N, Lüscher TF, Jahnke C. **Whole-heart dynamic three-dimensional magnetic resonance perfusion imaging for the detection of coronary artery disease defined by fractional flow reserve: determination of volumetric myocardial ischaemic burden and coronary lesion location.** *Eur Heart J.* 2012; **33:**2016–2024.
7. Jogiya R, Kozerke S, Morton G, De Silva K, Redwood S, Perera D, Nagel E, Plein S. **Validation of dynamic 3-dimensional whole heart magnetic resonance myocardial perfusion imaging against fractional flow reserve for the detection of significant coronary artery disease.** *J Am Coll Cardiol.* 2012; **60:**756–765.
8. Radjenovic A, Biglands JD, Larghat A, Ridgway JP, Ball SG, Greenwood JP, Jerosch-Herold M, Plein S. **Estimates of systolic and diastolic myocardial blood flow by dynamic contrast-enhanced MRI.** *Magn Reson Med.* 2010; **1703:**1696–1703.
9. Motwani M, Fairbairn TA, Larghat A, Mather AN, Biglands JD. **Systolic Versus Diastolic Acquisition in Myocardial Perfusion MR Imaging.** *Radiology.* 2012; **262:**816–23.
10. Shin T, Pohost GM, Nayak KS. **Systolic 3D first-pass myocardial perfusion MRI: Comparison with diastolic imaging in healthy subjects.** *Magn Reson Med.* 2010; **63:**858–64.
11. Huber A, Sourbron S, Klauss V, Schaefer J, Bauner KU, Schweyer M, Reiser M, Rummeny E, Rieber J. **Magnetic resonance perfusion of the myocardium: semiquantitative and quantitative evaluation in comparison with coronary angiography and fractional flow reserve.** *Invest Radiol.* 2012; **47:**332–338.
12. Jerosch-Herold M, Wilke N, Stillman AE, Wilson RF. **Magnetic resonance quantification of the myocardial perfusion reserve with a Fermi function model for constrained deconvolution.** *Med Phys.* 1998; **25:**73–84.
13. Costa MA, Shoemaker S, Futamatsu H, Klassen C, Angiolillo DJ, Nguyen M, Siuciak A, Gilmore P, Zenni MM, Guzman L, Bass TA, Wilke N. **Quantitative magnetic resonance perfusion imaging detects anatomic and physiologic coronary artery disease as measured by coronary angiography and fractional flow reserve.** *J Am Coll Cardiol.* 2007; **50:**514–522.
14. Cerqueira MD, Weissman NJ, Dilsizian V, Jacobs AK, Kaul S, Laskey WK, Pennell DJ, Rumberger JA, Ryan T, Verani MS. **Standardized myocardial segmentation and nomenclature for tomographic imaging of the heart: a statement for healthcare professionals from the Cardiac Imaging Committee of the Council on Clinical Cardiology of the American Heart Association.** *Circulation.* 2002; **105:**539–542.
15. Patel AR, Antkowiak PF, Nandalur KR, West AM, Salerno M, Arora V, Christopher J, Epstein FH, Kramer CM. **Assessment of Advanced Coronary Artery Disease Advantages of Quantitative Cardiac Magnetic Resonance Perfusion Analysis.** *J Am Coll Cardiol.* 2010; **56:**561–569.
16. Kajander SA, Joutsiniemi E, Saraste M, Pietilä M, Ukkonen H, Saraste A, Sipilä HT, Teräs M, Mäki M, Airaksinen J. **Clinical Value of Absolute Quantification of Myocardial Perfusion With 15O-Water in Coronary Artery Disease Clinical Perspective.** *Circ Cardiovasc Imaging.* 2011; **4:**678–684.
17. Christian TF, Rettmann DW, Aletras AH, Liao SL, Taylor JL, Balaban RS, Arai AE. **Absolute Myocardial Perfusion in Canines Measured by Using Dual-Bolus First-Pass MR Imaging.** *Radiology.* 2004; **232:**677–684.
18. Jerosch-Herold M, Swingen C, Seethamraju RT. **Myocardial blood flow quantification with MRI by model-independent deconvolution.** *Med Phys.* 2002; **29:**886–897.
19. Wilke N, Jerosch-Herold M, Wang Y, Huang Y, Christensen BV, Stillman AE, Ugurbil K, McDonald K, Wilson RF. **Myocardial perfusion reserve: assessment with multisection, quantitative, first-pass MR imaging.** *Radiology.* 1997; **204:**373–384.

20. Lockie T, Ishida M, Perera D, Chiribiri A, De Silva K, Kozerke S, Marber M, Nagel E, Rezavi R, Redwood S, Plein S. **High-resolution magnetic resonance myocardial perfusion imaging at 3.0-Tesla to detect hemodynamically significant coronary stenoses as determined by fractional flow reserve.** *J Am Coll Cardiol.* 2011; **57:**70–75.
21. Futamatsu H, Wilke N, Klassen C, Shoemaker S, Angiolillo DJ, Siuciak A, Morikawa-Futamatsu K, Suzuki N, von Ziegler F, Bass TA, Costa MA. **Evaluation of cardiac magnetic resonance imaging parameters to detect anatomically and hemodynamically significant coronary artery disease.** *Am Heart J.* 2007; **154:**298–305.
22. Sdringola S, Johnson NP, Kirkeeide RL, Cid E, Gould KL. **Impact of Unexpected Factors on Quantitative Myocardial Perfusion and Coronary Flow Reserve in Young, Asymptomatic Volunteers.** *J Am Coll Cardiol Img.* 2011; **4:**402–412.
23. Chareonthaitawee P, Kaufmann PA, Rimoldi O, Camici PG. **Heterogeneity of resting and hyperemic myocardial blood flow in healthy humans.** *Cardiovasc Res.* 2001; **50:**151–161.
24. Morton G, Chiribiri A, Ishida M, Hussain ST, Schuster A, Indermuehle A, Perera D, Knuuti J, Baker S, Hedström E, Schleyer P, O'Doherty M, Barrington S, Nagel E. **Quantification of absolute myocardial perfusion in patients with coronary artery disease: comparison between cardiovascular magnetic resonance and positron emission tomography.** *J Am Coll Cardiol.* 2012; **60:**1546–1555.
25. Larghat AM, Maredia N, Biglands J, Greenwood JP, Ball SG, Jerosch-Herold M, Radjenovic A, Plein S. **Reproducibility of first-pass cardiovascular magnetic resonance myocardial perfusion.** *J Magn Reson Imaging.* 2013; **874:**865–874.
26. Hiramatsu O, Goto M, Yada T, Kimura A, Chiba Y, Tachibana H, Ogasawara Y, Tsujioka K, Kajiya F. **In vivo observations of the intramural arterioles and venules in beating canine hearts.** *J Physiol.* 1998; **509:**619–628.
27. Rieber J, Huber A, Erhard I, Mueller S, Schweyer M, Koenig A, Schiele TM, Theisen K, Siebert U, Schoenberg SO, Reiser M, Klauss V. **Cardiac magnetic resonance perfusion imaging for the functional assessment of coronary artery disease: a comparison with coronary angiography and fractional flow reserve.** *Eur Heart J.* 2006; **27:**1465–1471.
28. Segal J, Kern MJ, Scott NA, King SB, Doucette JW, Heuser RR, Ofili E, Siegel R. **Alterations of phasic coronary artery flow velocity humans during percutaneous coronary angioplasty.** *J Am Coll Cardiol.* 1992; **20:**276–286.
29. Spaan JA, Breuls NP, Laird JD. **Diastolic-systolic coronary flow differences are caused by intramyocardial pump action in the anesthetized dog.** *Circ Res.* 1981; **49:**584–593.
30. Kramer CM, Barkhausen J, Flamm SD, Kim RJ, Nagel E. **Standardized cardiovascular magnetic resonance (CMR) protocols 2013 update.** *J Cardiovasc Magn Reson.* 2013; **15:**91.
31. Schulz-Menger J, Bluemke DA, Bremerich J, Flamm SD, Fogel MA, Friedrich MG, Kim RJ, von Knobelsdorff-Brenkenhoff F, Kramer CM, Pennell DJ, Plein S, Nagel E. **Standardized image interpretation and post processing in cardiovascular magnetic resonance: Society for Cardiovascular Magnetic Resonance (SCMR) Board of Trustees Task Force on Standardized Post Processing.** *J Cardiovasc Magn Reson.* 2013; **15:**35.
32. Pedersen H, Kozerke S, Ringgaard S, Nehrke K, Kim WY. **k-t PCA: temporally constrained k-t BLAST reconstruction using principal component analysis.** *Magn Reson Med.* 2009; **62:**706–716.
33. Sourbron S. **Technical aspects of MR perfusion.** *Eur J Radiol.* 2010; **76:**304–313.
34. Groothuis JG, Kremers FP, Beek AM, Brinckman SL, Tuinenburg AC, Jerosch-Herold M, van Rossum AC, Hofman MB. **Comparison of dual to single contrast bolus magnetic resonance myocardial perfusion imaging for detection of significant coronary artery disease.** *J Magn Reson Imaging.* 2010; **32:**88–93.

2

Targeted endomyocardial biopsy guided by real-time cardiovascular magnetic resonance

Christina Unterberg-Buchwald[1,3,6*†], Christian Oliver Ritter[3,6†], Verena Reupke[2], Robin Niklas Wilke[3,6], Christine Stadelmann[4], Michael Steinmetz[3,5], Andreas Schuster[1,3], Gerd Hasenfuß[1,3], Joachim Lotz[3,6] and Martin Uecker[3,6]

Abstract

Background: Endomyocardial biopsies (EMB) are an important diagnostic tool for myocarditis and other infiltrative cardiac diseases. Routinely, biopsies are obtained under fluoroscopic guidance with a substantial radiation burden. Despite procedural success, there is a large sampling error caused by missing the affected myocardium. Therefore, multiple (>6) biopsies are taken in the clinical setting. In cardiovascular magnetic resonance (CMR), late gadolinium enhancement (LGE) depicts areas of affected myocardium in myocarditis or in other infiltrative cardiomyopathies. Thus, targeted biopsy under real-time CMR image guidance might reduce the problem of sampling error.

Methods: Seven minipigs of the Goettingen strain underwent radiofrequency ablation in the left ventricle. At least two focal lesions were induced on the lateral wall in five and the apex in two animals. Each ablation lesion was created by two consecutive 30 sec ablations (max. 30 W, temperature 60–64 °C). Biopsies were taken immediately after lesion induction using a commercially available 7 F conventional bioptome under fluoroscopic guidance at the ablation site. Afterwards the animals underwent CMR and lesion visualization by LGE at 3T. The lesions were then targeted and biopsied under CMR-guidance using a MR-conditional bioptome guided by a steerable catheter. Interactive real-time (RT) visualization of the intervention on an in-room monitor was based on radial FLASH with nonlinear inverse reconstruction (NLINV) at a temporal resolution of 42 ms. All samples underwent a standard histological evaluation.

(Continued on next page)

* Correspondence: unterberg@med.uni-goettingen.de
†Equal contributors
[1]University Medical Center Goettingen, Clinic of Cardiology and Pneumology, Goettingen, Germany
[3]DZHK (German Centre for Cardiovascular Research), Partner Site Goettingen, Berlin, Germany
[6]University Medical Center Goettingen, Institute for Diagnostic and Interventional Radiology, Goettingen, Germany
Full list of author information is available at the end of the article

(Continued from previous page)

Results: Radiofrequency ablation was successful in all animals. Fluoroscopy-guided biopsies were performed with a success rate of 6/6 minipigs - resulting in a nonlethal pericardial effusion in one animal. Visualization of radiofrequency lesions by CMR was successful in 7/7 minipig, i.e. at least one lesion was clearly visible. Localization and tracking of the catheters and the bioptome using interactive control of the imaging plane was achieved in 6/6 MP; however in the animal with a large pericardial effusion after EMB under fluoroscopy no further EMB was attempted for safety reasons. Biopsies under interactive RT-CMR guidance were successfully performed in 5/6 animals, in one animal the bioptome reached the lesion, however the forceps did not cut out a sample. Specimens obtained under CMR guidance contained part of the lesion in 6/15 (40%) myocardial specimens and in 4/5 (80%) animals in which samples were achieved. Conventional biopsies revealed ablation lesions in 4/17 (23.5%) specimens in 3/6 minipigs (50%).

Conclusion: Focal lesions induced by radiofrequency ablation in a minipig model are a useful tool for CMR-guided biopsy studies. In contrast to fluoroscopy, CMR provides excellent visualization of lesions. Interactive real-time CMR allows excellent passive tracking of the instruments and EMB provides significantly superior sampling accuracy compared to fluoroscopy-guided biopsies. Nonetheless, further improvements of MR-compatible bioptomes and guiding catheters are essential before applying this method in a clinical setting.

Keywords: Endomyocardial biopsy, CMR, Targeted biopsy, Real-time MRI

Background

Endomyocardial biopsies (EMB) are an important diagnostic tool in myocarditis, arrhythmias, cardiac tumors, storage disease, cardiac allograft rejection and other cardiac diseases with unknown origin. With DNA and RNA detection EMB evolved into an important diagnostic tool [1, 2] proposed by the AHA and ACC [3] as well as ESC [4]. However, there are concerns about the large sampling error and the adequate clinical setting for biopsies is still in debate. Therefore, in today's clinical routine multiple (5–6) biopsies are taken from either the left or right ventricle under fluoroscopic guidance with a radiation burden for the patient and the interventionalist. Despite procedural success with overall (major and minor) complication rates from 0% [5] to 5% [6, 7] missing the affected myocardium results in a limited diagnostic value providing a diagnostic result in only 25.5% of clinical cases [6]. Thus, it seems desirable to use a method for visualization of the diseased parts of the heart in order to take directed samples from the affected myocardium. Cardiovascular magnetic resonance (CMR) has a superior soft-tissue contrast compared to X-ray [8, 9] and allows arbitrary orientation of the imaging plane in three dimensions without exposure to ionizing radiation. Hence, targeted EMB under real-time CMR guidance could solve the sampling problem by reducing the need for multiple biopsies. Nevertheless, interventional CMR has to solve several technical challenges. First, MR-safe and suitable guidewires as well as steerable guiding catheters with distal-tip visualization are mandatory to navigate and reliably reach the affected myocardium. Furthermore, the magnetic field does not allow the use of conventional metallic bioptomes due to heating, magnetization and massive metal artifacts. Until now, MR biopsies are mostly applied in non moving organs like breast [10], liver [11], kidney [12], prostate [13] or brain [14] using MR-compatible needles. MR-safe cardiac bioptomes are still not commonly available. Lossnitzer [15] evaluated a preclinical MR-conditional bioptome in an ex vivo animal heart model. The NIH group [16] recently demonstrated the feasibility of CMR-guided EMB in an in vivo swine model with extended infarct scars. However, clinically many cardiac conditions are associated with small circumscript lesions rendering targeted biopsies even more challenging. Therefore, we developed an animal model with distinct left ventricular lesions created by controlled radiofrequency ablation. The aim of our study was to show that targeted EMB of focal myocardial lesions is feasible by real-time CMR guidance using a clinical 3T scanner, i.e. that continuous real-time CMR in three dimensions enables a controlled positioning of the guidewire, the guiding catheter, the bioptome and the biopsy itself. Furthermore, we aimed at showing that targeted biopsy has a lower sampling error under real-time CMR compared to fluoroscopically controlled biopsies.

Methods

Animal model

Seven minipigs of the Goettingen strain weighing 30–46 kg and aged 12–24 months received diazepam at a dosage of 0.5 mg/kg oral and 2 mg/kg azaperone and 10 mg/kg ketamine i.m. as premedication. Anesthesia was induced by 40–60 mg of propofol and 100–150 μg of fentanyl. Anesthesia was maintained by 3–4 Vol% of sevoflurane in 50% oxygen and 50% air and 5–10 μg/kg/h fentanyl. Postoperative analgesia was provided by 50 mg/kg metamizole i.v. and 2.2 mg/kg flunixin i.m..

Blood gases were regularly monitored and ventilation was adjusted to maintain blood gases in the physiologic range. Surface electrocardiogram, concentration of carbon dioxide and oxygen level in the blood were monitored using MR-compatible LCD monitoring system (Precess 3160, Invivo, Orlando, Florida, USA).

All experiments consisted of five parts:

1. radiofrequency ablation in the left ventricle for creation of circumscript lesions under fluoroscopic guidance,
2. endomyocardial biopsy (aim: 3 specimens) under fluoroscopic guidance,
3. standardized CMR for characterization and lesion localization,
4. targeted endomyocardial biopsy using real-time MRI (aim: 3 specimens),
5. histology of the obtained endomyocardial biopsies.

A femoral artery ($n = 4$) or a carotid artery ($n = 3$) was punctured and a 10 French (F) introducer sheath was placed. A standard 7 F (in one case 5 F) deflectable ablation catheter (4-mm electrode without cooling, Marinr™, Medtronic, USA) was advanced into the left ventricle under fluoroscopic guidance. The intracardiac electrogram (ECG) was recorded by a dedicated electrophysiology system (Prucka, GE Healthcare, USA). Radiofrequency lesions were created on the endocardial surface with a clinical-grade radiofrequency generator (HAT 300 S, Osypka, Germany) using a power-controlled mode at 30 W for 30 s (once) or 2x30s at all other ablation sites. The ablation catheter was positioned to the lateral wall. Position was controlled via angulation of the c-arm x-ray in 30° RAO and 45° LAO (Siremobil, Siemens Healthineers, Erlangen, Germany). The intracardiac electrogram (bipolar with sharp ventricular potential and no atrial electrogram) was monitored. No other cardiac imaging – either echocardiogram, cardiac ventriculography or computer tomography - was performed prior to radiofrequency ablation and X-ray guided endomyocardial biopsy. At least 15 min. post ablation an 8.5 F deflectable guiding catheter was introduced into the left ventricle. The guiding catheter (St.Jude Medical, St. Paul, USA, Fast-Cath, SRO, 8.5 F) was advanced to the ablated myocardium under fluoroscopic guidance using the same angulations of the radiofrequency procedure with help of the stored pictures of the radiofrequency ablation sites as guidance. Endomyocardial biopsies were then taken utilizing a conventional 5.5 F cardiac bioptome (biopsy forceps Cordis, Cardinal Health, Dublin, Ireland; volume of samples approx. 2.46 mm^3) (Fig. 1). Time from introduction to extraction of the guiding catheter varied between 15–25 min for all biopsies. Ablations and biopsies under X-ray and under CMR were performed by one cardiologist with more than 20 years' experience in cardiac interventions (radiofrequency-ablations, angioplasties and biopsies) with the help of an interventional radiologist (>15 years' experience in interventions).

CMR

The animal was then placed into a 3T clinical MR scanner (Skyra, Siemens Healthineers, Erlangen, Germany). A cardiac 18-channel body array receive coil (Siemens Healthineers, Erlangen, Germany) was positioned on the chest. After standard T1-weighted scout images, images for function were obtained with standard bSSFP sequences in standard views (three long axis views and a stack of short axis views) followed by real-time movies using radial bSSFP with NLINV reconstruction (temporal resolution 33 ms; spatial resolution: 1.6 mm × 1.6 mm; slice thickness: 6 mm; FOV: 256 mm × 256 mm; matrix size: 160 × 160; TR = 2.56 ms; TE = 1.28 ms; flip angle: 26^0; bandwidth 1270 HZ/pixel; 13 projections per frame) [17]. For LGE 1 mmol/kg body weight gadobutrol (Gd-BT-DO3A, Gadovist®, Bayer

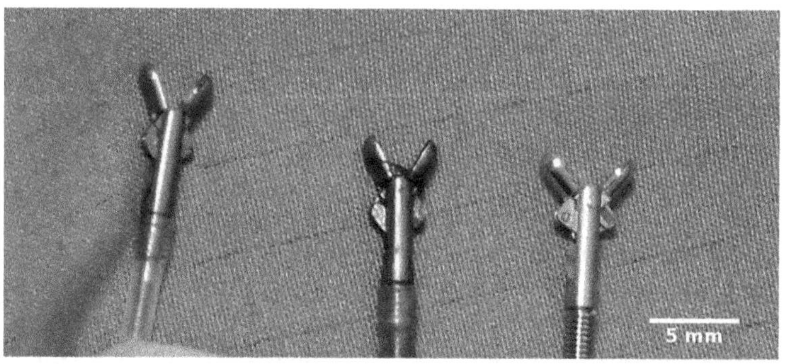

Fig. 1 Bioptomes. Bioptomes with forceps in the open state: the two bioptomes on the left are MR-conditional, the one on the right hand is a standard steel bioptome employed for EMB under fluoroscopic guidance. Notably, the standard bioptome achieves a maximum opening angle of about 90° whereas the MR-bioptomes only open at a maximum angle of about 50–70°

Schering Pharma AG, Leverkusen, Germany) was injected intravenously. Scars were depicted 15 mins after contrast injection using a standardized inversion recovery turboFLASH technique (spatial resolution 1.4 mm × 1.4 mm; slice thickness: 4 mm; FOV: 360 mm × 360 mm; matrix size: 256 × 256; retrospective gating; TR = 919 ms; TE = 1.41 ms, flip angle: 40^0; bandwidth 780 Hz/pixel).

An 8.5 F deflectable guiding catheter (Innovative Tomography Products, Bochum, Germany) with a 0.035 inch MR-conditional guidewire (MaRVis Medical, Hannover, Germany) was introduced into the left ventricle by a retrograde approach. The wire consists of glass and aramid fibers as well as epoxy resin. Metal particles are embedded in an envelope polymer and covered by a polytetrafluoroethylene shrink tube as the outer surface (information is provided on the website of the manufacturer [18]). The guiding catheter is comparable to a standard deflectable catheter but the braiding is replaced by special nonmetallic fibers. These are also part of the traction element. The distal tip is visible due to a very small ring made of nonmagnetic steel. This allows visualization under MRI as well as under X-ray. The artifacts under CMR are very small (see Additional file 1: Video). A multi-GPU computing system (BiomedNMR, Göttingen, Germany) designed for low-latency online image reconstruction was used with radial FLASH sequences for interactive real-time MRI [19]. This system allowed for immediate image display of real-time images and fast interactive sequence control. Here, a radial FLASH sequence with NLINV reconstruction optimized for interactive real-time MRI was used (temporal resolution: 42 ms; spatial resolution: 2 mm × 2 mm; slice thickness: 8 mm; FOV: 256 mm × 256 mm; matrix size: 128 × 128; TR = 2.02 ms, TE = 1.3 ms, flip angle: 8°, bandwidth: 1700 Hz/pixel, 21 projections per frame) [19]. In particular, images could be shown on the operating console of and on a MR-compatible in-room monitor (NordicNeuroLab, Bergen, Norway) with a time-delay of about 0.27 s providing an excellent visual feedback for the interventionalist. The time-delay includes the time for acquisition, data transfer, image reconstruction, post-processing and image display. It was measured by simultaneously tracking the motion of a moving water phantom using the real-time CMR sequence with the same parameters as during intervention and visible laser light. During an intervention, procedural adjustments of the image planes were performed by a trained technician at the console outside the scanner room cage based on communication with the interventionalist inside using the Imroc IR™ communication system (Optoacoustics, Mazov, Israel). Lesion size and location were clearly depicted by phase sensitive reconstructed turbo-FLASH inversion recovery late gadolinium enhancement imaging (PSIR-LGE). Images in three different planes were stored on the in-room monitor and were compared to the images simultaneously acquired by real time imaging. The MR-conditional bioptome (Innovative Tomography Products, Bochum, Germany) (Fig. 1) was introduced and guided towards the lesion under continuous visual control and interactive adjustment of the imaging plane. Papillary muscles, aortic valve as well as mitral valve served as landmarks. The final position of the bioptome was adjusted step by step: the tip of the device was kept in plane and directed to the target area that was visible on stored LGE images on the in-room monitor. The most difficult part of the procedure was the positioning of the deflectable guiding catheter due to its rigidity and diameter. The MR-conditional guiding catheter had more rigidity and less flexibility than the guiding catheter used under fluoroscopy.

Overall tracking was acquired with passive tracking via visible markers on the guidewire, on the distal tip of the guiding catheter (Innovative Tomography Products, Bochum, Germany) and via distal markers of the bioptome (Innovative Tomography Products, Bochum, Germany).

For later quantification of LGE a semiautomatic grayscale threshold technique (Qmass, Medis, Leiden, The Netherlands) was performed as published previously [20]. Areas of LGE were defined as a signal intensity of more than +4 standard deviations (SD) above the mean of remote healthy myocardium.

Histology

All samples were retained in a 10% buffered formalin solution and remained there for at least 24 h. Afterwards they were further processed including paraffin embedding and sectioning. Sections of 5 μm thickness were stained using hematoxylin-eosin, periodic acid-Schiff, elastic van Gieson staining as well as desmin immunohistochemistry to identify healthy and damaged myocardium, endocardium and hemorrhage. Blinded histologic evaluation was performed by two experienced physicians. Myocardial interstitial and intracellular edema and vacuolization, myocardial pallor, myocardial coagulation and hemorrhage were assessed and reported for each biopsy sample.

All animal protocols were reviewed and approved by the local animal ethics committee as well as the governmental animal care and use committee (Bezirksregierung Braunschweig, Germany).

Results

Radiofrequency ablation

Radiofrequency ablation was successful in all 7 MP and performed on the left ventricular lateral wall in five and the apex in two animals. Each (except one) ablation lesion (7-F catheter) was created by two consecutive 30-s ablations (max. 30 W, temperature 58-64 C^0). Ventricular fibrillation occurred twice in one animal (one minute after the first and 75 s after the second ablation that was limited to 30 s). Successful defibrillation resulted in sinus rhythm followed by stable hemodynamics. At least two ablation sites with sufficient endocardial contact (temperature continuously above 58 C^0) were achieved in all animals.

Endomyocardial biopsies

Fluoroscopic guidance

The conventional bioptome (Fig. 1) was guided under fluoroscopy (Siremobil, Siemens Healthcare, Erlangen, Germany) as in common clinical routine. Guiding towards the region of interest was accomplished by comparing the actual fluoroscopic image on the screen with the stored images of the ablation procedure using the same angulations of the c-arm x-ray. At least one sample was taken on what was judged to be within the ablation zone. A commercially available steel bioptome (5.5 F) was used in 6/7 animals. Time from introduction to extraction of the guiding catheter varied between 15–25 min for all biopsies. Further complications occurred in two animals: both suffered from pericardial effusion without major hemodynamic problems. Thus, samples were obtained from six animals (Table 1).

CMR guidance

7/7 animals survived and were transferred into the CMR suite. Detection of the lesion was achieved 100–150 min after ablation. Pre-contrast the lesions were invisible with the used sequences. For LGE, time of inversion (TI) value was between 250 and 300 ms. Images were acquired 15 ± 5 min after the body-weight adapted injection of gadubutrol. PSIR-LGE images provided good depiction of the lesions (Fig. 2). As the tip diameter of the ablation catheter was 4 mm, the induced lesions were rather small. As CMR imaging followed standard biopsies in all experiments we firstly ruled out that the biopsy itself led to a CMR detectable lesion in an additional animal. Left ventricular myocardium was analyzed with dedicated CMR software (Qmass, Medis, Leiden, The Netherlands). Lesion size defined as above varied between 3.8% (2.4 g) and 22.8% (12.8 g) of total myocardial mass (0.27 cm^2 and 4.64 cm^2 in the best available view), most probably depending on the contact and heating during the ablation. Lesions are given in table 1. Five lesions had a typical appearance with a contact point at the lesion core and an outer rim as described by Celik [21].

Localization and tracking of the guiding catheter with a distal tip marker (ITP, Bochum, Germany) (see Additional file 2) and an MR-safe 0.035 in. guidewire (MaRVis Technologies GmbH, Aachen, Germany) with passive tracking was successful in all animals. The guidewire was visible over the whole length with a distal extra ball-shaped tip marker increasing tip visibility.

Due to the availability of in-room real-time monitoring (as described above), the whole interventional procedure was trackable in all animals: advancing the guidewire into the aorta and the left ventricle followed by introduction of the guiding catheter could be safely performed using interactive navigation in different planes (Fig. 3). The MRbioptome's distal tip was clearly visible and the negative contrast (artifact) allowed simultaneous detection of the endocardial border (see Additional file 2). The most difficult part of the procedure was the positioning of the deflectable guiding catheter due to its rigidity and diameter. The MR-conditional guiding catheter had more rigidity and less flexibility than the guiding catheter used under fluoroscopy. Procedure time for real-time CMR guidance varied between 40–50 min (first introduction of the guiding catheter into the sheeth until extraction after the last biopsy) depending on the difficulty to place the bioptome. In 5/7 animals biopsies were successfully performed: in one minipig the bioptome reached the lesion; however the forceps didn't cut a sample, in one

Table 1 Numbers and pathologic findings in targeted endomyocardial biopsies gained under RT-CMR or fluoroscopic guidance (FI)

Ablation sites	No. of EMB RT-CMR/No. of trials	No. of EMB FI/No. of trials	No. of positive samples		Pathology correctly diagnosed/minipig		Lesion size	
			RT-CMR	FI	RT -CMR	FI	[g]	[% total LV mass]
3	3/6	0/0	3	0	yes	no	3.1	8.5
2	4/4	4/4	1	0	yes	no	12.8	22.8
3	2/6	1/1	1	0	yes	no	6.0	11
2	2/6	3/3	0	1	no	yes	11.4	20.6
3	0/5	2/2	0	0	no	no	3.5	7.7
3	4/6	3/3	2	1	yes	yes	2.7	5.0
3	0/0	4/4	0	2	no	yes	Not done	

Number (No) of tissue samples obtained by endomyocardial biopsy (EMB) under real-time CMR and under fluoroscopy (FI), number of trials of biopsies and lesion size in g and in % of total left ventricular (LV) mass are given. No EMB trials were done in the first animal under FL and in the last animal due to large pericardial effusion

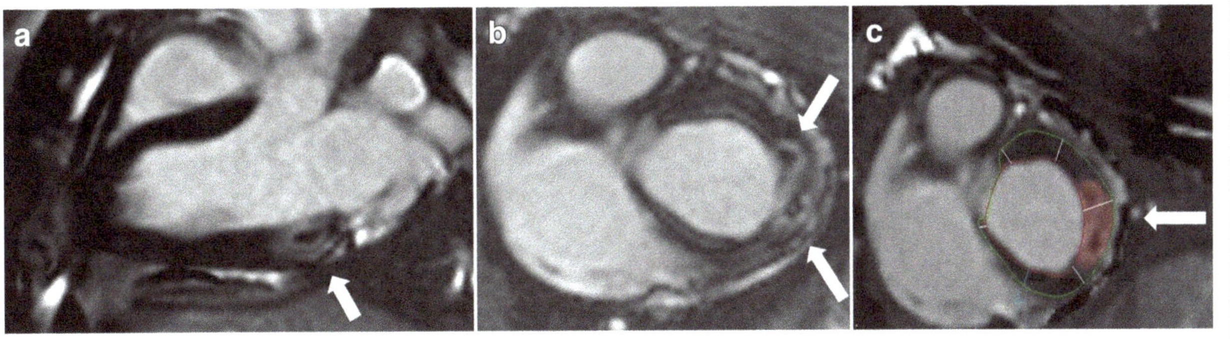

Fig. 2 a: Postcontrast visualization and assessment of acute lesions. Postcontrast two-dimensional PSIR-LGE (2D LGE) in two different animals after radiofrequency ablation. LGE images show good contrast between the lesion with its edematous core and the myocardium (white arrow). **a**: lesions targeted for biopsy are shown in an infero-basal segment in a long axis view and **b**: in a short axis view with **c**: the markers for quantitative segmentation of the lesion area (red area, see methods)

other MP pericardial effusion was major. In this animal the EMB under CMR guidance was skipped due to safety reasons. Handling of the catheters was tested by a carotid approach ($n = 3$) as well as by a femoral approach ($n = 4$). Continuous navigation was dependent on an optimal communication with the technician outside the scanner room to rotate image planes in the necessary position in a minimum of time. An additional movie file shows this in more detail (see Additional file 2). The handling from the carotid approach was uncomfortable for the interventionalist as geometric constraints required the interventionalist to move his or her head several times in and out of the scanner at the end of the bore which led to headache and slight nausea due to exposure to intense gradient fields

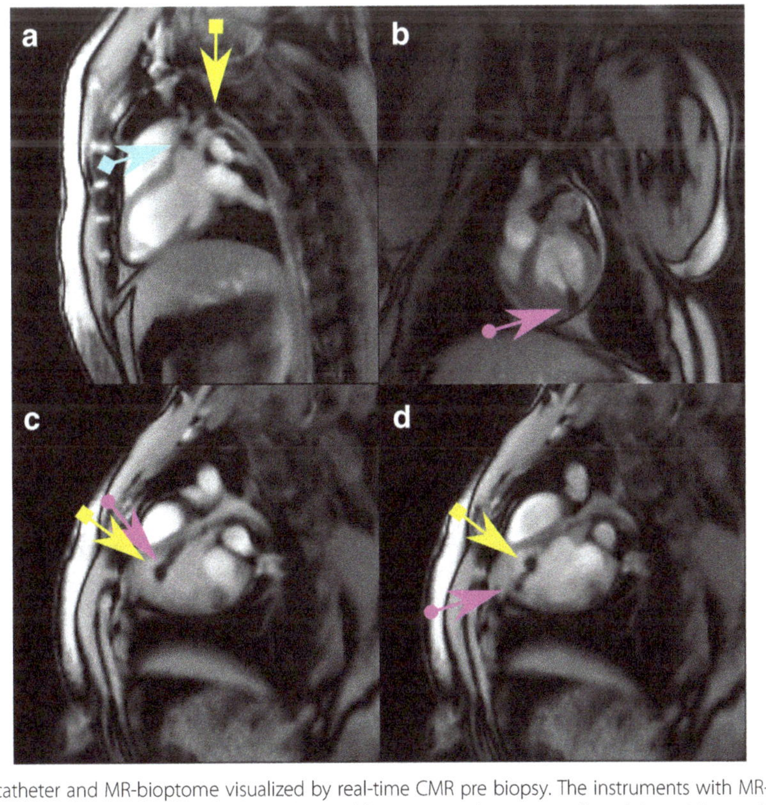

Fig. 3 Guidewire, guiding catheter and MR-bioptome visualized by real-time CMR pre biopsy. The instruments with MR-markers are visualized by interactive real-time CMR during a targeted biopsy. **a**: The guidewire (blue arrow with square end) and the guiding catheter (yellow arrow with square end) are advanced into the left ventricle through the aorta. **b**: The MR-conditional bioptome is used to perform a biopsy (violet arrow with round end) **c** and **d**: The bioptome (violet arrow with round end) is advanced inside (**c**) and then extruded out of (**d**) the guiding catheter (yellow arrow with square end)

during scans. On the other hand, the femoral approach allows for a position where the interventionalist can handle the catheter without having the head in the tunnel.

Histology of the myocardial specimen

Samples obtained under CMR guidance included ablation lesions in 6/15 (40%) samples and in 4/5 animals in which biopsies could be performed (Table 1) successfully. EMB obtained under fluoroscopy guidance revealed ablation lesions in 4/17 (23.5%) specimen and in 3/6 (50%) animals in hematoxylin-eosin stain (Fig. 4) or elastic van Gieson stain. Thus, biopsy of lesioned cardiac tissue was achieved with CMR-guided successful biopsies in 4/5 animals and in 3/6 animals taken under fluoroscopic guidance.

Discussion

Our work is a proof of concept for targeted EMB under real-time CMR guidance in a 3T environment. In a minipig model localized lesions were induced by radiofrequency ablation and visualized using CMR. In our study these lesions served as a useful tool for CMR-guided biopsy studies. We were able to show that biopsies of these lesions can be achieved under CMR guidance with a higher diagnostic yield compared to conventional fluoroscopic guidance in the same animals. We have used this dedicated animal model of defined circumscript lesions to mimic the clinical situation of unknown heart failure in which 6–8 specimens are taken for diagnostic purposes. The Lederman group [16] recently published targeted EMB using CMR guidance in an animal model with significantly larger infarct scars. Their results show a very good correlation to our observations: CMR guidance was superior to fluoroscopic guidance (82% vs 56%) in targeted EMB. Similar to our experience, specimens collected by the MR-conditional bioptome were smaller than those by the conventional steel bioptome. Moreover, we observed that success rates depend on the cutting force of the bioptome. However, this force was markedly less in the MR-bioptome compared to the steel bioptome. The use of the MR-bioptome resulted in a procedural success rate of 45% whereas conventional biopsies showed a rate of 100%. This illustrates a technical problem to be resolved in the future: the sharpness of the forceps was not optimal and inferior compared to a conventional steel bioptome with long metallic compounds and powerful traction of the forceps. The polymer design is optimal for elimination of heating problems but its mechanical rigidity still is not strong enough to transfer enough force to the forceps. Moreover, increasing the length from 80 cm (carotid access) to more than 150 cm (femoral access) resulted in decreased force on the forceps (personal communication of the manufacturer). Our aim was to cut at least three specimens in each setting but this was not achievable in all animals. For the steel bioptome we were successful in all cases, but we had two major complications in the minipigs: one animal suffered from small, hemodynamically non-fatal pericardial effusion and the other one from ventricular fibrillation. This complication rate was considerably higher than reported for left ventricular biopsies in clinical routine which may be explained by the combination of RF ablation immediately followed by EMB. Further, this complication might be the result of using monoplanar instead of biplanar fluoroscopy. Schäufele [5] reported on procedural success rates of 98% and a very low complication rate (0%) for left ventricular biopsies when using modern fluoroscopy and transradial equipment in humans in an elective clinical setting. In a larger clinical series of patients with unexplained heart failure left and right ventricular biopsies were associated with a complication rate of approx. 1.9% [6].

As LGE imaging provides a high contrast between healthy and altered myocardium we used it for visualization and targeting of the lesions before EMB in the CMR scanner. All lesions created with a 7 F ablation catheter were visible. Celik [21] suggested that native T1 contrast may be even more precise in separating the

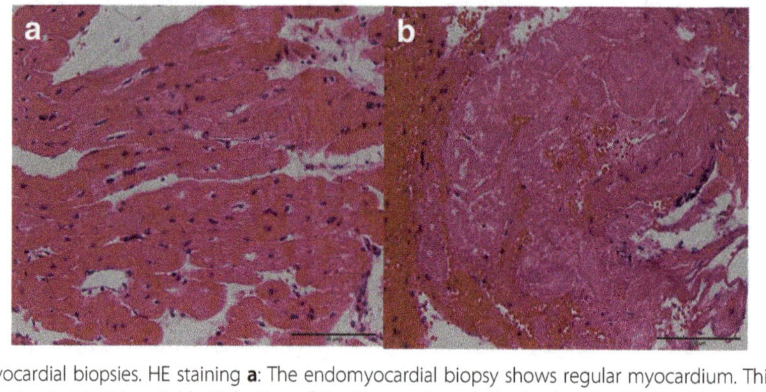

Fig. 4 Histology of endomyocardial biopsies. HE staining **a**: The endomyocardial biopsy shows regular myocardium. This specimen was gained under fluoroscopic guidance in minipig 1 (see Table 1). **b**: One of the two specimens obtained under CMR guidance. The ablated area reveals areas of myocardial coagulation with extensive hemorrhage

necrotic core from the surrounding edematous rims without waiting for the equilibrium after gadolinium injection. This specific aspect is of high interest for further studies using lesions induced by radiofrequency ablation as this can yield ablation zones early and without recurrent injection of gadolinium. It is suggested that this might be even more useful for localization of the center of the EMB target.

In our study, real-time CMR was applied for navigation of MR-compatible guidewires and catheters in a comparable manner to the procedure under fluoroscopy which is familiar to the interventionalists. In all cases the guiding catheters could be placed into the left ventricle under continuous real-time CMR guidance. Guidewires had an excellent visibility but their polymer-only construction results in a flexibility that was sufficient for the described purpose but not quite the same as that of metallic wires. Torquability and support were not measured and catheter exchange over the wire was not performed. However, the overall handling is inferior to wires that are routinely used in cardiac interventions. Wire shortcomings might be better solved by a segmented nitinol design as invented by the NIH group [22] but these wires are currently not available on the market. Although the use of commercially available nitinol wires is possible in the magnetic field without artifacts, these wires are not safe concerning heating and induction. By use of a prototype MR-guiding catheter the MR- bioptome could be introduced easily into the left ventricle in all cases. Again this is in good agreement with the study of the NIH group [16]. The size and intensity of the artifacts was unproblematic. However, exact placement towards the lesions was more challenging. Consequently required procedure time was more than doubled in the CMR scanner.

Most interventional MRI studies are currently performed using MRI at 1.5 T which has the general advantage of being less prone to artifacts and heating, and because equipment using active tracking is often only developed for this field strength. In our study, we use passive tracking using a real-time imaging method based on radial FLASH and highly accelerated by advanced parallel imaging (NLINV). This method is robust against field inhomogeneities (short TE), is not problematic with respect to heating (no wires and use of low-flip angles), and benefits from the higher SNR and improved parallel imaging at 3T. One major aspect of our study is the use of real-time CMR in a manner comparable to fluoroscopic guidance in a 1:1 imaging setting. Although the used real-time FLASH sequences with NLINV reconstruction allow a comparably high temporal resolution of 20 ms per frame [17], we have reduced the temporal resolution to 42 ms per frame in order to reduce computational load. This guaranteed excellent visual feedback for the interventionalist with a minimal time delay. We were also able to switch between different orientations within a few seconds. This makes the procedure less dependent on pre-scanned images or pre-defined imaging planes.

Limitations

Heating of the bioptome has not been assessed during imaging in the 3T environment. However, as the forceps are made of titanium and the shaft is made of plastic with aramid fibers these different components should have no major heating problems. In phantom dental implants made of titanium there is an increase of 0.6–0.8 °C in a 3T scanner [23]. As circulating blood has a cooling effect this heating should be no relevant problem. Safety studies will be required prior to clinical translation in regard to the problem of flex shaft, cutting jaw, safety and effectiveness of the MR-conditional bioptome. Compared to a 1.5 T scanner the 3T scanner offers better contrast of the myocardium with improved depiction of acute and chronic lesions but most MR-compatible catheters are approved for 1.5 T only. The mechanical features of MR-compatible guiding catheters such as flexibility, steerability, available different curvature and different sizes are problems still unresolved. We used a non CE approved flexible and deflectable guiding catheter in this work. Until now there is no adequate nonbraided femoral catheter on the market with deflectable tip and with a smaller outer diameter: in our case 8.0 F would have been wide enough, instead we had to use a 9.5 F guiding catheter that is more harmful for all structures. Nevertheless, our techniques should be translatable into clinical and commercially available products. Further improvements in real-time imaging will make the procedure more convenient, i.e. interactive control directly from the scanner room, interactive control of sequence parameters which control the contrast (e.g. saturation pulses), improved user-interface for interventional use with simultaneous 3D visualization of several imaging planes and an overlay of static images will facilitate CMR interventions. Finally, we cannot fully exclude that the pathologic assessment of endomyocardial biopsies may be influenced by the later sampling time point (approx. 120 min) of real-time CMR–guided biopsies.

Conclusion

Our work shows that focal myocardial lesions can be induced by radiofrequency ablation and afterwards visualized under CMR in a minipig model. These focal lesions can be successfully biopsied. Real-time CMR guidance show a higher rate of diagnostic success compared to biopsies obtained under fluoroscopic guidance. Visualization and passive tracking of the instruments using real-time CMR with interactive control is excellent. Further improvements of bioptomes and guiding catheters will contribute to the superior success of targeted CMR-guided biopsy compared to untargeted fluoroscopic EMB.

Abbreviations
ACC: American College of Cardiology; AHA: American Heart Association; bSSFP: Balanced steady state free precession; BW: Body weight ; CMR: Cardiovascular magnetic resonance; DZHK: German Center for Cardiovascular Research (Deutsches Zentrum für Herz-Kreislauf-Forschung); EMB: Endomyocardial biopsies; ESC: European Society of Cardiology; EVG: Elastic van Gieson; FLASH: Fast low-angle shot; HE: Hematoxylin-eosin; LGE: Late gadolinium enhancement; NLINV: Nonlinear inverse reconstruction ; PSIR: Phase-sensitive inversion recovery FOV, field of view; TE: Echo time; TR: Repetition time

Acknowledgement
We thank Jens Frahm and his team of the BiomedNMR (Goettingen, Germany) for the real-time MRI system, and in particular, we thank Dirk Voit for the interactive version of the real-time sequence. We are particularly grateful for the assistance given by Ulrike Köchermann and Tanja Otto.

Funding
This work was supported by the DZHK (Deutsches Zentrum für Herz-Kreislauf-Forschung eV).

Authors' contributions
CUB conception, design of the study, experimental workup, analysis and interpretation of data and writing of manuscript. CR experimental workup, analysis and interpretation of data and drafting of manuscript critically. VR overall animal handling, care and sedation. RNW support of experiments, data collection and critical revision of the manuscript. CS data collection and histologic analysis of the myocardial samples. MS assistance with experimental workup, critical revision of the manuscript. AS interpretation of data and critical revision of the manuscript. GH important and critical contributions to the major limitations. JL critical revision of the manuscript. MU development of real-time MRI methods, data collection and analysis and drafting the manuscript. All authors read and approved the final manuscript.

Authors' information
The manuscript is original and the manuscript, or substantial parts of it are not under consideration by any other journal.

Competing interests
The authors declare that they have no competing interests.

Author details
[1]University Medical Center Goettingen, Clinic of Cardiology and Pneumology, Goettingen, Germany. [2]Department of Experimental Animal Medicine, Georg-August University, Goettingen, Germany. [3]DZHK (German Centre for Cardiovascular Research), Partner Site Goettingen, Berlin, Germany. [4]Department of Neuropathology, University Medical Center Goettingen, Goettingen, Germany. [5]University Medical Center Goettingen, Clinic of Pediatric Cardiology and Intensive Care Medicine, Goettingen, Germany. [6]University Medical Center Goettingen, Institute for Diagnostic and Interventional Radiology, Goettingen, Germany.

References
1. Leone O, Veinot JP, Angelini A, Baandrup UT, Basso C, Berry G, Bruneval P, Burke P, Butany M, Calabrese F, D'Amati G, Edwards WD, Fallon JT, Fishbein MC, Gallagher PJ, Halushka MK, McManus B, Pucci A, Rodriguez ER, Saffitz JE, Sheppard MN, Steenbergen C, Stone JR, Tan C, Thiene G, van der Wal AC, Winters GL. 2011 consensus statement on endomyocardial biopsy from the Association for European Cardiovascular Pathology and the Society for Cardiovascular Pathology. Cardiovasc Pathol. 2012;21:245–74.
2. Thiene G, Bruneval P, Veinot J, Leone O. Diagnostic use of the endomyocardial biopsy: a consensus statement. Virchows Arch. 2013;463:1–5.
3. Cooper LT, Baughman KL, Feldman AM, Frustaci A, Jessup M, Kuhl U, Levine GN, Narula J, Starling RC, Towbin J, Virmani R, American Heart Association; American College of Cardiology; European Society of Cardiology. The role of endomyocardial biopsy in the management of cardiovascular disease: a scientific statement from the American Heart Association, the American College of Cardiology, and the European Society of Cardiology. Circulation. 2007;116:2216–33.
4. Caforio AL, Pankuweit S, Arbustini E, Basso C, Gimeno-Blanes J, Felix SB, Fu M, Heliö T, Heymans S, Jahns R, Klingel K, Linhart A, Maisch B, McKenna W, Mogensen J, Pinto YM, Ristic A, Schultheiss HP, Seggewiss H, Tavazzi L, Thiene G, Yilmaz A, Charron P, Elliott PM, European Society of Cardiology Working Group on Myocardial and Pericardial Diseases. Current state of knowledge on aetiology, diagnosis, management, and therapy of myocarditis: a position statement of the European Society of Cardiology Working Group on Myocardial and Pericardial Diseases. Eur Heart J. 2013;34: 2636–48.
5. Schäufele TG, Spittler R, Karagianni A, Ong P, Klingel K, Kandolf R, Marholdt H, Sechtem U. Transradial left ventricular endomyocardial biopsy: assessment of safety and efficacy. Clin Res Cardiol. 2015;104:773–81.
6. Bennett MK, Gilotra NA, Harrington C, Rao S, Dunn JM, Freitag TB, Halushka MK, Russell SD. Evaluation of the role of endomyocardial biopsy in 851 patients with unexplained heart failure from 2000–2009. Circ Heart Fail. 2013;6:676–84.
7. Yilmaz A, Kindermann I, Kindermann M, Mahfoud F, Ukena C, Athanasiadis A, Hill S, Marholdt H, Voehringer M, Schieber M, Klingel K, Kandolf R, Böhm M, Sechtem U. Comparative evaluation of left and right ventricular endomyocardiale biopsy: differences in complication rate and diagnostic performance. Circulation. 2010;122:900–9.
8. Hundley WG, Bluemke DA, Finn JP, Flamm SD, Fogel MA, Friedrich MG, Ho VB, Jerosch-Herold M, Kramer CM, Manning WJ, Patel M, Pohost GM, Stillman AE, White RD, Woodard PK. American College of Cardiology Foundation Task Force on Expert Consensus Documents, ACCF/ACR/AHA/ NASCI/SCMR 2010 expert consensus document on cardiovascular magnetic resonance: a report of the American College of Cardiology Foundation Task Force on Expert Consensus Documents. J Am Coll Cardiol. 2010;55:2614–62.
9. Lurz P, Luecke C, Eitel I, Föhrenbach F, Frank C, Grothoff M, de Waha S, Rommel KP, Lurz JA, Klingel K, Kandolf R, Schuler G, Thiele H, Gutberlet M. Comprehensive Cardiac Magnetic Resonance Imaging in Patients With Suspected Myocarditis: The MyoRacer-Trial. J Am Coll Cardiol. 2016;67:1800–11.
10. Fischbach F, Eggemann H, Bunke J, Wonneberger U, Ricke J, Strach K. MR-guided freehand biopsy of breast lesions in a 1.0-T open MR imager with a near-real-time interactive platform: preliminary experience. Radiology. 2012; 265:359–70.
11. Das CJ, Goenka AH. Srivastava DNMR-guided abdominal biopsy using a 1.5-Tesla closed system: a feasibility study. Abdom Imaging. 2010;35:218–23.
12. Garnon J, Schlier A, Buy X, Tsoumakidou G, de Mathelin M, Breton E, Gangi A. Evaluation of percutaneous biopsies of renal masses under MRI-guidance: a retrospective study about 26 cases. Eur Radiol. 2015;25:617–23.
13. Penzkofer T, Tempany-Afdhal CM. Prostate cancer detection and diagnosis: the role of MR and its comparison with other diagnostic modalities–a radiologist's perspective. NMR Biomed. 2014;27:3–15.
14. Chen AVM, Wininger FA, Frey S, Comeau RM, Bagley RS, Tucker RL, Schneider AR, Gay JM. Description and validation of a magnetic resonance imaging-guided stereotactic brain biopsy device in the dog. Vet Radiol Ultrasound. 2012;53:150–56.
15. Lossnitzer D, Seitz SA, Krautz B, Schnackenburg B, André F, Korosoglou G, Katus HA, Steen H. Feasibility of real-time magnetic resonance imaging-guided endomyocardial biopsies: An in-vitro study. World J Cardiol. 2015;26:415–22.
16. Rogers T, Ratnayaka K, Karmarkar P, Campbell-Washburn AE, Schenke WH, Mazal JR, Kocaturk O, Faranesh AZ, Lederman RJ. Real-time magnetic resonance imaging guidance improves the diagnostic yield of endomyocardial biopsy. JACC Basic Transl Sci. 2016;1:376–83.
17. Uecker M, Zhang S, Voit D, Karaus A, Merboldt K-D, Frahm J. Real-time magnetic resonance imaging at a resolution of 20 ms. NMR Biomed. 2010; 23:986–94.
18. http://www.marvistech.com/technology-products/mr-guidewires.html. Accessed 9 Apr 2017.
19. Schaetz P, Uecker M. A Multi-GPU Programming Library for Real-Time. Applications. In: Xiang Y, Stojmenovic I, Apduhan BO, Wang G, Nakano K, Zomaya A, editors. Algorithms and Architectures for Parallel Processing. Berlin, Heidelberg: Springer; 2012. p. 114–28.

20. Flett AS, Hasleton J, Cook C, Hausenloy D, Quarta G, Ariti C, et al. Evaluation of techniques for the quantification of myocardial scar of differing etiology using cardiac magnetic resonance. JACC. 2011;4:150–6.
21. Celik H, Ramanan V, Barry J, Ghate S, Leber V, Oduneye S, Gu Y, Jamali M, Ghugre N, Stainsby JA, Shurrab M, Crystal E, Wright GA. Intrinsic contrast for characterization of acute radiofrequency ablation lesions. Circ Arrhythm Electrophysiol. 2014;7:718–27.
22. Basar B, Rogers T, Ratnayaka K, Campbell-Washburn E, Mazal JR, Schenek WH, Sommez M, Faranesh AZ, Lederman RJ, Kocaturk O. Segmented nitinol guidewires with stiffness-matched connectors for cardiovascular magnetic resonance catheterization: preserved mechanical performance and freedom from heating. J Cardiovasc Magn Res. 2015;17:105.
23. Miyata K, Hasegawa M, Abe Y, Tabuchi T, Namiki T, Ishigami T. Radiofrequency heating and magnetically induced displacement of dental magnetic attachments during 3.0T MRI. Dentomaxillifac Radiol. 2012;41:668–74.

3

Hemorrhage promotes inflammation and myocardial damage following acute myocardial infarction: insights from a novel preclinical model and cardiovascular magnetic resonance

Nilesh R. Ghugre[1,2,3*], Mihaela Pop[1,2,3], Reuben Thomas[1], Susan Newbigging[4], Xiuling Qi[1], Jennifer Barry[1], Bradley H. Strauss[3] and Graham A. Wright[1,2,3]

Abstract

Background: Myocardial hemorrhage is a frequent complication following reperfusion in acute myocardial infarction and is predictive of adverse outcomes. However, it remains unsettled whether hemorrhage is simply a marker of a severe initial ischemic insult or directly contributes to downstream myocardial damage. Our objective was to evaluate the contribution of hemorrhage towards inflammation, microvascular obstruction and infarct size in a novel porcine model of hemorrhagic myocardial infarction using cardiovascular magnetic resonance (CMR).

Methods: Myocardial hemorrhage was induced via direct intracoronary injection of collagenase in a novel porcine model of ischemic injury. Animals ($N = 27$) were subjected to coronary balloon occlusion followed by reperfusion and divided into three groups ($N = 9$/group): 8 min ischemia with collagenase (+HEM); 45 min infarction with saline (I-HEM); and 45 min infarction with collagenase (I+HEM). Comprehensive CMR was performed on a 3 T scanner at baseline and 24 h post-intervention. Cardiac function was quantified by cine imaging, edema/inflammation by T2 mapping, hemorrhage by T2* mapping and infarct/microvascular obstruction size by gadolinium enhancement. Animals were subsequently sacrificed and explanted hearts underwent histopathological assessment for ischemic damage and inflammation.

Results: At 24 h, the +HEM group induced only hemorrhage, the I-HEM group resulted in a non-hemorrhagic infarction, and the I+HEM group resulted in infarction and hemorrhage. Notably, the I+HEM group demonstrated greater hemorrhage and edema, larger infarct size and higher incidence of microvascular obstruction. Interestingly, hemorrhage alone (+HEM) also resulted in an observable inflammatory response, similar to that arising from a mild ischemic insult (I-HEM). CMR findings were in good agreement with histological staining patterns.

(Continued on next page)

* Correspondence: nghugre@sri.utoronto.ca
[1]Physical Sciences Platform, Sunnybrook Research Institute, 2075 Bayview Avenue, Room M7-510, Toronto, ON M4N 3M5, Canada
[2]Department of Medical Biophysics, University of Toronto, Toronto, ON, Canada
Full list of author information is available at the end of the article

(Continued from previous page)

Conclusions: Hemorrhage is not simply a bystander, but an active modulator of tissue response, including inflammation and microvascular and myocardial damage beyond the initial ischemic insult. A mechanistic understanding of the pathophysiology of reperfusion hemorrhage will potentially aid better management of high-risk patients who are prone to adverse long-term outcomes.

Keywords: Myocardial infarction, Hemorrhage, Inflammation, Microvascular obstruction, T2, T2*, Ischemia reperfusion injury, cardiovascular magnetic resonance

Background

Acute Myocardial Infarction (AMI) occurs due to cessation of coronary blood flow to the heart muscle and the extent of injury follows a wavefront pattern of necrosis in proportion to the duration of occlusion [1]. While prompt reperfusion is favorable for myocardial salvage, ischemia-reperfusion injury (IRI) may often present itself as an adverse consequence. IRI has been associated with expansion of the prior ischemic damage and greater inflammation along with oxidative stress, apoptosis, stunning, free radicals and reperfusion arrhythmias [2, 3]. Lethal IRI may further result in myocardial hemorrhage [4] which, in association with microvascular no-reflow or obstruction (MVO), has been recognized to be a new independent predictor of adverse outcomes [5–8].

The presentation of myocardial hemorrhage as a consequence of IRI has been well documented in both humans [9] and animal models of AMI [10–12]. With recent advances in quantitative Cardiovascular Magnetic Resonance (CMR) techniques, hemorrhage-sensitive relaxation parameters - T2 and T2* have been instrumental in the in-vivo detection of hemorrhagic byproducts [7, 8, 13, 14], and have also made it possible to study the associated long-term consequences. A study by Mather et al. [6] demonstrated that hemorrhage was associated with large infarct size, reduced salvage, greater MVO and lower ejection fraction; it was also the strongest independent predictor of adverse left ventricular (LV) remodeling with an increased risk of arrhythmia and predictive power even greater than MVO. Recently, a much larger study in 286 patients by Carrick et al. [15] has shown that hemorrhage occurred in 40% of ST-segment elevation myocardial infarction (STEMI) patients and that it was independently responsible for adverse remodeling at 6 months. It was further found that hemorrhage was more associated with adverse remodeling and N-terminal pro-brain natriuretic peptide (surrogate outcomes) and cardiovascular death and heart failure following discharge (health outcomes) than MVO.

Although some of these observational clinical studies have reported the prognostic implications of myocardial hemorrhage utilizing the predictive power of CMR, the findings have not been consistent in the literature. Several other investigators have found hemorrhage to only be associated with infarct size and presence of MVO, but not offering prognostic significance beyond these parameters [7, 16]. Given these clinical observations, a systematic and mechanistic understanding of the underlying pathophysiological implications of hemorrhage are not fully understood, particularly as an individual and an additive phenomenon over an ischemic insult.

A critical question is whether hemorrhage is simply a bystander and a marker of severe microvascular injury or does it actively contribute to downstream myocardial and microvascular damage beyond the initial ischemic insult. Furthermore, hemorrhage has always been associated with MVO [6, 17]; however, the interaction and causality between the two is less understood. Our study was designed to probe the pathophysiological consequences of hemorrhage in a large animal model of AMI with CMR as the investigational tool. Our hypothesis was that hemorrhage is a mediator of inflammation, directly contributing to myocardial and microvascular damage in the setting of AMI.

Methods

Novel model of hemorrhagic injury

In order to evaluate the contribution of hemorrhage alone in ischemia-reperfusion injury, hemorrhage was artificially induced in porcine hearts by direct intracoronary injection of collagenase. A recent study has demonstrated that intracoronary collagenase is capable of inducing myocardial bleeding in a dose-dependent manner without any mortality attributed to collagenase [18]. This model was modified to study three groups of animals ($N = 27$) subjected to a coronary occlusion: 1) 8 min ischemia with collagenase resulting in only hemorrhage without infarction (+HEM group, $N = 9$) [18]; 2) 45 min ischemia with intracoronary injection of phosphate buffered saline (PBS) resulting in infarction without hemorrhage (I-HEM group, $N = 9$) [19]; and 3) 45 min ischemia with intracoronary injection of collagenase projected to cause infarction with hemorrhage (I+HEM group, $N = 9$).

Animal protocol

Female Yorkshire pigs (20-25 kg, Caughell Farms, ON) were employed in the study and all procedures were conducted in accordance with protocols approved by the Animal Care Committee of Sunnybrook Research Institute. Before catheterization, animals were sedated with an anesthetic cocktail comprising of atropine (0.05 mg/kg) and ketamine (30 mg/kg). Animals were then intubated, mechanically ventilated and maintained under anesthesia using isoflurane (1-5%). Complete coronary occlusion was achieved distal to the second diagonal branch of the left anterior descending (LAD) artery using an over-the-wire angioplasty balloon dilatation catheter (Sprinter OTW, Medtronic, MN); note that the same level of occlusion was maintained across all animals to ensure consistency. Blood flow was occluded for 8 min (+HEM group) or 45 min (I-HEM and I+HEM groups) and was followed by reperfusion; this was verified by X-ray fluoroscopy (Veradius C Arm, Philips Healthcare). One minute prior to balloon deflation (reperfusion), either 3.2 ml PBS (I-HEM group) or PBS containing collagenase (+HEM and I+HEM groups) (3.2 mg, Clostridium Histolyticum type VII-S, Sigma-Aldrich) was injected through the guide wire port. Cardiac events during ischemia-reperfusion were managed by antiarrhythmic drugs (75 mg over 5 min amiodarone bolus and lidocaine drip as needed) or defibrillation whenever necessary. Animals were then recovered and examined by CMR at 24 h post-intervention and subsequently sacrificed.

CMR protocol

CMR was performed on a 3 T whole body scanner (MR 750, General Electric Healthcare, Waukesha, Wisconsin, USA) at baseline (healthy state) and at 24 h post-intervention. Cardiac function was evaluated using a steady-state-free-precession (SSFP) sequence in cine mode: 12-15 short-axis slices, TR/TE = 4/1.7 ms, flip angle = 45°, FOV = 24x21.6 cm, matrix = 224x160, slice thickness = 5 mm, 8 views/segment, 20 phases/slice. Edema was quantified using a previously validated T2 mapping sequence [19]; spiral readout with T2 preparation, 10 spirals (12.3 ms, 3072 points), TE = 2.9, 24.3, 45.6, 88.2 and 184.2 ms, 10 short-axis slices, in-plane resolution ~1 mm. Hemorrhage was quantified by T2* mapping using a multi-echo gradient-echo acquisition: 8 echoes (1.4-15.8 ms), TR = 16.8 ms, flip angle = 30°, matrix = 128x128, 10 short-axis slices, in-plane resolution ~1.9 mm. Infarction and MVO were assessed by a T1-weighted inversion recovery gradient echo sequence (IR-GRE) sequence: TR/TE = 4.1/1.9 ms, flip angle = 15°, matrix = 224x192, 2RR intervals, 12-15 short-axis slices, inversion time was adjusted to null the myocardium (250-310 ms). Late gadolinium enhancement (LGE) imaging was initiated at 8-10 min post injection of contrast agent Gadolinium-DTPA (0.2 mmol/kg; Magnevist, Bayer Healthcare).

CMR data analysis

Cine SSFP images were analyzed using CVI42 software (Circle Cardiovascular Imaging, Calgary, CA) to quantify cardiac function parameters: ejection fraction (EF), end diastolic and end systolic volumes (EDV, ESV) and LV mass. Infarct volume was quantified by segmenting the LGE images using the full-width-half-maximum technique [20] and regions of hypoenhancement within the enhanced infarct were identified with a semi-automatic region growing algorithm using a level set method [21]. Myocardial T2 and T2* maps were generated by pixel-wise fitting with an exponential function using a least squares criterion. Hemorrhage was identified on T2* maps of each short axis slice using the criteria T2* < 20 ms [22] and the corresponding hemorrhage volume was computed. Edema volume was quantified by labeling pixels in the T2 maps whose values were 2 standard deviations (SD) above remote myocardial values [23]; if hemorrhage or MVO were present, then hypointense regions on T2 maps were labeled as edema using the same level set algorithm as mentioned earlier. LGE images and relaxation maps were analyzed using custom-written MATLAB® scripts (The Mathworks, Natick, MA). All volumes were represented as a percentage of the LV volume. Infarct zone T2 and T2* values were also noted in one mid-ventricular slice by copying the segmented infarct regions (from LGE) on to the relaxation maps; if no enhancement was observed on LGE images, then an anteroseptal (LAD) region was chosen. For comparison, baseline and remote myocardial T2 and T2* values were also recorded. Linear regression with goodness of fit analysis was performed between T2 and T2* values to determine relationship between inflammation and hemorrhage.

Histopathology

Animals were euthanized at 24 h following the CMR examination, hearts were explanted and the LV was sectioned into short-axis slices. Prior to sacrifice, a 4% solution of fluorescent dye thioflavin S (1 ml/kg, Sigma-Aldrich) was intravenously injected as a bolus to examine endothelial cell distribution and arterial patency in the heart [24]. Myocardial slices were immediately placed under an ultraviolet light and photographed to identify regions of no flow represented by Thioflavin S-negative regions. The slices were then immersed into a 1% solution of triphenyltetrazolium chloride (TTC) for 5 min at 37 °C and photographed under room light to identify the infarcted region (TTC-negative). Select slices containing the infarcted tissue were fixed in 10% neutral buffered formalin solution for histological staining. These sections were then dehydrated, embedded in paraffin blocks, sliced into 5 µm thick sections and treated with a) Hematoxylin and eosin (H&E) stain to qualitatively assess gross inflammation, hemorrhage, edema, and necrosis; and b) Immunohistochemistry with macrophage monoclonal antibody MAC387 (Thermo Scientific, Rockford, IL).

Statistics

All data (cardiac function; infarct, MVO, hemorrhage, and edema volumes; T2 and T2* relaxation parameters) were represented as continuous variables and expressed as mean ± SD. For data involving multiple time points i.e. baseline and 24 h, animal groups were compared using a repeated measures 2-way analysis of variance (ANOVA) statistical analysis with multiple comparisons carried out using the Sidak correction factor (GraphPad Prism®, La Jolla, CA); both within group and across group comparisons were performed. For comparisons across groups only at a single time point (24 h), a one way ANOVA statistical test was performed. Linear regression with goodness of fit analysis was performed between infarct zone T2 and T2* values to determine relationship between inflammation and hemorrhage. A p value <0.05 was considered statistically significant.

Results

Animal procedures

In the +HEM group, one animal died during the interventional procedure and one animal died post procedure and could not undergo a CMR examination. Two animals died during the infarct procedure in both the I-HEM and I+HEM groups, overall representing a 20% mortality rate associated with the ischemic event. The mortality and exclusions resulted in $N = 7$ animals in each group for further CMR and histological analysis. There were no adverse effects noted or any mortality attributed as a result of the collagenase administration.

Cardiac function

Cardiac function parameters by CMR (EF, EDV and ESV) were not significantly different across the three groups at 24 h post intervention (See Fig. 1a-c). However, LV mass was significantly increased at 24 h compared to baseline in the I-HEM (14.9%, $p < 0.01$) and I + HEM (14.5%, $p < 0.01$) groups, indicative of edematous swelling (Fig. 1d). In the + HEM group, mean LV mass was higher at 24 h compared to baseline but did not reach statistical significance (9.5%, p = NS).

Myocardial injury and microvascular obstruction

CMR revealed distinct patterns of injury across the three groups of animals at 24 h. Figure 2a shows representative short-axis sections using endogenous T2 and T2* contrast mechanisms beside corresponding LGE images. Hemorrhage was identified by low T2* signal intensity in the anteroseptal region supplied by the LAD coronary artery while edema was described by an elevated T2 signal. The +HEM group

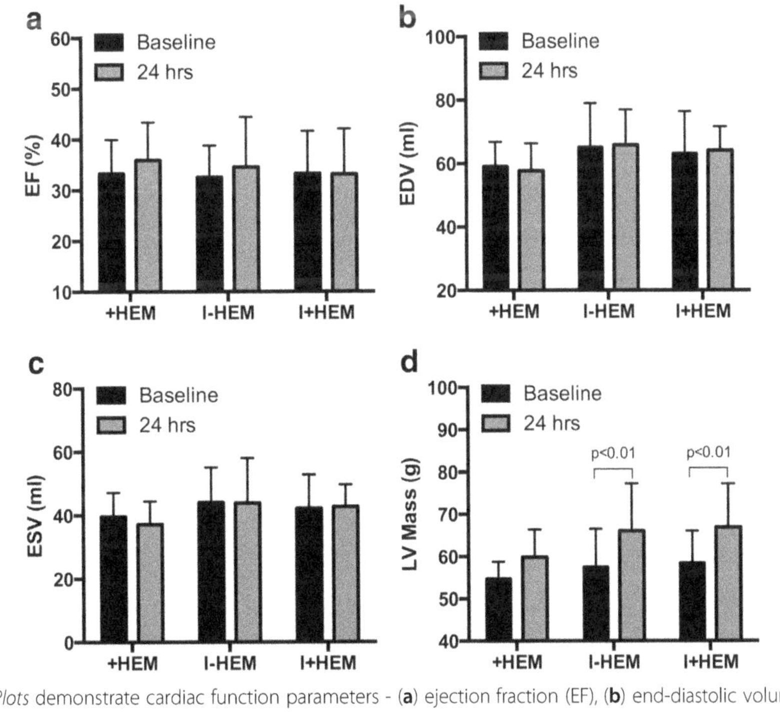

Fig. 1 Cardiac Function. *Plots* demonstrate cardiac function parameters - (**a**) ejection fraction (EF), (**b**) end-diastolic volume (EDV), (**c**) end-systolic volume (ESV) and (**d**) left ventricular (LV) mass at *baseline* and 24 h post intervention in the three animal groups. Only LV mass was significantly elevated at 24 h in the 45 min occlusion groups (I-HEM, I+HEM) indicative of inflammatory swelling

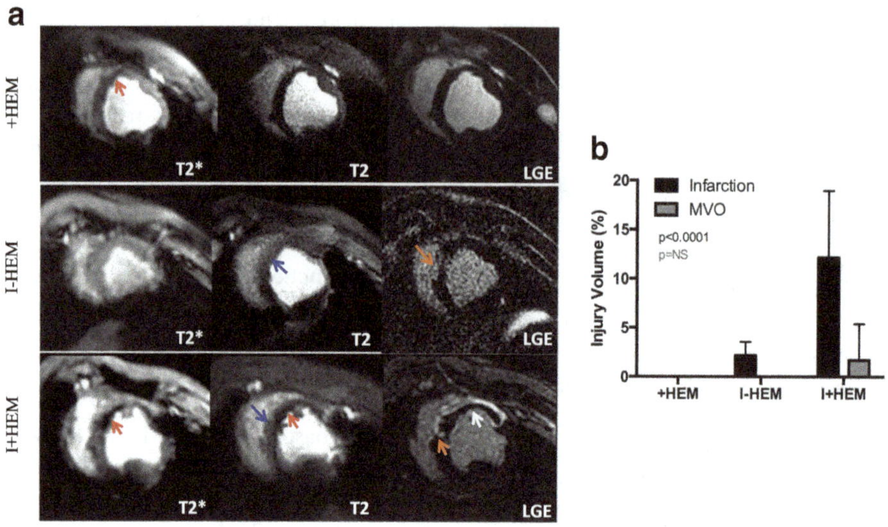

Fig. 2 Myocardial Injury and Microvascular Obstruction. **a** Representative T2*-weighted (TE = 16 ms), T2-weighted (TE = 88 ms) and LGE images from a representative animal in each of the three groups, demonstrating the tissue response at 24 h. The *arrows* are indicative of the following pathophysiological features: *Red* – Hemorrhage; *Blue* – Edema; *Orange* – Infarction; and *White* – MVO. Only +HEM and I+HEM groups demonstrated hemorrhage as indicated by low signal intensities on T2* images. The I-HEM group was non-hemorrhagic with a small infarction. High signal intensity on T2 images suggested the presence of edema in the LAD territory in all three groups. No infarction was detected in the hemorrhage only (+HEM) group, but when coupled with an ischemic insult (I+HEM group), it resulted in a large infarction with MVO. **b** *Plot* compares the cumulative infarct and MVO volumes across the three groups

demonstrated hemorrhage and some edema but without evidence of infarction or MVO. The I-HEM group was non-hemorrhagic with a small infarction (1.5 ± 1.3 g) and notable edema but no MVO. In contrast, the I+HEM group demonstrated considerable hemorrhage, larger infarction (8.1 ± 4.0 g) and the presence of MVO (1.1 ± 2.5 g; 3 of 7 animals or a 43% occurrence rate). Percent infarct volume was significantly different across the three groups ($p < 0.0001$); see bar plot in Fig. 2b.

Hemorrhage quantified by T2* mapping

Figure 3a shows representative T2* images at 24 h with a color overlay of regions identified as hemorrhage using the T2* < 20 ms criterion. The T2* value in the infarcted/injured territory was significantly depressed in both the +HEM (45%, $p < 0.0001$) and I + HEM (49%, $p < 0.0001$) groups compared to baseline values, indicating the presence of hemorrhage (Fig. 3b). The I-HEM group was non-hemorrhagic with the T2* value statistically unaltered (p = NS). Hemorrhage volume based on T2* mapping demonstrated that the extent of hemorrhage was significantly greater in the I+HEM group compared with the +HEM group (2.8 ± 1.8 g vs. 1.1 ± 0.4 g, $p < 0.0001$) (Fig. 3b).

Edema quantified by T2 mapping

Figure 4a shows representative T2 images from the three groups with a color overlay of regions identified as edema (elevated T2) at 24 h. In the +HEM group, intensity of edema in the anteroseptal region, determined by an elevated T2 value, was weak but detectable compared to baseline (19%, $p < 0.0001$). In the I-HEM group, edema in the infarcted tissue was also mild (20% elevation from baseline, $p < 0.0001$) and not significantly different than that in the +HEM group (p = NS). The severity of edema in the infarct zone was the greatest in the I+HEM group (35% elevation from baseline, $p < 0.0001$) and was significantly greater than the other two groups ($p < 0.001$) (Fig. 4b). Percent edema volume was also significantly different across the three groups ($p = 0.0027$) and was the greatest in I+HEM (15.8 ± 8.3%) compared to + HEM (1.7 ± 1.7%) and I-HEM (4.4 ± 2.4%) groups (Fig. 4c). In the animals with hemorrhage (+HEM and I+HEM groups), T2 values were highly correlated with T2* values ($Y = -0.58*X + 54.9$; $R^2 = 0.71$; $p < 0.0001$); see plot in Fig. 5.

Histopathology

Figure 6 shows the gross pathology of the heart sections stained with TTC and Thioflavin-S along with a corresponding panel of H&E stained sections from representative animals. In the infarct zone of the +HEM group, myocardium was distended with pools of red blood cells within wide interstitial spaces (edema), and a moderate number of inflammatory cells, particularly lymphocytes and neutrophils. No red blood cells were observed in the infarcted territory of the I-HEM group; however, this region was characterized by necrosis, degenerate myocytes,

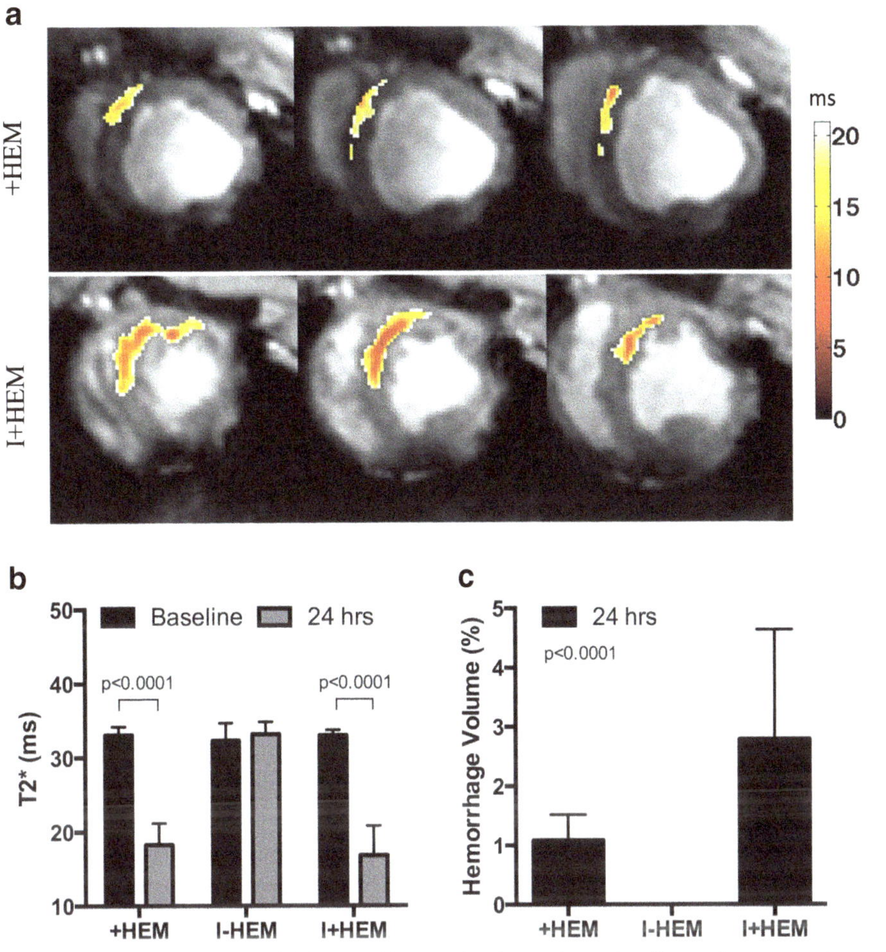

Fig. 3 Hemorrhage (T2*). **a** Representative T2*-weighted (TE = 16 ms) images showing a *color overlay* of hemorrhage extent, from animals in the +HEM and I+HEM groups; I-HEM group was non-hemorrhagic. Hemorrhagic sites were segmented using the T2* < 20 ms threshold. Each *row* shows multiple slices from the same animal. **b** Significantly low T2* values in the affected LAD territory in the +HEM and I+HEM groups quantified the occurrence of hemorrhage. **c** Resulting hemorrhage volume was greater when hemorrhage was coupled with an ischemic insult (I+HEM group) as opposed to the hemorrhage only group (+HEM)

small interstitial spaces (less edema) and small patchy areas of inflammatory cells. In contrast, the infarcted myocardium of the I+HEM group contained extensive red blood cells, necrosis, wide interstitial spaces (edema), basophilic granular material (calcium) and widespread presence of lymphocytes and macrophages and occasional fibroblasts. In both groups +HEM and I+HEM, sites of hemorrhage were spatially correlated with Thioflavin S-negative regions indicative of endothelial disruption whereas the I-HEM group demonstrated vessel patency in the infarct zone via Thioflavin S-positive signal. Qualitative observations indicated that macrophage staining was scarce and patchy in the non-hemorrhagic I-HEM group (Fig. 7). However, it was moderate to extensive in the +HEM and I+HEM groups. In these two hemorrhagic groups, it was noteworthy that macrophage activity was predominantly concentrated around the dispersed red blood cells.

Discussion

This is the first study to systematically and mechanistically demonstrate that hemorrhage is a critical component of ischemia-reperfusion injury. The novel preclinical model developed in this study was able to create three distinct patterns of ischemic injury – hemorrhage only, infarction without hemorrhage and infarction with hemorrhage. This offered a means of probing the contribution of myocardial hemorrhage in AMI in a progressive manner. Key findings of our study were as follows: 1) hemorrhage alone can induce a mild inflammatory response in the heart; 2) hemorrhage when combined with a mild ischemic insult, can further aggravate inflammation and result in greater myocardial injury beyond the initial ischemic insult; 3) hemorrhage can contribute towards the occurrence of an MVO; and 4) edema is correlated with the degree of hemorrhage and the hemorrhagic sites are targeted by infiltrating macrophages. Overall, these observations suggest

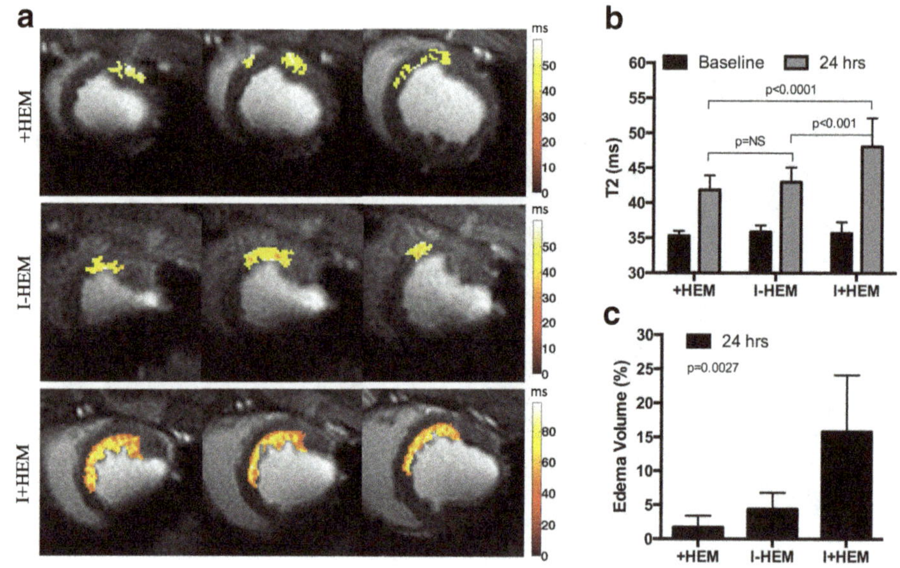

Fig. 4 Edema (T2). **a** Representative T2-weighted (TE = 88 ms) images showing a *color overlay* of edema extent, from animals in the three groups. Edematous tissue was segmented using the two standard deviation above remote T2 threshold criteria. Each *row* shows multiple slices from the same animal. Note that edema in the +HEM group was discontiguous (unlike an infarct) potentially due the non-uniform distribution of hemorrhage. **b** *Plot* shows that T2 values were significantly elevated (from baseline) in the affected LAD territory in all three groups, thus quantifying edematous development. **c** *Plot* demonstrates that edema volume was the greatest when hemorrhage and ischemia were coupled together in the I+HEM group

that a significant interaction occurs between hemorrhage, the inflammatory response and ischemic injury. Thus, hemorrhage is not simply a bystander, but an active modulator of cardiac injury and the reparative processes that follow mechanical reperfusion in AMI.

The pathophysiological mechanisms leading to reperfusion hemorrhage in humans are currently unclear. A comprehensive review on intramyocardial hemorrhage in AMI

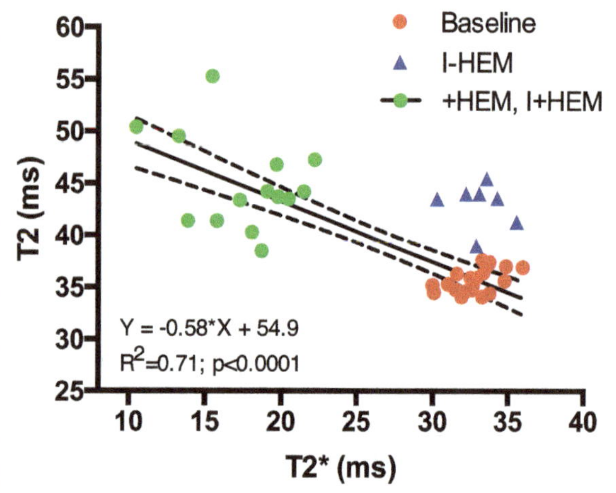

Fig. 5 Hemorrhage and Edema. *Plot* demonstrates that the inflammatory response (edema), represented by higher T2 values, was highly correlated with the presence of hemorrhage, represented by lower T2* values. The correlation was tested in animals presenting with myocardial hemorrhage (+HEM, I+HEM groups); non-hemorrhagic animals (I-HEM group) are shown in the *plot* but were excluded in the analysis

has been recently published by Betgem et al. [25]. In as early as 1960, Jennings et al. [26] identified hemorrhage as one of the key histological features of IRI in a canine model of myocardial infarction; hemorrhage always presented itself within the infarct core [24]. The primary mechanism for the development of hemorrhage appears to be via hypoxia-induced endothelial disruption. The absence of coronary blood flow might lead to increased endothelial stress, swelling and blebbing, further causing loss of interendothelial junction integrity. Beyond ischemia, reperfusion is thought to aggravate the endothelial junction leakiness and damage resulting in extravasation of red blood cells into the tissue interspaces. It has been also been demonstrated that permanent occlusions have resulted only in cellular swelling without hemorrhage and that reperfusion is a necessary condition for the occurrence of hemorrhage [4, 27–29]. Experimental studies have indicated that hemorrhage progressively increases with the duration of coronary occlusion; hemorrhage appears after 50-60 min occlusion in canines [26] and after 45 min occlusion in pigs [10, 19]. Hemorrhage is thus considered a hallmark of severe microvascular damage.

Clinical studies have shown that patients with durations of ischemia >4 h are at significantly high risk of experiencing major adverse cardiovascular events, such as re-infarction, repeat revascularization, heart failure and death [30]. These adverse outcomes appear to be highest in hemorrhagic infarcts [5, 6], although, it is still not clear whether hemorrhage has prognostic significance beyond infarct or MVO size. In a study involving STEMI

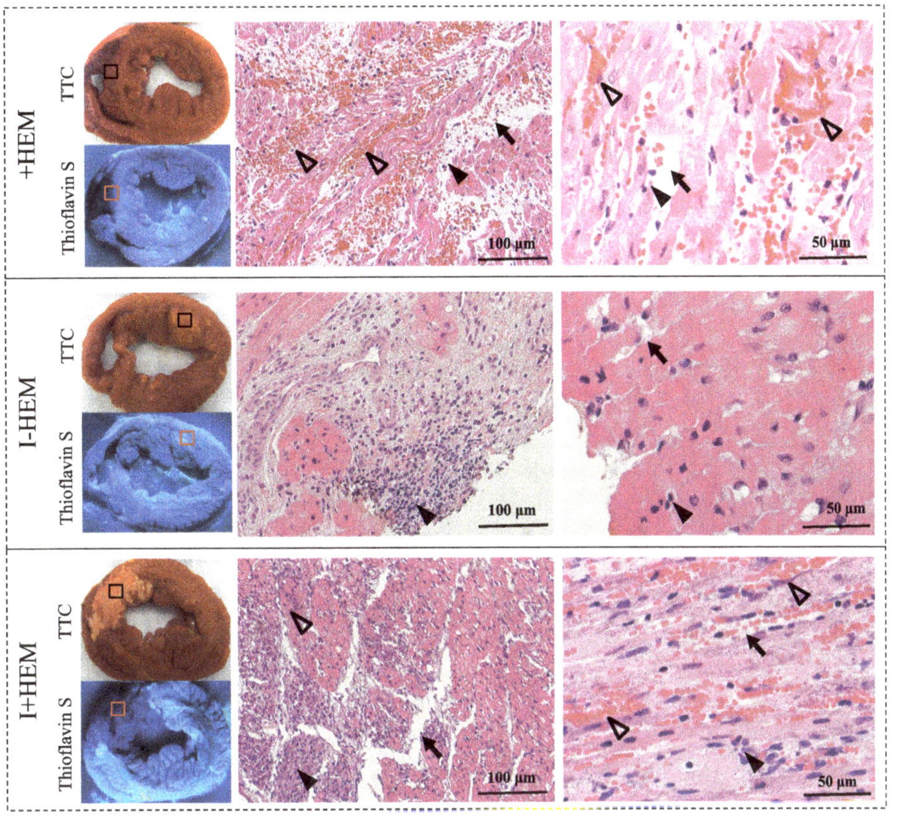

Fig. 6 *Injury Patterns* on Histology. Images show TTC, Thioflavin S and H&E stained *short axis* sections obtained from explanted hearts at 24 h post intervention. TTC sections indicate region on necrosis appearing white in the I-HEM group (no hemorrhage) and *reddish white* in I+HEM group (hemorrhage); the +HEM group did no show infarction. Under ultra-violet light, non-fluorescent regions on the Thioflavin S stain highlight areas of compromised endothelium as seen in the +HEM and I+HEM groups; this confirms presence of microvascular damage in the hemorrhage groups. The H&E images were obtained from the region of interest shown on the TTC stained sections. Hemorrhage was apparent in the +HEM and I+HEM groups as evidenced from the interstitial distribution of red blood cells (*open arrow heads*) in the affected LAD territory; red blood cells were absent in the I-HEM group. Edematous development was observed in all three groups (*arrows*) along with the presence of inflammatory cells (*closed arrow heads*)

patients, Beek et al. [16] found hemorrhage to be closely associated with infarct size, presence of MVO and cardiac function, however with no prognostic significance beyond MVO. In a study with reperfused AMI patients, Bekkers et al. [7] further concluded that MVO and hemorrhage together only represent a consequence of a severely damaged microvasculature in large infarction and that only infarct size is an independent predictor of adverse remodeling. Thus, the true role of hemorrhage remains less understood.

To understand the consequences of hemorrhage, animal models have been utilized to show differences between hemorrhagic and non-hemorrhagic infarcts using either fixed or variable occlusion times [14, 19]. For example, in the porcine model, it has been shown that 45 min coronary occlusions result in a non-hemorrhagic infarct [19] and that 45 min appears to be a threshold for the presentation of intramyocardial hemorrhage [10]; hence this model was our choice to serve as the control group. However the presence or absence of hemorrhage in these models is dependent on the physiological response of the animal to ischemia coupled with coronary architecture. Moreover, routine occlusion models cannot assess the effect of hemorrhage alone as they are always associated with ischemic injury. This is the case with clinical studies as well – clinical studies are able to determine outcomes of hemorrhage in association with infarction and MVO but cannot isolate the contribution of hemorrhage post-AMI or assess its active interaction with the healing process. In contrast, our proposed collagenase model offers a more controlled and systematic framework to interrogate the effect of hemorrhage in a progressive manner.

Collagenases are a group of metalloproteinases that can disrupt the interstitial and basal membrane collagen matrix [31]; when injected in a blood vessel this results in an increase in wall permeability and thus spillage of blood into the extravascular space. Collagenase-induced bleeding has been widely used in small animal models of intracerebral hemorrhage and the method has been

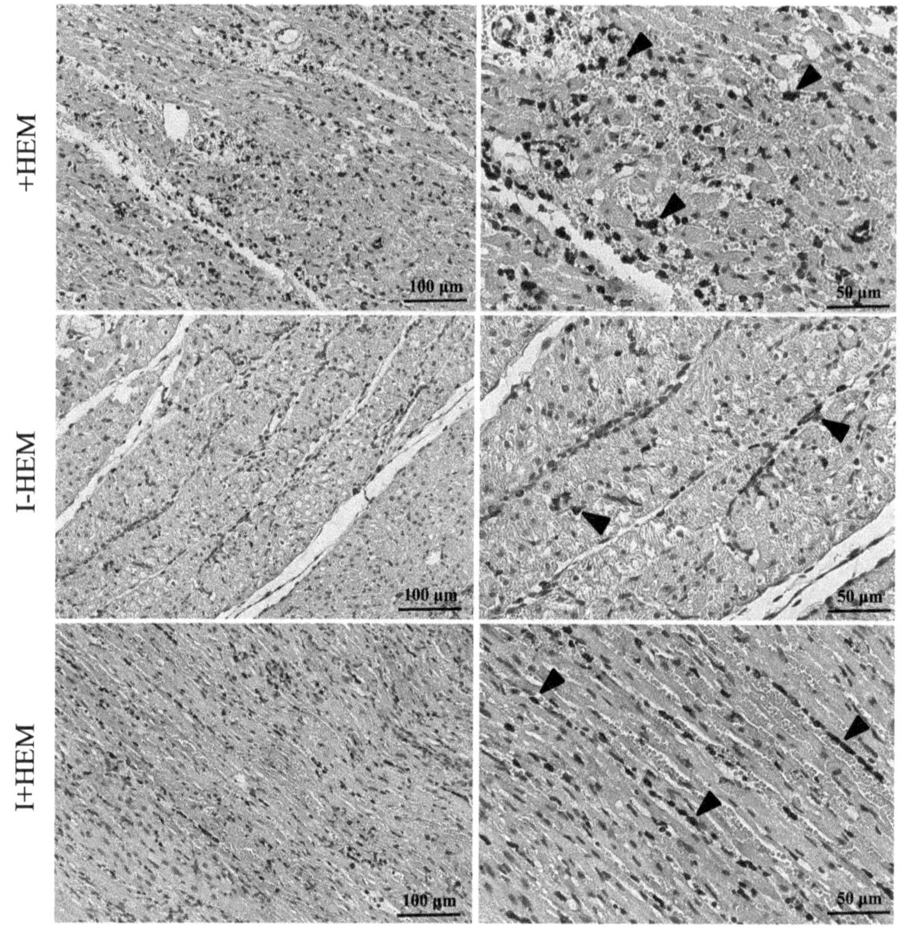

Fig. 7 Macrophage Activity. Images show MAC387 macrophage stained sections from the LAD territory. Macrophage infiltration was extensive in both the hemorrhagic groups (+HEM and I+HEM) while it was scarce in the non-hemorrhagic infarct (I-HEM). *Arrowheads* indicate sites with macrophage activity. Notably, macrophages were predominantly concentrated beside the spilled red blood cells in the interstitial spaces. (*Left* column: 20x; *Right* column: 40x)

shown to be reproducible without causing tissue necrosis [32]. Osherov et al. [18] were the first to show the effect of collagenase in the heart. They demonstrated that a single bolus injection of bacterial collagenase into a normal coronary artery was able to induce localized myocardial hemorrhage in a dose-dependent manner. For the +HEM group, we utilized an 8 min occlusion model, similar to that used by Osherov et al., to avoid any backflow of the infusate and to ensure the collagenase effects were confined to the territory of occlusion. At high dose levels, moderate sized hemorrhages were present in both epicardial and intramyocardial tissue. In our study we chose a high dose regimen of 3.2 mg bolus to ensure the consistent occurrence of intramyocadial hemorrhage in all animals. Utilizing this model, the pattern of distribution of myocardial hemorrhage observed in our study closely approximated previously observed changes following a 90 min LAD occlusion model [33].

Although the occurrence of myocardial hemorrhage following AMI has been known from human autopsy studies from the 1980s and preclinical tissue specimens [9, 10, 34], this feature was neglected due to lack of sensitive imaging techniques for in vivo detection. The in vivo identification of hemorrhage with CMR is a relatively new finding, especially in humans. Shortening of T2 and T2* relaxation times have been exploited to detect and quantify hemorrhage degradation products post-AMI [5, 6, 8, 13, 14, 17, 35, 36]; these parameters have further been validated against histopathological ground truth as well as tissue iron stores [14, 17, 35]. Visualization of hemorrhage with CMR has established the link between hemorrhage and compromised function, major cardiac events, re-hospitalization and death [37, 38]. Thus, there has been renewed interest in reperfusion hemorrhage due to its adverse consequences presented in the clinic.

The sole effect of hemorrhage in tissue has been extensively studied in the brain for understanding the implication of intracerebral hemorrhage [39–41]. CMR relaxation parameters (T1, T2, T2*) have also been well characterized in the case of brain hemorrhage along with the alterations during hemorrhagic transformation [42]. Animal models of brain hemorrhage have been instrumental in correlating the effects of hemorrhage alone on inflammation and adverse neurological effects [32]. Our study is the first to utilize this collagenase model to demonstrate that hemorrhage itself may have similar detrimental effects in the heart as well. Our findings indicate that the presence of hemorrhage attracts abundant macrophages (MAC387 positive cells) to the site of injury and interestingly, the recruitment is qualitatively many fold greater than that seen with a mild ischemic insult where macrophage infiltration is scarce, even in the acute setting. This indicates that hemorrhagic byproducts themselves are inherently pro-inflammatory in the heart and that greater hemorrhage (lower T2*) is associated with a larger inflammatory response (higher T2). Note that the low inflammatory status offered by the 45 min occlusion model (I-HEM), as demonstrated earlier [19], provided a reference for the other two groups, with which we could observe that if a small ischemic insult were coupled with hemorrhage, then the inflammatory response is further amplified. This overdriven inflammatory response may possibly be the first-stage mechanism for downstream adverse consequences in hemorrhagic infarcts.

Following successful reperfusion, the 'no-reflow' phenomenon is often encountered, characterized by ischemia-induced microvascular obstruction (MVO) and has been correlated with adverse left ventricular (LV) remodeling and poor patient outcome [43]. Recent studies have indicated that the clinical presentation of MVO and myocardial hemorrhage can be as high as 25%-63% in patients with ST-segment elevation myocardial infarction (STEMI) [5–8], and represents a high-risk group. It is well known now that hemorrhage and MVO are related; however, the causal relationship between the two has been less explored. It is uncertain whether MVO causes endothelial damage resulting in blood leakage, making hemorrhage simply a marker of severity, or whether pools of hemorrhagic sites compress the vessels leading to or worsening an MVO. Kumar et al. have demonstrated in a dog model that degree of hemorrhage increases with the size of infarction and also with extent of MVO [44]. Recent findings in STEMI patients by Carrick et al. [15, 45] demonstrate that MVO almost always precedes hemorrhage in the evolution of reperfused ischemic injury. It was shown that the temporal evolution of hemorrhage was different than that of MVO, where MVO volume peaked maximally between 4-12 h post-AMI and decreased thereafter while hemorrhage volume gradually increased from 4-12 h post-AMI, peaked at 72 h and then decreased thereafter. This study concluded that hemorrhage is a downstream consequence of MVO. This study also indicated that it is possible to observe an MVO without hemorrhage in some patients. However, it is important to note that the degree of hemorrhage is highly variable spatially within the MVO region as well as across patients i.e. it is possible to have a very small hemorrhagic region with in a very large MVO. In this regard, Carrick et al. utilized only three T2* slices in their study to detect hemorrhage, which has been acknowledged as a limitation, as a result of which regions of hemorrhage could have been missed in patients identified as having MVO but no hemorrhage.

Hence, mechanistic studies are still lacking, particularly related to complex interaction of hemorrhage with the ischemic tissue bed and vasculature. Specifically, once hemorrhage is present, does it contribute to worsening the ischemic injury and aggravating the MVO (causality)? Our study was designed to address this aspect and we speculate that vascular compression by hemorrhage and the associated inflammatory response (edema) could potentially worsen an MVO. In the +HEM group, we did not observe the classic MVO, however histology confirmed the presence of a perfusion deficit with the Thioflavin S stain. A possible explanation for this could that the regions of perfusion abnormality were too small and subtle to be detected on CMR given that this group did not present with a classical infarct. However, our findings indicate that ischemia in association with hemorrhage (I+HEM group) leads to a greater incidence of MVO suggesting a potential causal relationship between the two. Furthermore, a secondary inflammatory response arising from hemorrhage could also contribute to the no-reflow phenomenon as suggested in the literature [46]. We would also like to note that in the clinical situation, hemorrhage is not seen in the absence of an MVO post-AMI, as observed in animals in the +HEM group and some in the I+HEM group. Our animal model was not aimed to directly replicate the clinical scenario but rather identify the pathophysiological implications of hemorrhage itself, given that it is now confirmed to be a better predictor of adverse outcome than MVO.

We did not note any significant difference in cardiac function parameters, particularly EF at 24 h post-intervention across the three groups. This could potentially be attributed to the relatively small infarct sizes observed in the I-HEM and I+HEM groups with mean infarct size of 2% and 12% (of LV mass) respectively; +HEM group did not show an infarction on CMR. Based on our previous study utilizing a 90 min occlusion model [19], an infarct size greater than 20% might be necessary to see a significant alteration in cardiac function parameters in the early sub-acute phase. Nevertheless, further chronic studies are necessary to evaluate cardiac remodeling as a consequence of the hemorrhage induced by the collagenase model.

Limitations

We acknowledge several limitations. Firstly, the collagenase-based model for artificially induced hemorrhage is not a true representation of reperfusion hemorrhage resulting from injured/leaky microvasculature. Nevertheless, the model was able to achieve a similar microvascular response. Histological findings clearly identified the extravasation of blood in the interstitial spaces, creating a blood distribution pattern identical to that seen in a 90 min LAD occlusion hemorrhagic model of porcine AMI [17, 19]. Thus the goal of the collagenase model was not to mimic all aspects of reperfusion hemorrhage, but rather to introduce hemorrhage in a manner similar to that seen in IRI, i.e. through injured microvasculature.

Our study also cannot address or distinguish the effects (eg. inflammatory response) of collagenase itself from that arising from hemorrhage, which occurs as a result of its administration; this is an inherent limitation of the model. Nevertheless, the collagenase model does offer an elegant methodology for creating hemorrhagic tissue, similar to that utilized in brain hemorrhage studies [47, 48]. Our findings are in good agreement with the extensive studies investigating collagenase-induced bleeding in the brain; these studies have demonstrated that the features and consequence (edema, inflammation) of this model closely represent that seen in the case of human intracerebral hemorrhage. The collagenase model was able to achieve the intended result of blood spilling into the interstitial spaces of the myocardium. Furthermore, we would like to highlight that irrespective of the other possible effects of collagenase (if any), our study does demonstrate that hemorrhage itself induces an inflammatory response as evidenced by the presence of macrophages near red blood cells under histology, identical to that observed in the collagenase-based studies in the brain [49].

Despite a fixed dose of intracoronary collagenase, the amount of myocardial hemorrhage induced was variable across animals; in some animals hemorrhage was predominantly epicardial with some right ventricular involvement. This would be expected in a cohort of animals since the degree of microvascular response to enzymatic action and ischemia is not predictable. Nevertheless, the selection of a high dose collagenase regimen ensured a consistent induction of myocardial hemorrhage within a given group.

Lastly, T2 measurements can be influenced by both edema and hemorrhage; T2 is elevated in edematous conditions whereas it is lowered by hemorrhage and its by products [17, 33, 42]. Hence our study may have underestimated the intensity and extent of edema, as measured by the T2 parameter, in the hemorrhagic cases. In addition, given the absence of an infarct and uneven distribution of hemorrhage in the +HEM group, the T2-based regions of edema appeared to be non-contiguous given the nature of the injury. Yet, histology patterns agreed well with T2 in representing the inflammatory response with areas of wide interstitial spaces and inflammatory cell aggregation correlating well with regions of elevated T2 values; this has also been verified in our prior porcine study [17].

Conclusions

Hemorrhage is not simply a bystander but an active contributor to cellular and microvascular damage and inflammation beyond the initial ischemic insult. CMR is a powerful investigational tool that was able to reveal the underlying interactions of hemorrhage and thus demonstrate its critical role in ischemia-reperfusion injury. Future studies can be designed to address the chronic effects of hemorrhage using this novel animal model. A mechanistic understanding of the pathophysiology of reperfusion hemorrhage in the setting of AMI will potentially aid better management of the high-risk patients who are prone to adverse long-term outcomes.

Abbreviations

+HEM: Hemorrhage without Infarction; AMI: Acute Myocardial Infarction; ANOVA: Analysis of Variance; CMR: Cardiovascular Magnetic Resonance; EDV: End Diastolic Volume; EF: Ejection Fraction; ESV: End Systolic Volume; H&E: Hematoxylin and Eosin; I+HEM: Infarction with Hemorrhage; I-HEM: Infarction without Hemorrhage; IR-GRE: Inversion Recovery Gradient Echo Sequence; IRI: Ischemia-Reperfusion Injury; LAD: Left Anterior Descending coronary artery; LGE: Late Gadolinium Enhancement; LV: Left Ventricle; MVO: Microvascular Obstruction; PBS: Phosphate Buffered Saline; SD: Standard Deviation; SSFP: Steady State Free Precession; STEMI: ST-Segment Elevation Myocardial Infarction; TTC: Triphenyltetrazolium Chloride

Acknowledgements

Not Applicable.

Funding

The study was supported by the Grants-in-Aid award #000334 from the Heart and Stroke Foundation of Ontario.

Authors' contributions

NG, BS and GW contributed to the conception and study design. JB performed the animal procedures and was responsible for animal handling and care. NG, MP and XQ contributed to CMR data acquisition. NG analyzed and interpreted the CMR data and drafted the manuscript. MP, RT and SN performed the histopathological analysis and immunohistochemistry and associated interpretation. BS and GW critically revised the manuscript. All authors read and approved the final manuscript.

Competing interests

The authors declare that they have no competing interests.

Author details
[1]Physical Sciences Platform, Sunnybrook Research Institute, 2075 Bayview Avenue, Room M7-510, Toronto, ON M4N 3M5, Canada. [2]Department of Medical Biophysics, University of Toronto, Toronto, ON, Canada. [3]Schulich Heart Research Program, Sunnybrook Health Sciences Centre, Toronto, ON, Canada. [4]The Toronto Centre for Phenogenomics, Mount Sinai Hospital, Toronto, ON, Canada.

References

1. Reimer KA, Lowe JE, Rasmussen MM, Jennings RB. The wavefront phenomenon of ischemic cell death. 1. Myocardial infarct size vs duration of coronary occlusion in dogs. Circulation. 1977;56:786–94.
2. Yellon DM, Hausenloy DJ. Myocardial reperfusion injury. N Engl J Med. 2007; 357:1121–35.
3. Jennings RB, Schaper J, Hill ML, Steenbergen CJ, Reimer KA. Effect of reperfusion late in the phase of reversible ischemic injury. Changes in cell volume, electrolytes, metabolites, and ultrastructure. Circ Res. 1985;56:262–78.
4. Fishbein MC, Y-Rit J, Lando U, Kanmatsuse K, Mercier JC, Ganz W. The relationship of vascular injury and myocardial hemorrhage to necrosis after reperfusion. Circulation. 1980;62:1274–9.
5. Ganame J, Messalli G, Dymarkowski S, Rademakers FE, Desmet W, Van de Werf F, et al. Impact of myocardial haemorrhage on left ventricular function and remodelling in patients with reperfused acute myocardial infarction. Eur Heart J. 2009;30:1440–9.
6. Mather AN, Fairbairn TA, Ball SG, Greenwood JP, Plein S. Reperfusion haemorrhage as determined by cardiovascular MRI is a predictor of adverse left ventricular remodelling and markers of late arrhythmic risk. Heart. 2011; 97:453–9.
7. Bekkers SC, Smulders MW, Passos VL, Leiner T, Waltenberger J, Gorgels AP, et al. Clinical implications of microvascular obstruction and intramyocardial haemorrhage in acute myocardial infarction using cardiovascular magnetic resonance imaging. Eur Radiol. 2010;20:2572–8.
8. Eitel I, Kubusch K, Strohm O, Desch S, Mikami Y, de Waha S, et al. Prognostic value and determinants of a hypointense infarct core in T2-weighted cardiac magnetic resonance in acute reperfused ST-elevation-myocardial infarction. Circ Cardiovasc Imaging. 2011;4:354–62.
9. Fishbein MC, Maclean D, Maroko PR. The histopathologic evolution of myocardial infarction. Chest. 1978;73:843–9.
10. Garcia-Dorado D, Theroux P, Solares J, Alonso J, Fernandez-Aviles F, Elizaga J, et al. Determinants of hemorrhagic infarcts. Histologic observations from experiments involving coronary occlusion, coronary reperfusion, and reocclusion. Am J Pathol. 1990;137:301–11.
11. Roberts CS, Schoen FJ, Kloner RA. Effect of coronary reperfusion on myocardial hemorrhage and infarct healing. Am J Cardiol. 1983;52:610–4.
12. Reimer KA, Jennings RB. The changing anatomic reference base of evolving myocardial infarction. Underestimation of myocardial collateral blood flow and overestimation of experimental anatomic infarct size due to tissue edema, hemorrhage and acute inflammation. Circulation. 1979;60:866–76.
13. O'Regan DP, Ahmed R, Karunanithy N, Neuwirth C, Tan Y, Durighel G, et al. Reperfusion hemorrhage following acute myocardial infarction: assessment with T2* mapping and effect on measuring the area at risk. Radiology. 2009; 250:916–22.
14. Kali A, Kumar A, Cokic I, Tang RLQ, Tsaftaris SA, Friedrich MG, et al. Chronic manifestation of postreperfusion intramyocardial hemorrhage as regional iron deposition: a cardiovascular magnetic resonance study with ex vivo validation. Circ Cardiovasc Imaging. 2013;6:218–28.
15. Carrick D, Haig C, Ahmed N, McEntegart M, Petrie MC, Eteiba H, et al. Myocardial hemorrhage after acute reperfused ST-segment-elevation myocardial infarction: relation to microvascular obstruction and prognostic significance. Circ Cardiovasc Imaging. 2016;9:e004148.
16. Beek AM, Nijveldt R, van Rossum AC. Intramyocardial hemorrhage and microvascular obstruction after primary percutaneous coronary intervention. Int J Cardiovasc Imaging. 2010;26:49–55.
17. Ghugre NR, Ramanan V, Pop M, Yang Y, Barry J, Qiang B, et al. Quantitative tracking of edema, hemorrhage, and microvascular obstruction in subacute myocardial infarction in a porcine model by MRI. Magn Reson Med. 2011;66: 1129–41.
18. Osherov AB, Lim SY, Qiang B, Jaffe R, Erlich I, Strauss BH. Effects of intracoronary collagenase injection in a porcine model: a safety dose-finding study. J Clin Exp Cardiol. 2014;5:323. doi:10.4172/2155-9880.1000323.
19. Ghugre NR, Pop M, Barry J, Connelly KA, Wright GA. Quantitative magnetic resonance imaging can distinguish remodeling mechanisms after acute myocardial infarction based on the severity of ischemic insult. Magn Reson Med. 2013;70:1095–105.
20. Amado LC, Gerber BL, Gupta SN, Rettmann DW, Szarf G, Schock R, et al. Accurate and objective infarct sizing by contrast-enhanced magnetic resonance imaging in a canine myocardial infarction model. J Am Coll Cardiol. 2004;44:2383–9.
21. Li C, Huang R, Ding Z, Gatenby JC, Metaxas DN, Gore JC. A level set method for image segmentation in the presence of intensity inhomogeneities with application to MRI. IEEE Trans Image Process. 2011;20:2007–16.
22. Anderson LJ, Holden S, Davis B, Prescott E, Charrier CC, Bunce NH, et al. Cardiovascular T2-star (T2*) magnetic resonance for the early diagnosis of myocardial iron overload. Eur Heart J. 2001;22:2171–9.
23. Ugander M, Bagi PS, Oki AJ, Chen B, Hsu L-Y, Aletras AH, et al. Myocardial edema as detected by pre-contrast T1 and T2 CMR delineates area at risk associated with acute myocardial infarction. JACC Cardiovasc Imaging. 2012; 5:596–603.
24. Kloner RA, Ganote CE, Jennings RB. The "no-reflow" phenomenon after temporary coronary occlusion in the dog. J Clin Invest. 1974;54:1496–508.
25. Betgem RP, de Waard GA, Nijveldt R, Beek AM, Escaned J, van Royen N. Intramyocardial haemorrhage after acute myocardial infarction. Nat Rev Cardiol. 2015;12:156–67.
26. Jennings RB, Sommers HM, Smyth GA, Flack HA, Linn H. Myocardial necrosis induced by temporary occlusion of a coronary artery in the dog. Arch Pathol. 1960;70:68–78.
27. Bresnahan GF, Roberts R, Shell WE, Ross JJ, Sobel BE. Deleterious effects due to hemorrhage after myocardial reperfusion. Am J Cardiol. 1974;33:82–6.
28. Reffelmann T, Kloner RA. Microvascular reperfusion injury: rapid expansion of anatomic no reflow during reperfusion in the rabbit. Am J Physiol Heart Circ Physiol. 2002;283:H1099–107.
29. Basso C, Thiene G. The pathophysiology of myocardial reperfusion: a pathologist's perspective. Heart Br Card Soc. 2006;92:1559–62.
30. Hudson MP, Armstrong PW, O'Neil WW, Stebbins AL, Weaver WD, Widimsky P, et al. Mortality implications of primary percutaneous coronary intervention treatment delays: insights from the assessment of pexelizumab in acute myocardial infarction trial. Circ Cardiovasc Qual Outcomes. 2011;4:183–92.
31. Robert AM, Godeau G. Action of proteolytic and glycolytic enzymes on the permeability of the blood-brain barrier. Biomedicine. 1974;21:36–9.
32. Rosenberg GA, Mun-Bryce S, Wesley M, Kornfeld M. Collagenase-induced intracerebral hemorrhage in rats. Stroke. 1990;21:801–7.
33. Zia MI, Ghugre NR, Connelly KA, Strauss BH, Sparkes JD, Dick AJ, et al. Characterizing myocardial edema and hemorrhage using quantitative T2 and T2* mapping at multiple time intervals post ST-segment elevation myocardial infarction. Circ Cardiovasc Imaging. 2012;5:566–72.
34. Higginson LA, Beanlands DS, Nair RC, Temple V, Sheldrick K. The time course and characterization of myocardial hemorrhage after coronary reperfusion in the anesthetized dog. Circulation. 1983;67:1024–31.
35. Robbers LFHJ, Eerenberg ES, Teunissen PFA, Jansen MF, Hollander MR, Horrevoets AJG, et al. Magnetic resonance imaging-defined areas of microvascular obstruction after acute myocardial infarction represent microvascular destruction and haemorrhage. Eur Heart J. 2013;34:2346–53.
36. Ochiai K, Shimada T, Murakami Y, Ishibashi Y, Sano K, Kitamura J, et al. Hemorrhagic myocardial infarction after coronary reperfusion detected in vivo by magnetic resonance imaging in humans: prevalence and clinical implications. J Cardiovasc Magn Reson. 1999;1:247–56.
37. Amabile N, Jacquier A, Shuhab A, Gaudart J, Bartoli J-M, Paganelli F, et al. Incidence, predictors, and prognostic value of intramyocardial hemorrhage lesions in ST elevation myocardial infarction. Catheter Cardiovasc Interv Off J Soc Card Angiogr Interv. 2012;79:1101–8.
38. Husser O, Monmeneu JV, Sanchis J, Nunez J, Lopez-Lereu MP, Bonanad C, et al. Cardiovascular magnetic resonance-derived intramyocardial hemorrhage after STEMI: Influence on long-term prognosis, adverse left ventricular remodeling and relationship with microvascular obstruction. Int J Cardiol. 2013;167:2047–54.
39. Schlunk F, Greenberg SM. The pathophysiology of intracerebral hemorrhage formation and expansion. Transl Stroke Res. 2015;6:257–63.
40. Williamson MR, Colbourne F. Evidence for decreased brain parenchymal volume after large intracerebral hemorrhages: a potential mechanism limiting intracranial pressure rises. Transl Stroke Res. 2017. doi:10.1007/ s12975-017-0530-x. [Epub ahead of print].

41. Yang J, Li Q, Wang Z, Qi C, Han X, Lan X, et al. Multimodality MRI assessment of grey and white matter injury and blood-brain barrier disruption after intracerebral haemorrhage in mice. Sci Rep. 2017;7:40358.
42. Bradley WGJ. MR appearance of hemorrhage in the brain. Radiology. 1993; 189:15–26.
43. Wu KC, Zerhouni EA, Judd RM, Lugo-Olivieri CH, Barouch LA, Schulman SP, et al. Prognostic significance of microvascular obstruction by magnetic resonance imaging in patients with acute myocardial infarction. Circulation. 1998;97:765–72.
44. Kumar A, Green JD, Sykes JM, Ephrat P, Carson JJL, Mitchell AJ, et al. Detection and quantification of myocardial reperfusion hemorrhage using T2*-weighted CMR. JACC Cardiovasc Imaging. 2011;4:1274–83.
45. Carrick D, Haig C, Ahmed N, Rauhalammi S, Clerfond G, Carberry J, et al. Temporal evolution of myocardial hemorrhage and edema in patients after acute ST-segment elevation myocardial infarction: pathophysiological insights and clinical implications. J Am Heart Assoc. 2016; 23;5(2):e002834. doi:10.1161/JAHA.115.002834.
46. Jaffe R, Charron T, Puley G, Dick A, Strauss BH. Microvascular obstruction and the no-reflow phenomenon after percutaneous coronary intervention. Circulation. 2008;117:3152–6.
47. Chesney JA, Kondoh T, Conrad JA, Low WC. Collagenase-induced intrastriatal hemorrhage in rats results in long-term locomotor deficits. Stroke. 1995;26:312–6. discussion 317.
48. MacLellan CL, Silasi G, Auriat AM, Colbourne F. Rodent models of intracerebral hemorrhage. Stroke. 2010;41:S95–98.
49. Wang J, Doré S. Inflammation after intracerebral hemorrhage. J Cereb Blood Flow Metab Off J Int Soc Cereb Blood Flow Metab. 2007;27:894–908.

4

Myocardial perfusion is impaired in asymptomatic renal and liver transplant recipients: a cardiovascular magnetic resonance study

Susie Parnham[1,3], Jonathan M. Gleadle[2,3], Darryl Leong[3,5], Suchi Grover[1], Craig Bradbrook[1], Richard J. Woodman[4], Carmine G. De Pasquale[1,3] and Joseph B. Selvanayagam[1,3*]

Abstract

Background: Myocardial ischemia is a major cause of death in chronic kidney disease (CKD) patients, which can be caused by either epicardial or microvascular coronary artery disease (CAD). Although renal transplantation improves survival, cardiovascular disease remains a major cause of mortality in post renal transplant recipients, including those with no significant epicardial CAD pre-transplant. We aim to utilize stress cardiovascular magnetic resonance (CMR) and MR coronary angiography (MRCA) to assess silent myocardial ischemia and epicardial CAD in renal transplant recipients.

Methods: Forty-five subjects: twenty renal transplant (RT) with no known CAD, fifteen liver transplant (LT) controls without prior CKD and no known CAD, and ten hypertensive (HT) controls underwent stress perfusion CMR and MRCA.

Results: A total of 1308 myocardial segments (576 of RT, 468 of LT, and 264 of HT) were compared using mixed linear modeling. Left ventricular mass index, septal diameter and presence of diabetes mellitus were similar between the groups. The mean transmural MPRI was significantly lower in the RT and LT groups compared to HT controls (1.19 ± 0.50 in RT versus 1.23 ± 0.36 in LT versus 2.04 ± 0.32 in HT controls, $p < 0.0001$), in the subepicardium (1.33 ± 0.57 in RT versus 1.30 ± 0.33 in LT versus 2.01 ± 0.30 in HT controls, $p < 0.001$), and in the subendocardium (1.19 ± 0.54 in RT versus 1.11 ± 0.31 in LT versus 1.85 ± 0.34 in HT controls, $p < 0.0001$). Seven (35 %) RT and five (33 %) LT had significant epicardial CAD compared to none in HT controls, $p = 0.12$. One RT and one LT had LGE suggesting sub-endocardial infarction.

Conclusions: RT recipients have impaired myocardial perfusion independent of LVH or diabetes mellitus. The impaired myocardial perfusion in RT is similar to LT without prior renal disease, thus unlikely related to previous CKD. It is not fully explained by the presence of significant epicardial CAD, and therefore most likely represents microvascular CAD.

Keywords: Magnetic resonance, Renal transplant, Coronary artery disease, Myocardial perfusion, Liver transplant

Background

Cardiovascular disease is the leading cause of mortality and morbidity in the chronic kidney disease (CKD) population, accounting for 50 % of all deaths [1]. CKD patients have a 10 to 20 fold increased risk of cardiac death than the normal population, although the mechanism is uncertain [1]. Furthermore, despite the risk of cardiovascular mortality being significantly reduced by renal transplantation [2], cardiovascular disease remains a major cause of mortality in post-renal transplant recipients with an annual event rate of 3.5 to 5 % [3]. Renal transplant recipients carry a multitude of risk factors including traditional atherosclerotic (dyslipidemia, hypertension, diabetes), myocardial (hypertension and fluid overload pre transplant), microvascular (diabetes, renal failure), and immunosuppression.

Current diagnostic investigations of myocardial ischemia in renal population lack sensitivity and specificity or may have adverse effects [4]. Multi-parametric Cardiovascular Magnetic Resonance (CMR) enables concurrent assessment

* Correspondence: Joseph.Selva@health.sa.gov.au
[1]Department of Cardiovascular Medicine, Flinders Medical Centre, Bedford Park, Adelaide, SA 5042, Australia
[3]School of Medicine, Flinders University, Bedford Park, Adelaide, SA, Australia
Full list of author information is available at the end of the article

of myocardial function, perfusion and irreversible injury with high spatial resolution [5]. In particular, stress perfusion CMR has high sensitivity and negative predictive value for detecting myocardial ischemia with a sensitivity of 89 % and a specificity of 80 % [6]. In addition, two large prospective controlled trials,-CE-MARC and MR-IMPACT II-demonstrated higher diagnostic accuracy of stress perfusion CMR compared to SPECT [7, 8]. Huber et al. found that semi-quantitative evaluation provides identical diagnostic performance for coronary artery disease (CAD) to quantitative evaluation if both stress and rest examinations were used [9]. Recently, magnetic resonance coronary angiography (MRCA) has emerged as an imaging alternative for coronary artery anatomy, especially for the proximal and mid coronary segments [10]. Finally, CMR allows accurate quantification of ventricular function and mass as well as tissue characterization, thereby uniquely positioning it as a powerful modality to explore the high cardiovascular event rate in renal transplant patients.

We sought to investigate the mechanism of cardiovascular morbidity and mortality in otherwise well post renal transplant recipients using multi-parametric CMR. Our primary aim was to assess the presence and degree of myocardial ischemia utilizing stress perfusion CMR and the presence of significant epicardial disease using non-contrast whole-heart MRCA. Majority (50–90 %) of renal transplant recipients have hypertension [11] and the high (75 %) prevalence of left ventricular hypertrophy (LVH) in CKD population [12] likely persists post transplantation [13]. In contrast to the advanced CKD pre-renal transplant population, the prevalence of CAD in the end-stage liver disease patients is similar or only slightly greater than the normal population, ranging from 2.5 % to 27 %, however, cardiovascular disease is a major cause of mortality post liver transplantation [14]. We used 2 control groups- an aged matched population of hypertensive controls (to control for LVH commonly seen in the renal transplant recipients) and a post-liver transplant group (to allow differentiation of transplant milieu effects from prior renal failure effects).

Methods

Study population

Renal transplant (RT) recipients who were well and with stable renal function between three months and five years post transplantation were invited to participate to have CMR imaging at Flinders Medical Centre, a tertiary teaching hospital in South Australia, in 2012–2014. RT subjects had the following inclusion criteria: no established CAD (no history of myocardial infarction, angina, coronary artery stent or bypass surgery or angiographically documented significant CAD > 70 %, and no significant inducible myocardial ischemia pre-transplant), and no previous systolic heart failure. Liver transplant (LT) recipients with the same inclusion criteria were recruited. Ten people with a clinical diagnosis of hypertension (HT) and who were asymptomatic with no known CAD were prospectively recruited from the hospital's Hypertension Clinic.

Exclusion criteria for each group were severe claustrophobia, metallic implants, contraindications to adenosine (second or third degree atrioventricular block, obstructive pulmonary disease, dipyridamole use), and contraindications to gadolinium chelate (anaphylaxis, estimated glomerular filtration rate (eGFR) < 45 ml/min/1.73 m^2).

We identified a total of 171 RT patients from the hospital's renal database within the calendar year 2012. Exclusions were: >60 months post renal transplantation (102), ischaemic heart disease or known coronary artery disease (11), CMR contraindication (20), <3 months post renal transplantation (2), declined participation (13), language barrier (2) and pregnancy (1). Following exclusion, a total of 20 RT patients were enrolled into the study.

All participants gave written informed consent, and the study was approved by Southern Adelaide Clinical Human Research Ethics Committee (SAC HREC).

CMR protocol

All participants were instructed to refrain from caffeine 24 h prior to the scan. Subjects on beta blockers continued with their medications.

Cine imaging was acquired using standard method [15]. Stress imaging with adenosine infusion 140 μg/kg/min for 3–4 min was performed of the basal, mid, and apical myocardial segments, using an ECG-gated T1-weighted fast gradient echo sequence (echo time, 1.04 ms; repetition time, 2 ms; voxel size, 29×2.3×8 mm, flip angle 17°), and a peripheral bolus injection of a gadolinium-based agent (0.1 mmol/kg; gadolinium-based contrast agent, Gadovist, Bayer, Australia), followed by a 15 ml bolus of normal saline (rate 5 ml/s), as previously described [16, 17]. All slices were imaged during each heart beat, for a total of 50 heart beats. Blood pressure and heart rate were recorded by an automated recording machine at baseline and at 1 min intervals during adenosine infusion. After discontinuing adenosine for 15 min, the same sequence was repeated without intravenous adenosine to obtain resting perfusion images. For late enhancement imaging, an additional bolus of Gadovist (0.05 mmol/kg) was injected, and after 6 min, images were acquired in the 3 long axes and in the short axis plane to obtain coverage of the entire left ventricle using a gated T1-weighted segmented inversion recovery turbo fast low-angle shot sequence (echo time, 4.8 ms; voxel size, 1.4×2.4×8 mm; flip angle, 20°). The inversion time was adjusted to achieve optimal nulling of non-infarcted myocardium, as previously described [18].

MRCA images were obtained as a separate scan by using an 18-channel flex coil 1.5 T clinical MR scanner

(Siemens Sonata, Erlangen, Germany). A four-lead ECG was obtained for cardiac gating. Glyceryl trinitrate 400 micrograms/metered dose was administered prior to MRCA. The navigator-gated, free-breathing, non-contrast whole-heart CMRA was acquired using a 3D segmented Steady-State Free Precession sequence protocol as previously described [19, 20].

CMR image analysis

CMR analysis was performed with CMR[42] Version 4.1, Circle Cardiovascular Imaging Inc. Left ventricular mass, left and right ventricular volumes and functions were calculated using 3D short axis stack by tracing of the endocardial and epicardial contours in end-diastole and end-systole, as previously described [15]. Each parameter was indexed to body surface area (BSA). The septal and lateral wall diameters were measured in end-diastole at mid-ventricular level from short-axis view.

For perfusion analysis, semi-quantitative analysis using CMR[42] software was used. Transmural, subepicardial and subendocardial contours were traced and manually corrected for breathing displacement (Fig. 1). Each basal, mid and apical myocardial slice were divided into 6 segments with the right ventricular insertion as the reference point [21]. Since basal myocardial blood flow is closely related to the rate-pressure product (RPP), and index of left ventricular oxygen consumption, values for rest flow in each patient were also corrected for rate-pressure product [22]: Corrected Rest perfusion = (Rest perfusion/RPP) × 10^4. Myocardial Perfusion Reserve Index (MPRI) was calculated as the ratio of perfusion during adenosine-induced hyperemia to perfusion at rest corrected for RPP [23].

For late enhancement analysis, areas of subendocardial hyperenhancement were assessed visually as present or absent. The fibrosis was quantified using CMR[42] software as a percentage of myocardial mass [24, 25].

MRCA images were transferred to a 4D viewer image reconstruction CMR[42] software. Three-dimensional volume-rendered images were generated by the software. The left main, left anterior descending artery (LAD), left circumflex (LCx) and right coronary artery (RCA) were manually traced and followed for their course in axial, coronal, sagittal, cranial left anterior oblique, lateral, caudal right anterior oblique and caudal left anterior oblique views. The coronary arteries were analysed and segmented

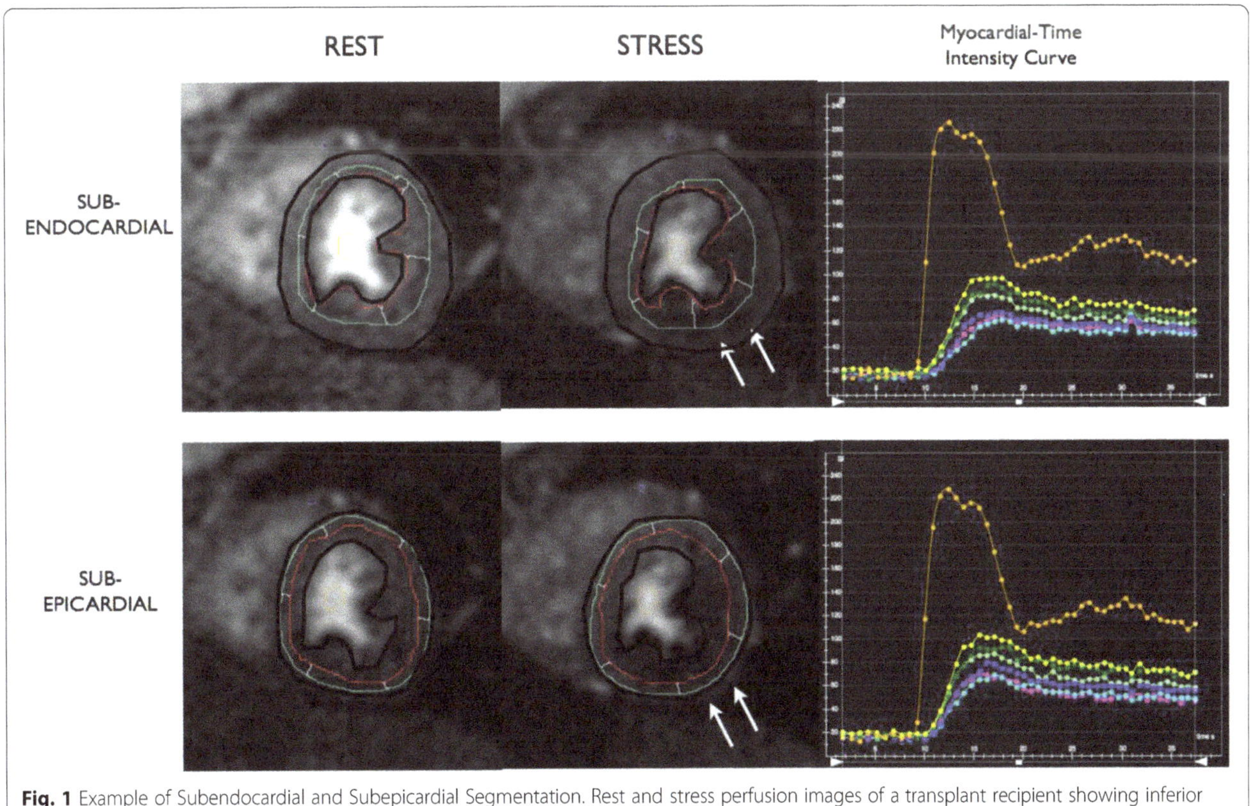

Fig. 1 Example of Subendocardial and Subepicardial Segmentation. Rest and stress perfusion images of a transplant recipient showing inferior and anterolateral perfusion defect (white arrows). Basal, mid, and apical short axis slices were acquired (a mid short axis slice was shown as representative). Transmural, subepicardial (bottom) and subendocardial (top) contours were traced. The left ventricular myocardium was segmented into six segments (anterior, anterolateral, inferolateral, inferior, inferoseptal, anteroseptal) with right ventricular insertion point as a reference. Segmental myocardial-time intensity curves at stress (shown on the right) and at rest were measured by the CMR[42] software

according to the American College of Cardiology/ American Heart Association classification [26].

One CMR experienced cardiologist (JBS) blinded to the clinical information and stress perfusion results, evaluated the left main, LAD, LCx and RCA arteries using sliding thin-slab maximum intensity projection. Significant coronary artery stenoses were defined as luminal narrowing greater than 50 % [20]. Minor coronary artery disease was defined as luminal narrowing of less than 50 %. The coronary artery was classified normal if it was smooth without any plaque occupying lumen.

Statistical analysis

Statistical analysis was performed with STATA version 13.0. Parametric data is expressed as mean ± SD and non-parametric values as median (inter-quartile range). Independent t-tests and ANOVA was used to compare the clinical characteristics of the study groups. Fisher's exact test was used for comparison of categorical variables. MPRI evaluation of coronary artery level data was analysed using linear mixed modeling (LMM) with a random intercept used for each subject to account for the within-subject correlation present from measuring at 3 different artery sites. Both unadjusted and adjusted LMM was performed with adjustment for medication use (where significant in univariate analysis) and left ventricular mass a priori. Statistical tests were 2-tailed and a p value <0.05 was considered statistically significant.

Results

Subject characteristics

Forty-five subjects participated in the study: twenty RT, fifteen LT controls, and ten HT controls participated in the study. Clinical characteristics are presented in Table 1. Using Bonferroni correction for multiple group comparison, the eGFR was lower in the renal transplant group compared to hypertensive control ($p = 0.012$), but similar compared to liver transplant group ($p = 0.67$). The eGFR was similar between the liver transplant and hypertensive control groups ($p = 0.21$). The presence of hypertension was similar between the renal transplant and hypertensive groups. The liver transplant group had less degree of hypertension compared to the hypertensive group ($p = 0.027$). The presence of hypertension in the renal transplant and liver transplant groups was not statistically different ($p = 0.06$). The use of statin between the renal transplant and hypertensive groups was similar ($p = 0.95$).

The etiology of renal diseases in the RT group were: polycystic kidney disease ($n = 7$), glomerulonephritis ($n = 9$), diabetic nephropathy ($n = 1$), medication related ($n = 1$), reflux nephropathy ($n = 1$), Alport's syndrome ($n = 1$), and unknown ($n = 1$). The etiology of liver diseases in the LT group were: alcoholic liver disease ($n = 7$), hepatitis C ($n = 5$, 1 of which was combined hepatitis C and B), primary sclerosing cholangitis ($n = 1$), non-alcoholic steatohepatitis ($n = 1$), and unknown ($n = 1$). The mean post-transplant duration between the RT and LT groups were similar (33 ± 17 versus 36 ± 18 months, $p = 0.44$). The immunosuppressant medications received by the RT and LT groups are outlined in Table 2. Their exposures were similar apart from LT patients only receiving prednisolone in the first three months post transplantation and the use of mycophenolate, which was more prevalent in RT patients.

Assessment of left ventricular mass, volumes and function

The CMR results are summarized in Table 3. Left ventricular mass index, septal and lateral wall diameter were similar between the groups.

Assessment of Myocardial Perfusion Reserve Index (MPRI)

A total of 1308 out of 1452 (90 %) myocardial segments were analyzable. A total of 576 of RT, 468 of LT, and 264 of HT) were analyzed and compared using mixed linear modeling.

Figures 2, 3 and 4 show the distribution of the MPRI across the three groups and within each of the three coronary artery sites. Across all 3 artery sites combined, the mean transmural MPRI was significantly reduced in RT subjects compared to HT controls but was similar between RT and LT subjects (1.19 ± 0.50 in RT versus 1.23 ± 0.36 in LT versus 2.04 ± 0.32 in HT controls, $p < 0.0001$). The subepicardial MPRI was 1.33 ± 0.57 in RT versus 1.30 ± 0.33 in LT versus 2.01 ± 0.30 in HT controls, $p < 0.001$. The subendocardial MPRI was 1.19 ± 0.54 in RT versus 1.11 ± 0.31 in LT versus 1.85 ± 0.34 in HT controls, $p < 0.0001$. In the renal transplant and liver transplant subgroups, the transmural MPRI was 0.97 ± 0.54 in those with significant CAD >50 % versus 1.05 ± 0.00 in those without, $p = 0.02$. Fifteen out of 20 (75 %) RT versus eleven out of 15 (73 %) LT versus one out of 10 (10 %) HT had transmural MPRI < 1.5 in at least one coronary artery territory, $p < 0.0001$.

Results remained similar in mixed model regression analysis after adjustment for statin use, aspirin use and left ventricular mass index with MPRI lower in RT subjects compared to HT controls ($\beta = 0.85$, $p < 0.0001$) but similar to LT subjects ($\beta = 0.04$, $p = 0.79$).

Significantly, in the RT group, the mean MPRI was associated with eGFR ($\beta = 0.014$, 95 % CI = 0.0023 to 0.026, p = 0.0019).

Assessment of myocardial fibrosis

One RT subject had late gadolinium enhancement indicating sub-endocardial infarction in the inferoseptal wall (1.7 g of infarct mass (0.8 % of LV mass)), while one LT subject had late gadolinium enhancement indicating

Table 1 Clinical characteristics

	Renal transplant subjects ($n = 20$)	Liver transplant subjects ($n = 15$)	Hypertensive controls ($n = 10$)	*p*-value*
Age, years (mean ± SD)	55 ± 11	61 ± 6	55 ± 11	0.17
Male sex, *n* (%)	11 (55)	12 (80)	5 (50)	0.18
BMI[a], kg/m^2 (mean ± SD)	29 ± 5	30 ± 4	33 ± 3	0.26
eGFR[b], mL/min/1.73 m^2 (mean ± SD)	78 ± 19	89 ± 29	108 ± 30	0.009
Systolic Blood Pressure (mmHg)	131 ± 19	130 ± 14	140 ± 11	0.26
Diastolic Blood Pressure (mmHg)	77 ± 14	80 ± 9	80 ± 11	0.74
Heart Rate (beats per minute)	71 ± 11	64 ± 9	77 ± 15	0.02
Cardiovascular Risk Factors, *n* (%)				
Hypertension	18 (90)	9 (60)	10 (100)	0.03
Diabetes Mellitus	3 (15)	4 (27)	2 (20)	0.62
Total cholesterol (mmol/L)	4.8 ± 1.2	4.5 ± 1.1	5.7 ± 1.0	0.06
Low-density lipoprotein (mmol/L)	2.1 ± 1.1	2.6 ± 1.0	3.6 ± 0.9	0.005
Triglyceride (mmol/L)	2.3 ± 1.4	1.5 ± 0.6	1.5 ± 0.7	0.08
Smoking History	7 (35)	6 (40)	3 (30)	1.00
Cardiac Medications, n (%)				
Aspirin	1 (5)	0 (0)	2 (20)	0.14
Beta blocker	9 (45)	3 (20)	2 (20)	0.29
ACE[c] inhibitor	5 (25)	1 (7)	2 (20)	0.41
Angiotensin Receptor Blocker	3 (15)	1 (7)	5 (50)	0.07
Calcium channel blocker	5 (25)	5 (33)	5 (50)	0.54
Statin	7 (35)	0 (0)	2 (20)	0.03

Data are presented as n (%) or mean ± SD
*Assessed using ANOVA or Fisher's exact as appropriate
[a]BMI indicates body mass index
[b]eGFR, estimated Glomerular Filtration Rate
[c]ACE, angiotensin-converting enzyme

sub-endocardial infarction in the lateral wall (2.9 g of infarct mass (2.1 % of LV mass)).

Assessment of epicardial coronary artery disease

Seven out of 20 (35 %) RT, five out of 15 (33 %) LT, and 0 out of 10 (0 %) HT controls had coronary artery stenosis >50 % in at least one coronary artery territory, $p = 0.12$. There was no significant relationship between epicardial CAD and transmural MPRI as per coronary artery territories ($\beta = -0.14$, 95 % CI −0.30 to 0.23, $p = 0.09$). Figure 5 shows representative MRCA images of the transplant recipients.

Table 2 Prescribed immunosuppressant medications in the renal and liver transplant groups

	Renal transplant subjects ($n = 20$)	Liver transplant subjects ($n = 15$)	*p*-value*
Immunosuppressant, *n* (%)			
Azathioprine	2 (10)	4 (27)	0.37
Mycophenolate	16 (80)	4 (27)	0.002
Prednisolone	18 (90)	0 (0)	<0.0001
Cyclosporine	1 (45)	1 (7)	0.68
Tacrolimus	16 (80)	14 (93)	0.37
Everolimus	1 (5)	0 (0)	0.57
Sirolimus	1 (5)	0 (0)	0.57

*Asessed using Fisher's exact

Discussion

Stress perfusion CMR and MRCA provide valuable insight into the cardiac phenotype. To our knowledge, this is the first study to investigate myocardial perfusion in asymptomatic post renal transplantation patients using stress perfusion CMR and MRCA. We have demonstrated that myocardial perfusion is significantly reduced in asymptomatic post renal transplant patients independently of the degree of left ventricular hypertrophy and diabetes mellitus. Furthermore, MRCA abnormalities do not seem to explain the perfusion abnormalities. Our findings suggest that myocardial perfusion abnormalities in renal transplant patients are predominantly due to coronary microvascular dysfunction possibly secondary to post-transplant milieu rather than significant epicardial disease. Our study findings may assist in understanding

Table 3 Left ventricular mass, septal and lateral wall thickness, ventricular volumes and ejection fraction

	Renal transplant subjects ($n = 20$)	Liver transplant subjects ($n = 15$)	Hypertensive controls ($n = 10$)	*p*-value*
LV[a] Mass index, g/m^2	64 ± 13	65 ± 11	60 ± 10	0.60
LV Septal Wall thickness, cm	1.2 ± 0.3	1.2 ± 0.2	1.1 ± 0.3	0.22
LV Lateral Wall thickness, cm	0.9 ± 0.3	0.9 ± 0.2	0.9 ± 0.2	0.81
LV End Diastolic Volume index, ml/m^2	68 ± 12	62 ± 13	70 ± 13	0.43
LV End Systolic Volume index, ml/m^2	18 ± 8	19 ± 8	22 ± 9	0.75
LV Stroke Volume index, ml/m^2	50 ± 12	45 ± 9	46 ± 10	0.26
LV Ejection Fraction, %	74 ± 9	71 ± 8	69 ± 8	0.45
RV[b] End Diastolic Volume index, ml/m^2	70 ± 11	67 ± 14	71 ± 18	0.73
RV End Systolic Volume index, ml/m^2	27 ± 8	24 ± 6	26 ± 9	0.47
RV Stroke Volume index, ml/m^2	43 ± 8	41 ± 11	46 ± 12	0.77
RV Ejection Fraction, %	62 ± 10	63 ± 7	63 ± 6	0.92

All data are presented as mean ± SD
*Assessed using ANOVA
[a]LV indicates Left Ventricle
[b]RV, Right Ventricle

the contributors to cardiac mortality and morbidity in the post- renal transplant population, thus, may lead to better management of coronary microvascular disease in this population.

CMR stress perfusion has been well validated in the assessment of epicardial coronary disease and/or coronary microvascular dysfunction. A recent meta-analysis showed stress perfusion CMR to have a high sensitivity of 89 % and a specificity of 80 % for diagnosis of significant obstructive coronary artery disease [6]. The sensitivity and specificity of stress CMR performed with a semi-quantitative measure of myocardial perfusion reserve index (MPRI) with a cutoff value of 1.5 for the detection of functionally significant (by Fractional Flow Reserve) coronary heart disease were 91 % and 94 %, respectively, with positive and negative predictive values of 91 % and 94 % [27]. Impaired coronary flow reserve suggestive of microvascular dysfunction has been reported in pre-

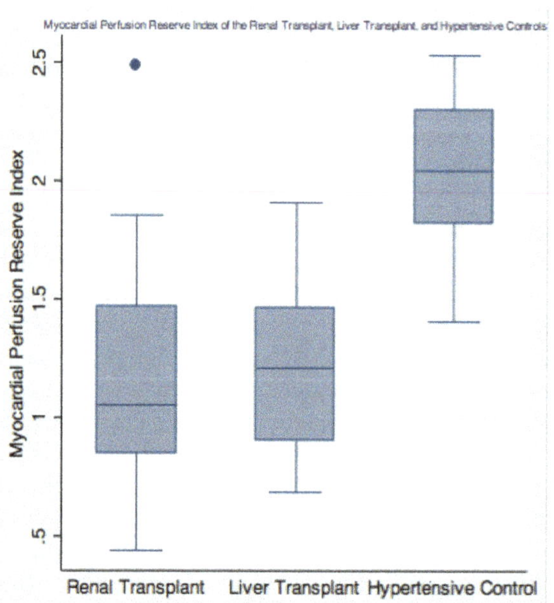

Fig. 2 Mean Myocardial Perfusion Reserve Index (MPRI) of the Renal Transplant, Liver Transplant, and Hypertensive Controls (1.19 ± 0.50 in RT versus 1.23 ± 0.36 in LT versus 2.04 ± 0.32 in HT controls, $p < 0.0001$)

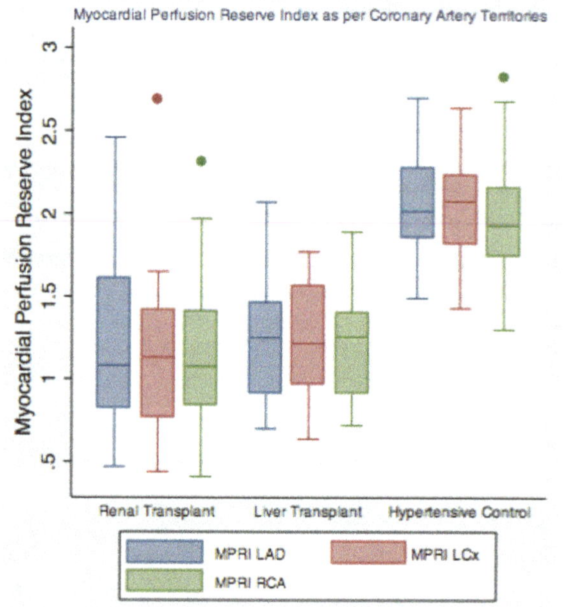

Fig. 3 Myocardial Perfusion Reserve Index (MPRI) of the Renal Transplant, Liver Transplant, and Hypertensive Controls within each of the three coronary artery territories LAD indicates Left Anterior Descending; LCx, Left Circumflex; RCA, Right Coronary Artery

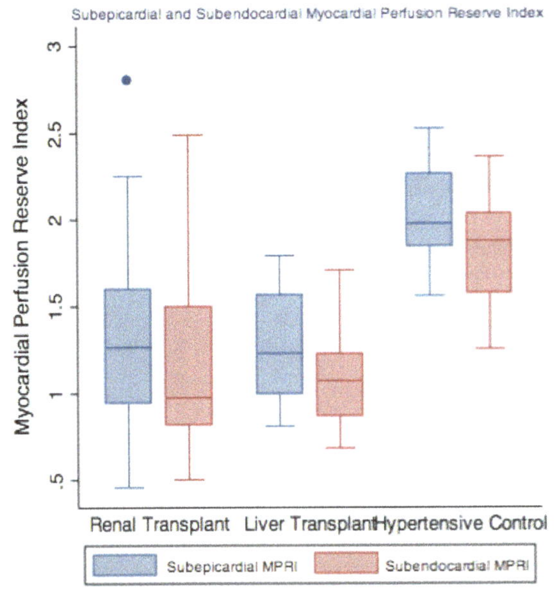

Fig. 4 Subepicardial and Subendocardial Myocardial Perfusion Reserve Index (MPRI) of the Renal Transplant, Liver Transplant, and Hypertensive Controls (Subepicardial MPRI 1.33 ± 0.57 in RT versus 1.30 ± 0.33 in LT versus 2.01 ± 0.30 in HT controls, $p < 0.001$; Subendocardial MPRI 1.19 ± 0.54 in RT versus 1.11 ± 0.31 in LT versus 1.85 ± 0.34 in HT controls, $p < 0.0001$)

transplant end-stage renal disease patients without coronary artery disease [28]. Impaired coronary flow reserve, similarly, has been observed in post renal transplant patients, even at a young age [29–31]. Given the association between LVH and reduced MPRI [32], it was important that we controlled for the degree of LVH when assessing myocardial perfusion in the renal cohort. Our HT, RT and LT groups were well matched in respect of degree of LVH, LV mass, and diabetes mellitus. Hence, our finding of reduced MPRI in the RT group is unlikely to solely reflect LVH or the degree of diabetes, and likely reflects additional abnormalities in coronary microvascular function and/or asymptomatic ('occult') epicardial coronary artery disease.

In order to further identify the mechanisms of MPRI reduction we compared the RT group with a second control group of liver transplant patients. Pre-renal transplant CKD patients have high prevalence of cardiovascular disease, in contrast, pre-liver transplant chronic liver disease (CLD) patients have low prevalence of cardiovascular disease [33]. Whilst most CKD patients have hypertension, CLD patients have portal hypertension, which causes vasodilatation and decreased in arterial blood pressure. An et al. studied 1045 liver cirrhosis patients matched with 6283 controls and showed that asymptomatic cirrhotic patients had similar prevalence of obstructive CAD compared to controls with healthy livers [33]. However, cardiovascular disease is one of the leading cause of death in post liver transplant patients [34]. A retrospective study of 455 liver transplant recipients by Fussner et al. showed that cardiovascular disease developed in 10.6 %, 20.7 % and 30.3 % of liver transplant recipients within one, five and eight years respectively [35]. In our study, the LT and RT groups were well matched in terms of the time post-transplant, age, and duration and importantly exposure to immunosuppressive medications (except for corticosteroids and mycophenolate). Intriguingly, we found that myocardial perfusion reserve was reduced in asymptomatic post renal transplant patients similar to post liver transplant patients, despite the relatively low prevalence of CAD in chronic liver disease compared to CKD patients, and despite early discontinuation of steroid use in the latter. This finding tends to absolve corticosteroid exposure as responsible for the myocardial perfusion abnormality. In our renal transplant cohort 75 % had an MPRI < 1.5 in any coronary artery territory versus 73 % of the liver transplant cohort. Although our numbers are small, there is a strong

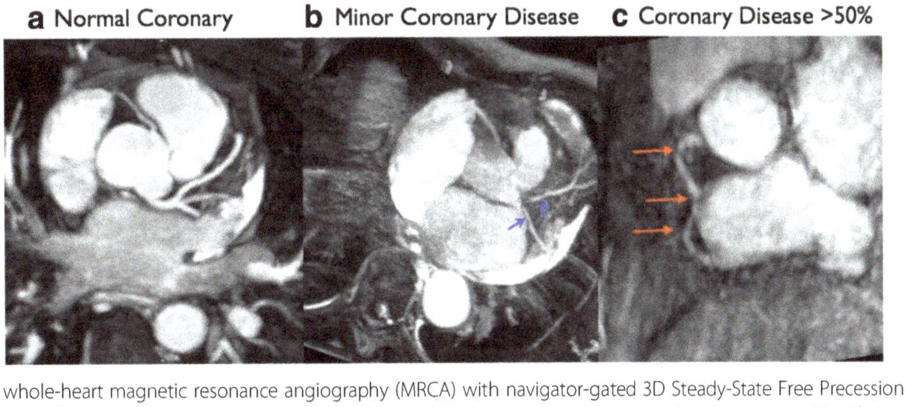

Fig. 5 Reformatted whole-heart magnetic resonance angiography (MRCA) with navigator-gated 3D Steady-State Free Precession sequence in (**a**) transplant recipient with normal coronary arteries, (**b**) transplant recipient with minor coronary artery disease <50 % with irregularities (arrows), and (**c**) transplant recipient with coronary artery disease >50 % stenosis in RCA (arrows)

biologic plausibility to this finding, given the well recognized effect of immunosuppressants in potentiating an increased prevalence of traditional cardiovascular risk factors in this population. Tacrolimus may cause vasoconstriction of the afferent and efferent glomerular arterioles, similar to cyclosporine [36]. The same mechanism may also induce coronary vasoconstriction or "spasm".

In order to investigate the presence of asymptomatic epicardial CAD, we further assessed both the RT and LT groups with MRCA. This showed that 31 % of patients post transplant (both liver and renal) had significant coronary artery disease in at least one territory. We do not routinely perform invasive coronary angiography before renal or liver transplantation in our centre. Thirty-one out of thirty-five renal transplant recipients had negative stress imaging pre-transplantation. The remaining four transplant recipients had inconclusive stress imaging and underwent coronary angiography greater than five years previously that showed only minor coronary artery disease (less than 50 % in major epicardial vessel). There was no significant difference between the presence of significant CAD between RT and LT patients. Furthermore, there was no significant relationship between the presence of significant epicardial coronary artery disease and impaired myocardial perfusion reserve, implying that the mechanism of MPRI reduction is small vessel related ("coronary microvascular") rather than epicardial disease. Microvascular CAD has been shown to be associated with reduced survival, although the rate of survival is better than for epicardial CAD [37].

Our study has several limitations. Firstly, the sample size for each group of patients was relatively small, consistent with being a pilot study. Secondly, the MRCA has lower diagnostic accuracy in the distal vessels compared with CT coronary angiography but is a safer option for post transplant recipients who have increased risk of malignancy even with small dose of radiation. Thirdly, a semi-quantitative method was used to analyze myocardial perfusion reserve since we do not have quantitative method in our center. Quantitative perfusion using CMR [17] would have permitted distinction between impaired MPRI from reduced stress myocardial blood flow (MBF) versus increased resting MBF in post transplant population. Non-contrast T1 mapping was also not available at the time of the study. Our study demonstrates the utility of multi-parametric CMR in renal transplant recipients, and confirmation in larger scale studies is warranted.

Conclusion

Asymptomatic renal transplant recipients have a global reduction in myocardial perfusion, independent of the degree of LVH and the presence of diabetes mellitus. Myocardial perfusion is also impaired in liver transplant recipients, thus unlikely due to previous CKD. In our transplant cohort, the impaired myocardial perfusion is incompletely accounted for by epicardial coronary artery disease suggesting a pathophysiologic role for coronary microvascular dysfunction in this clinical setting.

Abbreviations

CAD: Coronary artery disease; CKD: Chronic kidney disease; CMR: Cardiovascular magnetic resonance; eGFR: Estimated glomerular filtration rate; HT: Hypertensive; LVH: Left ventricular hypertrophy; LT: Liver transplant; MPRI: Myocardial Perfusion Reserve Index; RT: Renal transplant.

Competing interests

The authors declare that they have no competing interests.

Authors' contributions

SP recruited the patients, undertook data collection, analysis, interpretation of the results and drafted the manuscript. SG wrote the initial study application. RJW and DPL provided statistical analysis and made critical review of the manuscript. CB acquired the CMR images. CDP made critical review of the manuscript. JMG and JBS conceived the original study design, made an interpretation of the data and critically reviewed the manuscript. All authors read and approved the final manuscript.

Acknowledgements

Dr. Parnham was supported by the Flinders University PhD Scholarship. Dr. Grover was supported by the MFand MH Joyner scholarship in Medicine.

Author details

[1]Department of Cardiovascular Medicine, Flinders Medical Centre, Bedford Park, Adelaide, SA 5042, Australia. [2]Department of Renal Medicine, Bedford Park, Adelaide, SA, Australia. [3]School of Medicine, Flinders University, Bedford Park, Adelaide, SA, Australia. [4]Flinders Centre for Epidemiology and Biostatistics, School of Medicine, Flinders University, Bedford Park, Adelaide, SA, Australia. [5]Population Health Research Institute, Hamilton, ON, Canada.

References

1. Foley RN, Murray AM, Li S, Herzog CA, McBean AM, Eggers P. Chronic kidney disease and the risk for cardiovascular disease, renal replacement, and death in the United States Medicare population, 1998 to 1999. JASN. 2005;16(2):489–95.
2. Meier-Kriesche HU, Baliga R, Kaplan B. Decreased renal function is a strong risk factor for cardiovascular death after renal transplantation. Transplantation. 2003;75(8):1291–5.
3. Ojo AO. Cardiovascular complications after renal transplantation and their prevention. Transplantation. 2006;82(5):603–11.
4. Parnham S, Gleadle J, De Pasquale C, Selvanayagam J. Myocardial ischemia assessment in chronic kidney disease: challenges and pitfalls. Front Cardiovasc Med. 2014;1:13.
5. Karamitsos TD, Dall'Armellina E, Choudhury RP, Neubauer S. Ischemic heart disease: comprehensive evaluation by cardiovascular magnetic resonance. Am Heart J. 2011;162(1):16–30.
6. Hamon M, Fau G, Nee G, Ehtisham J, Morello R, Hamon M. Meta-analysis of the diagnostic performance of stress perfusion cardiovascular magnetic resonance for detection of coronary artery disease. J Cardiovasc Magn Reson. 2010;12(1):29.
7. Greenwood JP, Maredia N, Younger JF, Brown JM, Nixon J, Everett CC. Cardiovascular magnetic resonance and single-photon emission computed tomography for diagnosis of coronary heart disease (CE-MARC): a prospective trial. Lancet. 2012;379(9814):453–60.
8. Schwitter J, Wacker CM, Wilke N, Al-Saadi N, Sauer E, Huettle K. MR-IMPACT II: Magnetic Resonance Imaging for Myocardial Perfusion Assessment in Coronary artery disease Trial: perfusion-cardiac magnetic resonance vs. single-photon emission computed tomography for the detection of

coronary artery disease: a comparative multicentre, multivendor trial. Eur Heart J. 2012;34(10):775–81.
9. Huber A, Sourbron S, Klauss V, Schaefer J, Bauner KU, Schweyer M. Magnetic resonance perfusion of the myocardium: semiquantitative and quantitative evaluation in comparison with coronary angiography and fractional flow reserve. Investig Radiol. 2012;47(6):332–8.
10. Schuijf JD, Bax JJ, Shaw LJ, de Roos A, Lamb HJ, van der Wall EE. Meta-analysis of comparative diagnostic performance of magnetic resonance imaging and multislice computed tomography for noninvasive coronary angiography. Am Heart J. 2006;151(2):404–11.
11. Wadei HM, Textor SC. Hypertension in the kidney transplant recipient. Transplant Rev (Orlando). 2010;24(3):105–20.
12. Foley RN, Parfrey PS, Sarnak MJ. Epidemiology of cardiovascular disease in chronic renal disease. JASN. 1998;9(12 Suppl):S16–23.
13. Patel RK, Mark PB, Johnston N, McGregor E, Dargie HJ, Jardine AG. Renal transplantation is not associated with regression of left ventricular hypertrophy: a magnetic resonance study. CJASN. 2008;3(6):1807–11.
14. Lentine KL, Costa SP, Weir MR, Robb JF, Fleisher LA, Kasiske BL, et al. Cardiac disease evaluation and management among kidney and liver transplantation candidates: a scientific statement from the American Heart Association and the American College of Cardiology Foundation. J Am Coll Cardiol. 2012;60(5):434–80.
15. Karamitsos TD, Hudsmith LE, Selvanayagam JB, Neubauer S, Francis JM. Operator induced variability in left ventricular measurements with cardiovascular magnetic resonance is improved after training. J Cardiovasc Magn Reson. 2007;9(5):777–83.
16. Karamitsos TD, Leccisotti L, Arnold JR, Recio-Mayoral A, Bhamra-Ariza P, Howells RK. Relationship between regional myocardial oxygenation and perfusion in patients with coronary artery disease: insights from cardiovascular magnetic resonance and positron emission tomography. Circ Cardiovasc Imaging. 2010;3(1):32–40.
17. Selvanayagam JB, Jerosch-Herold M, Porto I, Sheridan D, Cheng AS, Petersen SE. Resting myocardial blood flow is impaired in hibernating myocardium: a magnetic resonance study of quantitative perfusion assessment. Circulation. 2005;112(21):3289–96.
18. Cheng AS, Robson MD, Neubauer S, Selvanayagam JB. Irreversible myocardial injury: assessment with cardiovascular delayed-enhancement MR imaging and comparison of 1.5 and 3.0 T–initial experience. Radiology. 2007;242(3):735–42.
19. Sakuma H, Ichikawa Y, Suzawa N, Hirano T, Makino K, Koyama N. Assessment of coronary arteries with total study time of less than 30 minutes by using whole-heart coronary MR angiography. Radiology. 2005;237(1):316–21.
20. Yoon YE, Kitagawa K, Kato S, Ishida M, Nakajima H, Kurita T. Prognostic value of coronary magnetic resonance angiography for prediction of cardiac events in patients with suspected coronary artery disease. J Am Coll Cardiol. 2012;60(22):2316–22.
21. Cerqueira MD, Weissman NJ, Dilsizian V, Jacobs AK, Kaul S, Laskey WK. Standardized myocardial segmentation and nomenclature for tomographic imaging of the heart: a statement for healthcare professionals from the Cardiac Imaging Committee of the Council on Clinical Cardiology of the American Heart Association. Circulation. 2002;105(4):539–42.
22. Czernin J, Muller P, Chan S, Brunken RC, Porenta G, Krivokapich J. Influence of age and hemodynamics on myocardial blood flow and flow reserve. Circulation. 1993;88(1):62–9.
23. Nagel E, Klein C, Paetsch I, Hettwer S, Schnackenburg B, Wegscheider K. Magnetic resonance perfusion measurements for the noninvasive detection of coronary artery disease. Circulation. 2003;108(4):432–7.
24. Selvanayagam JB, Porto I, Channon K, Petersen SE, Francis JM, Neubauer S. Troponin elevation after percutaneous coronary intervention directly represents the extent of irreversible myocardial injury: insights from cardiovascular magnetic resonance imaging. Circulation. 2005;111(8):1027–32.
25. Flett AS, Hasleton J, Cook C, Hausenloy D, Quarta G, Ariti C. Evaluation of techniques for the quantification of myocardial scar of differing etiology using cardiac magnetic resonance. J Am Coll Cardiol Img. 2011;4(2):150–6.
26. Kuettner A, Kopp AF, Schroeder S, Rieger T, Brunn J, Meisner C. Diagnostic accuracy of multidetector computed tomography coronary angiography in patients with angiographically proven coronary artery disease. J Am Coll Cardiol. 2004;43(5):831–9.
27. Watkins S, McGeoch R, Lyne J, Steedman T, Good R, McLaughlin MJ. Validation of magnetic resonance myocardial perfusion imaging with fractional flow reserve for the detection of significant coronary heart disease. Circulation. 2009;120(22):2207–13.
28. Bozbas H, Pirat B, Demirtas S, Simsek V, Yildirir A, Sade E. Evaluation of coronary microvascular function in patients with end-stage renal disease, and renal allograft recipients. Atherosclerosis. 2009;202(2):498–504.
29. Caliskan Y, Oflaz H, Demirturk M, Yazici H, Turkmen A, Cimen A. Coronary flow reserve dysfunction in hemodialysis and kidney transplant patients. Clin Transplant. 2008;22(6):785–93.
30. Turiel M, Sitia S, Tomasoni L, Cicala S, Vigano SM, Menegotto A. Subclinical impairment of coronary flow velocity reserve assessed by transthoracic echocardiography in young renal transplant recipients. Atherosclerosis. 2009;204(2):435–9.
31. Vigano SM, Turiel M, Martina V, Meregalli E, Tomasoni L, De Blasio G. Reduced coronary flow reserve in young adults with renal transplant. Nephrol Dial Transplant. 2007;22(8):2328–33.
32. Nakajima H, Onishi K, Kurita T, Ishida M, Nagata M, Kitagawa K. Hypertension impairs myocardial blood perfusion reserve in subjects without regional myocardial ischemia. Hypertens Res. 2010;33(11):1144–9.
33. An J, Shim JH, Kim SO, Lee D, Kim KM, Lim YS, et al. Prevalence and prediction of coronary artery disease in patients with liver cirrhosis: a registry-based matched case–control study. Circulation. 2014;130(16):1353–62.
34. Pruthi J, Medkiff KA, Esrason KT, Donovan JA, Yoshida EM, Erb SR, et al. Analysis of causes of death in liver transplant recipients who survived more than 3 years. Liver Transpl. 2001;7(9):811–5.
35. Fussner LA, Heimbach JK, Fan C, Dierkhising R, Coss E, Leise MD, et al. Cardiovascular Disease After Liver Transplantation. When, what and who is at risk. Liver Transplantation: official publication of the American Association for the Study of Liver Diseases and the International Liver Transplantation Society. 2015;21(7):889–896.
36. Lanese DM, Conger JD. Effects of endothelin receptor antagonist on cyclosporine-induced vasoconstriction in isolated rat renal arterioles. J Clin Invest. 1993;91(5):2144–9.
37. Lin T, Rechenmacher S, Rasool S, Varadarajan P, Pai RG. Reduced survival in patients with "coronary microvascular disease". Int J Angiol. 2012;21(2):89–94

5

Unrecognized myocardial infarctions assessed by cardiovascular magnetic resonance are associated with the severity of the stenosis in the supplying coronary artery

Per Hammar[1,5*], Anna M. Nordenskjöld[2], Bertil Lindahl[3,4], Olov Duvernoy[5], Håkan Ahlström[5], Lars Johansson[6], Nermin Hadziosmanovic[3] and Tomas Bjerner[5]

Abstract

Background: A previous study has shown an increased prevalence of late gadolinium enhancement cardiovascular magnetic resonance (LGE CMR) detected unrecognized myocardial infarction (UMI) with increasing extent and severity of coronary artery disease. However, the coronary artery disease was evaluated on a patient level assuming normal coronary anatomy. Therefore, the aims of the present study were to investigate the prevalence of UMI identified by LGE CMR imaging in patients with stable angina pectoris and no known previous myocardial infarction; and to investigate whether presence of UMI is associated with stenotic lesions in the coronary artery supplying the segment of the myocardium in which the UMI is located, using coronary angiography to determine the individual coronary anatomy in each patient.

Methods: In this prospective multicenter study, we included patients with stable angina pectoris and without prior myocardial infarction, scheduled for coronary angiography. A LGE CMR examination was performed prior to the coronary angiography. The study cohort consisted of 235 patients (80 women, 155 men) with a mean age of 64.8 years.

Results: UMIs were found in 25 % of patients. There was a strong association between stenotic lesions (≥70 % stenosis) in a coronary artery and the presence of an UMI in the myocardial segments supplied by the stenotic artery; it was significantly more likely to have an UMI downstream a stenosis ≥ 70 % as compared to < 70 % (OR 5.1, CI 3.1-8.3, $p < 0.0001$). 56 % of the UMIs were located in the inferior and infero-lateral myocardial segments, despite predominance for stenotic lesions in the left anterior descending artery.

Conclusion: UMI is common in patients with stable angina and the results indicate that the majority of the UMIs are of ischemic origin due to severe coronary atherosclerosis. In contrast to what is seen in recognized myocardial infarctions, UMIs are predominately located in the inferior and infero-lateral myocardial segments.

Keywords: Angiography, Coronary disease, Imaging, Infarction, Cardiovascular magnetic resonance

* Correspondence: per.hammar@ltv.se
[1]Västmanland County Hospital Västerås, Department of Radiology, Västerås S-72189, Sweden
[5]Department of Radiology, Oncology and Radiation Science, Uppsala University, S-75185 Uppsala, Sweden
Full list of author information is available at the end of the article

Background

Myocardial infarction (MI) is typically associated with symptoms (e.g. chest pain) that cause the patient to seek medical care. However, MI might be asymptomatic or have atypical symptoms that are not recognized by either the patient or the health professionals as indicating MI. These silent myocardial infarctions or more correctly, unrecognized myocardial infarctions (UMIs), have traditionally been detected as pathological Q-waves on electrocardiography (ECG) taken after the acute event. UMIs represent between 22 and 44 % of all myocardial infarctions [1]. In the general population the prevalence of UMI detected by Q-waves is strongly related to age. It is extremely rare under the age of 40, while the prevalence is > 5 % in men >75 years of age [2]. The mortality rates after unrecognized and recognized myocardial infarctions are similar [3].

Late gadolinum enhancement cardiac magnetic resonance (LGE CMR) is a recent technique that can identify even very small MIs [4]. Using this technique previous studies have shown a prevalence of UMIs among 65–75 -year-olds in the general population of 17–30 % [5–7]. UMI was more than four times more common than recognized myocardial infarctions (RMIs), 19.8 % and 4.4 %, respectively, in the study of Barbier et al. [7].

Kim et al. have recently shown that the prevalence of LGE CMR detected UMI increased with the extent and severity of coronary disease in the patient [8]. However, to the best of our knowledge, the association between the severity of atherosclerosis in a specific coronary artery and occurrence of an UMI in the myocardial segments supplied by that very same artery has not previously been investigated. Therefore, the aims of the present study were twofold: to investigate the prevalence of UMI detected by LGE CMR imaging in patients with stable angina pectoris and no known previous MI; and to elucidate whether UMI is associated with stenotic lesions in the coronary artery supplying the segment of the myocardium in which the UMI is located.

Methods

Study population

In the prospective multicenter study, Prevalence and Prognostic Value of Unrecognized Myocardial Injury in Stable Coronary Artery Disease (PUMI), we included patients with angina pecoris scheduled for coronary angiography. The diagnosis of angina pectoris was made by the treating physician based on symptoms compatible with stable angina pectoris. The decision to perform coronary angiography was made prior to study recruitment. In all patients included in the study a LGE CMR examination was scheduled for research purpose only prior to the coronary angiography. In the normal clinical work-up of patients with symptoms of stable angina pectoris at our institutions, no LGE CMR examinations are usually done. Exclusion criteria were: pathological Q-wave on 12-lead ECG, previously known myocardial infarction, previous percutaneous coronary intervention (PCI) or coronary artery bypass graft (CABG), history of congestive heart failure, estimated glomerular filtration rate (GFR) < 30 ml/min/1,73 m^2, conventional conditions contraindicating an CMR examination (e.g. pacemaker, claustrophobia, intracranial clips) or lack of suitability for participation in the study for any reason as judged by the investigator. Patients were enrolled from 6 Swedish sites: Danderyd County Hospital ($n = 13$), Falun County Hospital ($n = 68$), Gävle County Hospital ($n = 22$), Linköping University Hospital ($n = 32$), Uppsala University Hospital ($n = 87$) and Örebro University Hospital ($n = 43$) during the period January 2008 to March 2011.

Of the 265 included patients in the study, the 235 patients that had both a coronary angiography and a CMR possible to analyse constituted the study cohort in the present report (Fig. 1). Five patients did not perform

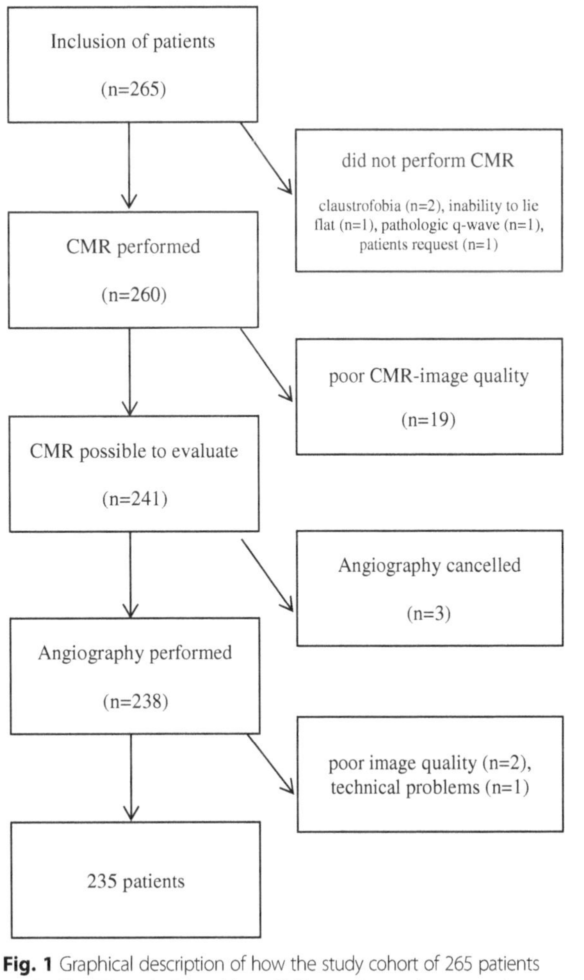

Fig. 1 Graphical description of how the study cohort of 265 patients resulted in 235 evaluable subjects. CMR = cardiovascular magnetic resonance

CMR, 19 patients were excluded because of poor MR quality, six patients either did not perform coronary angiography or was not possible to evaluate.

The study was approved by the regional ethics committee in Uppsala (U-07-001 PUMI) and all patients provided written informed consent. The PUMI study is registered at ClinicalTrials.gov (NCT01257282).

Study procedure

Patients referred for coronary angiography to the participating hospitals were screened for inclusion and exclusion criteria. In eligible patients enrolled, after obtaining the clinical history and a physical examination, LGE CMR was performed. In the study population we performed LGE CMR imaging prior to, but not more than 4 weeks before, the scheduled coronary angiography.

During the study the patients received treatment at the discretion of the responsible physician.

Image acquisition

CMR was performed on clinical 1,5-T scanners (Philips Intera, Best, the Netherlands; Philips Achieva, Best, the Netherlands or Siemens Symphony, Erlangen, Germany) using a general scanning protocol. This consisted of survey scans to plan further scanning, cine short axis images and a viability sequence in short axis (SA), long axis 2-chamber, 3-chamber and 4-chamber views using ECG-triggering and breath-holding. Patients were given an injection of 0.15 ml/kg bodyweight (maximum dose 15 ml) of gadobutrol (Gadovist®, Bayer, Leverkusen, Germany) and viability imaging was performed with a minimum delay of 15 minutes. In the waiting time cine short axis was performed. This consisted of a steady state free precession (SSFP) sequence with the following parameters: repetition time (TR) shortest, echo time (TE) shortest, flip angle 70°, image matrix 176x190 reconstructed to a voxel size 1.37x1.37x6 mm with a slice gap of 4 mm, 18 heart phases acquired, 2 slices per breath hold. The viability sequence was a 3D inversion recovery gradient echo sequence with the following parameters: TR set to shortest (typically 4.0-4.2 ms), TE set to shortest (typically 1.18-1.28 ms), inversion time (TI) chosen by the operator to null normal myocardium, flip angle 15°, image matrix 256x100, FOV 375 x 281 mm, acquired voxel size 1.46x2.81x10 mm reconstructed to a voxel size 0.73x0.73x5 mm. Eleven slices were acquired per breath hold for the long axis slices (2CH, 3CH and 4CH) and 22 slices divided in two breath holds for the short axis. Each breath hold were 16 seconds at heart rate 60 bpm. A 3D sequence was used instead of 2D contiguous slices. This strategy allows imaging in 4 different planes with good patient compliance due to less breath-holds and shorter examination time. This protocol was acquired in the majority of the subjects. A few sites had to adapt the protocol (e.g. due to hardware constraints) to ensure best possible image quality to demarcate LGE. In the single site with Siemens equipment 2D imaging with contiguous slices was used due to difficulties with applying 3D imaging at that site. When this had to be done the adaption was chosen to be as minor as possible compared to the standard protocol.

Coronary angiography was performed after (more than 12 hours but less than 4 weeks) the CMR in a routine way with standard projections.

Image analysis, CMR

At CMR, areas of LGE that were visible in at least two imaging planes were noted and localized using the American Heart Association (AHA) 17-segment model, proposed by Cerqueira et al. [9]. The images were analysed at the core lab by two radiologists (T.B. and P.H.) in consensus. Areas of LGE could engage one or several adjacent segments. If there were distinctly separate areas of LGE, each of those was assessed individually. Presence of LGE in each subject was noted. If a LGE had a subendocardial component it was categorized as "transmural" or "subendocardial" depending on whether the contrast enhancement was reaching the epicardium or not [10]. In the following, subjects within those two groups are labelled unrecognized myocardial injury ("UMI"). Areas of LGE without a subendocardial component, i.e. located only subepicardially or in the center of the myocardium, were labelled as "no MI" together with subjects with no LGE. The myocardium displaying LGE was analysed using manual contouring of the area in each short axis slice on a clinical PACS-system (Carestream Health, Rochester, NY, USA) and the volumes of the enhanced myocardium were calculated. Finally UMI mass was calculated by multiplying the volume by the density of the myocardial tissue (1.05 g mL^{-1}).

The treating physician had no access to the results of the analysis of the CMR examination with the exception of calculated ejection fraction (EF) and any observed wall motion abnormalities.

Image analysis, coronary angiography

CMR was followed by coronary angiography. In accordance with the Swedish Coronary Angiography and Angioplasty Registry (SCAAR) the coronary vessels were divided in 19 segments, derived from the 16 segment model proposed by Austen et al. [11].

The degree of narrowing of the diameter in each of the 19 coronary segments was visually categorized as 0-29 %, 30-49 %, 50-69 %, 70-99 % or 100 % (occlusion) in accordance with the SCAAR-registry. This methodology is in accordance with previous published studies on the SCAAR-registry [12].

In the proposed AHA 17-segment model by Cerqueira et al. [9] individual myocardial segments are assigned to specific coronary arteries. However, this assumption has been challenged and has been shown to be inaccurate [13, 14], e.g. Ortiz-Pérez showed in a CMR-study that only four segments were completely specific for the left anterior descending artery (LAD), but no segments were completely specific for the right coronary artery (RCA) or for the circumflex artery (LCX) [14]. Therefore, in each patients we assessed visually for all coronary arteries with a stenosis of ≥30 %, which of the myocardial segments in the 17-segment model that were supplied by that particular artery downstream the stenosis, taking the individual coronary anatomy in consideration. This assessment was done at the core lab by two radiologists (P.H. and O.D.) blinded for the result on CMR, first individually, then in consensus.

Analysis of association between coronary artery stenosis and LGE

The association between coronary artery stenosis and presence of LGE was analysed in two ways. In the primary analysis, a perfect match was required between the myocardial segments deemed to be supplied by a coronary artery with stenosis, and the myocardial segment(s) with LGE. However, because of the obvious difficulties in some cases to correctly assess which myocardial segments are supplied by a certain coronary artery we also performed a secondary, less conservative "near match" analysis. Near match was considered to exist even when LGE occurred in any adjacent segment to segments that were deemed to be supplied by a coronary artery with stenosis, with one exception. The border between septum and the free wall was angiographically clear and therefore the segments on different sides of this border were not considered near. The list of segments used when converting "exact match" to "near match" is shown in Additional file 1: Table S1.

Statistical analysis

For statistical analysis SAS 9.3 was used. Level of significance set at $p < 0.05$. Fishers exact test was used to compare categorical values for patients. Data by segment were analysed with a generalized estimating equation (GEE) model [15] that fully accounts for any dependence between segments for the same patient. This approach approximately addresses error estimates in the context of correlated observations. In addition to the univariate model, the relation between severity of stenosis and UMI was also analysed in a multivariate model adding age, gender, diabetes and hypertension as covariates. Age was analysed as a continuous variable. Gender, diabetes and hypertension were analysed as categorical variables. Results were presented as odds ratios (OR) with 95 % confidence intervals (CIs) and p-values. When describing clinical characteristics number (%), mean and standard deviation or median and interquartile range (IQR) were used as appropriate.

Results

Clinical characteristics and prevalence of UMI

UMIs were found in 58 patients (24.7 %), out of whom 3 patients had two distinctly separate areas of UMI. The background characteristics of the study population stratified in those with and without UMIs are shown in Table 1. UMIs tended to be more common among men compared to women, 44/155 (28 %) vs. 14/80 (18 %) ($p = 0.08$); and in patients with compared to without diabetes mellitus, 17/49 (35 %) vs. 41/186 (22 %) ($p = 0.09$). There was no significant difference in left ventricular ejection fraction, 66 % vs. 67 % ($p = 0{,}55$).

Areas of LGE without a subendocardial component, i.e. not fulfilling the criteria for UMI, were present in 25 patients (11 %).

Table 1 Background characteristics

	No UMI ($n = 177$)	UMI ($n = 58$)	*P*-value
Age at inclusion, years	64.2 ± 8.8	66.6 ± 8.2	0.07
Women (%)	66 (37 %)	14 (24 %)	0.08
Current smoker (%)	16 (9 %)	6 (10 %)	0.80
Previous smoker (%)	89 (50 %)	32 (55 %)	0.55
Family history of IHD (%)	87 (49 %)	30 (52 %)	0.76
Hypertension (%)	94 (53 %)	38 (66 %)	0.13
Diabetes mellitus (%)	32 (18 %)	17 (29 %)	0.09
Previous stroke/TIA (%)	7 (4.0 %)	6 (10 %)	0.09
PVD (%)	6 (3.4 %)	6 (10 %)	0.08
COPD (%)	13 (7.3 %)	3 (5.2 %)	0.77
BMI	27.3 ± 3.5	27.7 ± 4.0	0.49
Waist circumference, cm	99.1 ± 10.0	101.8 ± 11.7	0.55
Systolic BP, mmHg	139 ± 17	143 ± 19	0.22
Diastolic BP, mmHg	79 ± 10	79 ± 10	0.96
Ejection fraction, % median (IQR)	66 (61–71)	67 (62–72)	0.55
Symptoms of angina pectoris			
<2 months (%)	6 (3 %)	1 (2 %)	0.75
2-12 months (%)	80 (45 %)	25 (43 %)	
>12 months (%)	91 (51 %)	32 (55 %)	
Medications			
Aspirin (%)	158 (89 %)	53 (91 %)	0.81
Clopidogrel (%)	4 (2 %)	3 (5 %)	0.37
Statin/other lipid lowering agent (%)	121 (68 %)	46 (79 %)	0.13

IHD Ischemic Heart Disease, *TIA* Transient Ischemic Attack, *PVD* Peripheral Vascular Disease, *COPD* Chronic Obstructive Pulmonary Disease, *BMI* Body Mass Index, *BP* Blood Pressure, *IQR* InterQuartileRange

Some representative images of UMIs and corresponding coronary angiographies are shown in Fig. 2. Additional files 2, 3 and 4 contains moving images, Additional file 2: short axis 3D CMR, Additional file 3: coronary angiography of LCA, Additional file 4: coronary angiography of RCA.

Size and localization of the UMIs

The LGE was transmural in 21 patients, and subendocardial in 37 patients. The three patients with two distinct UMIs had in two cases two separate subendocardial UMIs and in one case one subendocardial UMI and one transmural UMI. The majority of the UMIs were small, the median size of the UMI was 2.1 g (IQR 0.7 – 4.5 g), and the maximum size was 27.8 g (Additional file 5: Figure S1).

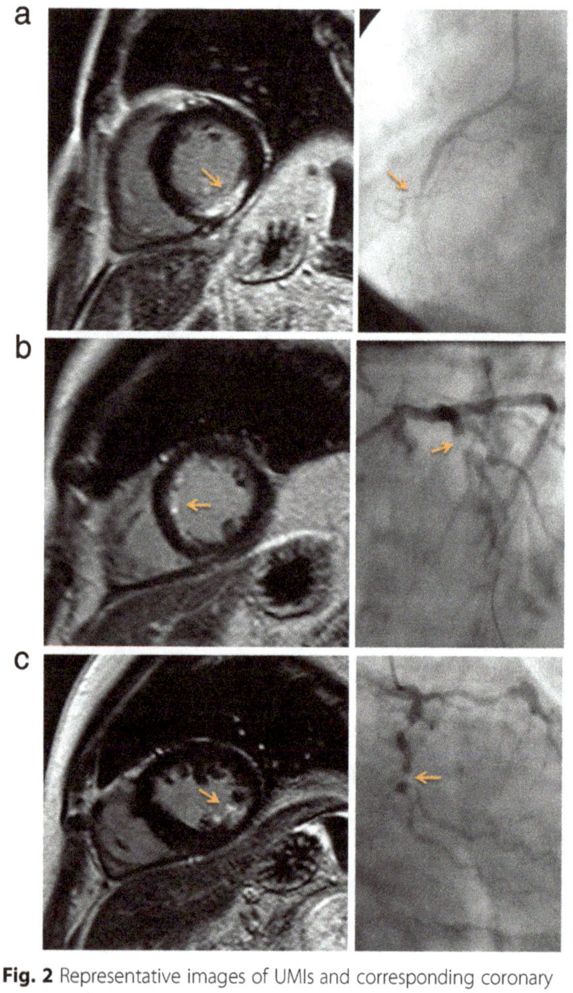

Fig. 2 Representative images of UMIs and corresponding coronary angiographies. **a** transmural UMI in AHA segment 4 but also partly in segment 3 and 5 with corresponding RCA occlusion on coronary angiography, **b** subendocardial UMI in AHA segment 8 and 9 with corresponding high grade stenosis in proximal LAD, **c** subendocardial UMI in AHA segment 11 with corresponding high grade stenosis in proximal LCX. Three supplemental moving images of example (**c**) are also provided; Additional files 2, 3 and 4

In total 110 myocardial segments were affected in the 58 patients with UMI. The localization of the segments with UMI is shown in Fig. 3. The UMIs were predominately located in the inferior and inferior-lateral myocardial segments (AHA segments 4, 5, 10, 11, 15, 16) with 56 % of the UMIs located in those areas.

Findings at coronary angiography

At coronary angiography 32 patients (13.6 %) had a total occlusion of at least one coronary branch, 103 patients (43.8 %) had a maximal stenosis of ≥70-99 %, 8 patients (3.4 %) a maximal stenosis ≥50-69 %, 63 patients (30.2 %) a maximal stenosis of ≥30-49 %, and 29 patients (12.3 %) had no stenosis or a maximal stenosis grade of less than 30 %. In men, 64 % had a maximal stenosis ≥ 70 %, whereas only 45 % in women ($p = 0.008$). In patients with diabetes 80 % had a maximal stenosis ≥ 70 %, compared with 52 % in patients without diabetes ($p < 0.0001$). The distribution of the lesions causing a stenosis ≥70 % showed predominance for lesions in the LAD territory (Fig. 4), except for patients with diabetes where there was an equal predominance for LAD and LCX territories.

Relation between coronary stenosis and UMI on patient level and on segment level

UMIs were more prevalent in the 135 patients with at least one coronary artery stenosis ≥ 70 %, as compared to the 100 patients with coronary artery stenosis <70 %, 47 (34.8 %) vs. 11 (11.0 %) ($p < 0.0001$).

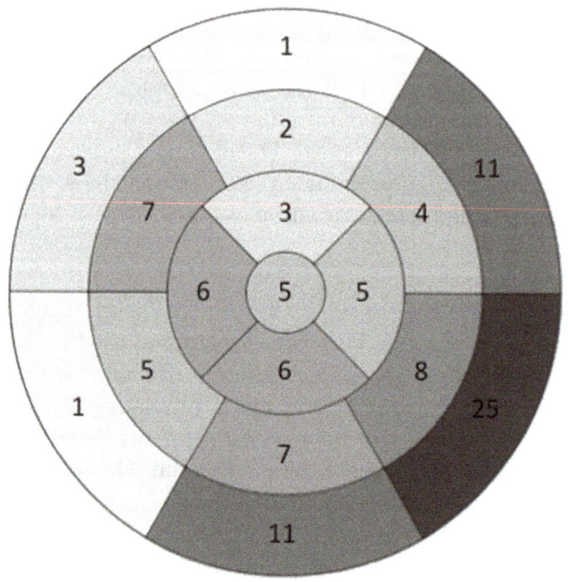

Fig. 3 The localization of the infarctions found by CMR in the 58 patients with unrecognized myocardial infarctions (UMIs). The number in each of the 17 different myocardial segments gives how often a certain segment was affected. In total, 110 segments were affected in the 58 patients

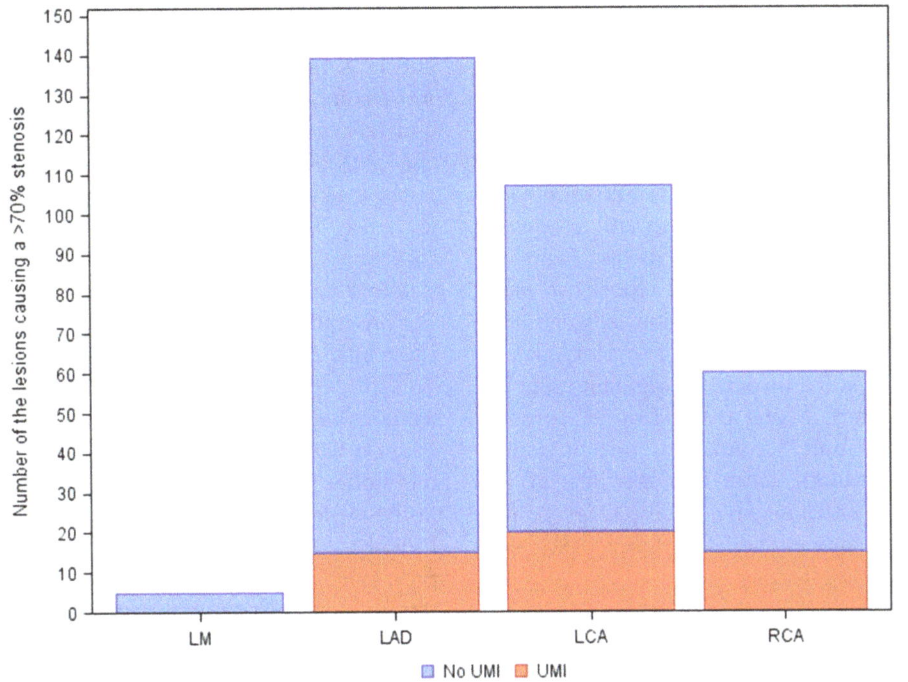

Fig. 4 Distribution of segments supplied by a coronary artery with a stenosis ≥70 % on coronary angiography. The red part of the bars are segments with a UMI and the remaining blue bars are segments without UMI. LM = left main artery, LAD = left anterior descending artery, LCA = left circumflex artery, RCA = right coronary artery

When assessing the prevalence of UMI in myocardial segments downstream a coronary stenosis, taking the individual coronary anatomy in consideration and requiring "perfect match" (see method section) a significant relation between the stenosis grade in the supplying artery and the prevalence of UMI was found (Table 2). The prevalence of UMIs in segments supplied by an artery with <30 % stenosis was 1.3 % compared to 20.1 % in those segments supplied by an artery with total occlusion. It was significantly more likely to have an UMI downstream a stenosis ≥70 % as compared to <70 % (OR 5.1, CI 3.1-8.3, $p < 0.0001$). The strong association remained almost unchanged after adjustment for age, gender, diabetes and hypertension (OR 4.7, CI 2.8-7.7, $p < 0.0001$). If the segments supplied by an artery with total occlusion were excluded, it was still significantly more likely to have an UMI downstream a stenosis ≥70-99 % as compared to <70 % (adjusted OR 2.88, CI 1.6-5.1, $p = 0.0002$).

Table 2 Myocardial segments with and without UMI grouped by degree of coronary artery stenosis

	No UMI	UMI	Total no of segments
Stenosis < 30 %	1331	18	1349
	98,7 %	1.3 %	
Stenosis ≥ 30 % - < 50 %	1194	14	1208
	98.8 %	1.2 %	
Stenosis ≥ 50 % - < 70 %	310	3	313
	99.0 %	1.0 %	
Stenosis ≥ 70 % - 99 %	927	44	971
	95.5 %	4.5 %	
Stenosis 100 %	123	31	154
	79.9 %	20.1 %	
Total no of segments	3885	110	3995

Small numbers indicate number of segments and the percentage is calculated towards the total number in the right-most column. The percentage in bold indicate the percentage of affected segments with UMI

UMI Unknown Myocardial Infarction, *No UMI* No Unknown Myocardial Infarction

The proportions of UMI downstream a stenosis ≥70 % tended to be unevenly distributed between RCA, LCX and LAD, 25.0 %, 18.7 % and 10.8 %, respectively ($p = 0.08$), Fig. 4. However, the size of the UMIs downstream a stenosis ≥70 % was not significantly different between the three coronary arteries (median 3.9, 3.9 and 2.9 g, respectively).

Of all myocardial segments with UMI, 68 % occurred in segments downstream a stenosis ≥70 %; no difference in proportions was found between men and women or between patients with and without diabetes.

In a sensitivity analysis, the relation between coronary stenosis and UMI requiring "near match", but not "perfect match", between the supplying artery with stenosis and the myocardial segment with UMI was assessed. In that analysis the proportion of myocardial segments with UMI downstream a stenosis ≥70 % rose from 68 % to 88 %. In contrast to the UMIs, areas of LGE without a subendocardial component had no clear relation to the findings at the coronary angiogram (data not shown).

Discussion

In this multicenter study performed to prospectively evaluate the prevalence of UMI in patients with symptoms of angina pectoris and the association between UMIs and significant coronary artery disease, we could confirm a high prevalence of UMI and report two major novel findings. First, a strong association between stenotic lesions (≥70 % stenosis) in a coronary artery and the presence of an UMI in the myocardial segments supplied by that stenotic artery, taking the individual coronary anatomy in consideration. Second, a striking predominance for the UMIs to be located in the inferior and inferior-lateral myocardial segments, despite predominance for stenotic lesions in the left anterior descending artery (LAD) territory.

Prevalence of UMI and its relation to clinical characteristics

The prevalence of UMI of 25 % in the present study is close to the 27 % found in a previous study of UMI in a similar population [8], but higher than the prevalence of 20 % [7] and 17 % [5] found in general populations, which is not surprising given the higher pre-test probability of ischemic heart disease in our study population with symptoms of angina pectoris. Consequentially, we found an association between conventional cardiovascular risk factors and occurrence of UMI (Table 1) in contrast to in the study in the general population of Barbier et al. [7].

The large difference numerically (but only reaching borderline significance) in prevalence of UMI between men and women; and patients with and without diabetes, is in line with previous studies [6, 16]. One likely explanation for these findings is the clear differences in occurrence and severity of underlying coronary atherosclerosis in the present study between men and women, and patients with and without diabetes, respectively.

Size and localization of the UMIs

The UMIs were predominantly subendocardial infarctions and rather small, which is in accordance with previous findings [7]. However, it is important to notice that a Q-wave in the qualifying ECG was an exclusion criteria, regardless of whether the Q-wave was associated with a known previous MI or not. Nevertheless, a significant proportion of the UMIs were transmural infarctions.

In striking contrast to what is seen in recognized MIs [17], the UMIs were located predominantly in the inferior and inferolateral areas of the myocardium, in line with the findings in the study of Barbier et al. [7], but somewhat in contrast to the study by Kim et al. [8]. This distribution occurred despite that a ≥70 % stenosis was more common in the LAD territory than in the RCA and LCX territories. Hence, UMI tended to be relatively more common downstream a ≥70 % stenosis in the RCA and LCX compared to downstream a ≥70 % stenosis in the LAD (Fig. 4). The reason for this paradox is unclear, but it is likely that ischemia in the inferior and inferolateral areas of the myocardium leading to small infarctions may cause less severe, and more often atypical (e.g. abdominal pain or discomfort), symptoms and therefore not prompt the patient to seek medical attention. Hence, these infarctions may more often go undetected.

Relation between coronary stenosis and UMI

Patients with a ≥70 % coronary stenosis had significantly more often UMI than patients without coronary stenosis in the present study, which is in line with the findings of Kim et al. [8]. Likewise, have Choi et al. [18] shown high prevalence of not only RMI, but also of UMI, downstream a chronically occluded coronary artery. However, a unique and novel feature of the present study was the attempt to evaluate in each patient individually the relation between presence of UMI and the occurrence and severity of atherosclerotic lesions in the coronary artery supplying the affected myocardial segment. Thereby, we could demonstrate a strong association between occurrence of a ≥70 % stenosis in the coronary artery and presence of UMI in the myocardial segments supplied by that coronary artery downstream of the stenosis. One could argue that this finding is driven largely by the occluded arteries since 20.1 % of segments in these territories were associated with UMI compared with only 4.5 % in those with lesions of >70-99 % and 1.0-1.3 % for less severe disease. However, a significant association remained, albeit weaker, also if the segments supplied by an artery with total occlusion were excluded. Therefore, a "dose response" effect seems to exist between the severity of stenosis and presence of UMI.

Since it is difficult to exactly match the coronary artery with the corresponding myocardial segment it supplies due to the large individual differences in coronary anatomy our finding that 68 % of the UMIs were supplied by an artery with ≥70 % stenosis is probably an underestimation. We therefore performed a secondary sensitivity analysis requiring only "near match"; in that analysis, which most likely is an overestimation, 88 % of the UMIs were supplied by a coronary artery with ≥70 % stenosis.

There is an ongoing discussion in the extent to which myocardial infarctions occur downstream an unstable plaque in a moderate stenosis or if the stenosis underlying myocardial infarctions usually are severe [19]. A recent study [20] showed fewer myocardial infarctions on follow-up in a group of patients with non-significant (FFR >0.8) coronary artery stenosis compared to a group of patients with significant coronary artery stenosis (FFR ≤ 0.8) supporting the importance of the severity of the stenosis. The results of the present study also support the importance of stenosis severity, at least for the development of UMI. The relative importance of atherosclerotic plaque rupture (myocardial infarction type 1) [21] versus supply–demand mismatch (myocardial infarction type 2) [21] as the cause of the infarction may well vary between clinically recognized MIs and UMIs. A substantial proportion of the UMIs may well be due to supply–demand mismatch, as patients with a hemodynamically significant stenosis undoubtedly are at risk of having episodes with supply–demand mismatch in the presence of a triggering factor, e.g. tachycardia. Furthermore, the small size of the UMIs may also indicate that supply–demand mismatch may not be an uncommon cause of UMI, since myocardial infarctions type 2 are usually substantially smaller than myocardial infarctions type 1 [22].

Limitations

This is a multicenter study with sites using different CMR scanners. The examination protocols were therefore not exactly the same for all examinations. However, all CMR scans were evaluated at the core lab; only 19 CMR studies had to be excluded due to poor image quality, the remaining studies were of satisfactory quality and could be evaluated. The lesions described had to be seen in at least two planes to be accepted as representing a true finding and not an artefact.

The coronary artery stenoses were assessed visually and not using quantitative coronary angiography (QCA) grading of the lumen narrowing, nor were the stenosis evaluated by fractional flow reserve measurements, a method which has been shown to more accurately predict the hemodynamic significance of coronary stenosis [23]. Other factors that might be of importance for the risk of myocardial infarction such as the complexity of the coronary artery [24] or the coronary microcirculation [25] were not evaluated.

The assessment of which myocardial segments were affected by a coronary artery stenosis was determined subjectively taking the individual coronary anatomy into account. Unfortunately, there exist no objective or universally accepted criteria for how this should be done. However, we believe that our approach was more accurate than assuming the standardized distribution suggested by Cerqueira et al. [9] which has been shown not always to be accurate [13, 14].

Conclusions

UMIs are common in patients with stable angina and the results indicate that the majority of the UMIs are of ischemic origin due to severe coronary atherosclerosis and in contrast to what is seen in recognized myocardial infarctions, to be predominately located in the inferior and infero-lateral myocardial segments.

Additional files

Additional file 1: Table S1. List of segments used when converting "exact match" to "near match".

Additional file 2: Moving images, short axis 3D CMR.

Additional file 3: Coronary angiography of left coronary artery.

Additional file 4: Coronary angiography of right coronary artery.

Additional file 5: Figure S1. All UMIs plotted according to size in grams (g).

Abbreviations

LGE: Late gadolinium enhancement; CMR: Cardiovascular magnetic resonance; UMI: Unrecognized myocardial infarction; MI: Myocardial infarction; ECG: Electrocardiography; PUMI: Prevalence and prognostic value of unrecognized myocardial injury in stable coronary artery disease (study); PCI: Percutaneous coronary intervention; CABG: Coronary artery bypass graft; GFR: Glomerular filtration rate; SSFP: Steady state free precession; TR: Repetition time; TE: Echo time; CH: Chamber, as in 2CH, 3CH, 4CH; AHA: American Heart Association; PACS: Picture archiving and communications system; SCAAR: Swedish Coronary Angiography and Angioplasty Registry; LAD: Left anterior descending artery; RCA: Right coronary artery; LCX: Left circumflex artery; GEE: Generalized estimating equation; OR: Odd's ratio; CI: Confidence interval; IQR: Interquartile range.

Competing interests

Tomas Bjerner is on the advisory board of Carestream Health. Lars Johansson is employed by Astra Zeneca. The other authors declare that they have no competing interests.

Authors' contributions

PH analyzed the coronary angiograms and CMR scans and drafted the manuscript. AN and BL participated in the study design, helped to analyze the data and helped to draft the manuscript. OD analyzed the coronary angiograms. HA participated in the study design and helped to analyze the data. LJ participated in the study design. NH performed the statistical analysis. TB participated in the study design, analyzed the CMR-examinations, helped to analyze the data and helped to draft the manuscript. All authors read and approved the final manuscript.

Acknowledgements

The PUMI-investigators responsible for data collection on the participating sites:
Kai Eggers, Department of Cardiology, Uppsala University Hospital, Sweden; Stella Cizinsky, Department of Cardiology, Örebro University Hospital, Sweden; Pär-Lennart Ågren, Department of Cardiology, Falu Hospital, Sweden; Lars Svennberg, Department of Cardiology, Gävle Hospital, Sweden; Peter Wodlin, Department of Cardiology, Linköping University Hospital, Sweden; Pia Lundman, Department of Cardiology, Danderyd Hospital, Sweden.
Design of MR protocols and adaption of protocols to different sites: Anders Lundberg, Department of Radiology, Oncology and Radiation Science, Uppsala, Sweden.
Data collection: Margareta Forsman and Maria Axetun, Uppsala Clinical Research Centre, Uppsala, Sweden.
This work was supported by Regional Research Council, Uppsala-Örebro region; Center for Clinical Research , County of Västmanland (PH); Bayer Pharmaceuticals Sweden; Swedish Research Counsil (HA).

Author details

[1]Västmanland County Hospital Västerås, Department of Radiology, Västerås S-72189, Sweden. [2]Department of Cardiology, Örebro University Hospital,

S-70182 Örebro, Sweden. [3]Uppsala Clinical Research Centre, S-75237 Uppsala, Sweden. [4]Department of Medical Sciences, Cardiology, Uppsala University, Uppsala S-75105, Sweden. [5]Department of Radiology, Oncology and Radiation Science, Uppsala University, S-75185 Uppsala, Sweden. [6]Astra Zeneca, Molndal, Sweden.

References

1. Sheifer SE, Manolio TA, Gersh BJ. Unrecognized myocardial infarction. Ann Intern Med. 2001;135:801–11.
2. Sigurdsson E, Thorgeirsson G, Sigvaldason H, Sigfusson N. Unrecognized myocardial infarction: epidemiology, clinical characteristics, and the prognostic role of angina pectoris. The Reykjavik Study. Ann Intern Med. 1995;122:96–102.
3. Kannel WB, Sorlie P, McNamara PM. Prognosis after initial myocardial infarction: the Framingham study. Am J Cardiol. 1979;44:53–9.
4. Kim RJ, Chen EL, Lima JA, Judd RM. Myocardial Gd-DTPA kinetics determine MRI contrast enhancement and reflect the extent and severity of myocardial injury after acute reperfused infarction. Circulation. 1996;94:3318–26.
5. Schelbert EB, Cao JJ, Sigurdsson S, Aspelund T, Kellman P, Aletras AH, et al. Prevalence and prognosis of unrecognized myocardial infarction determined by cardiac magnetic resonance in older adults. JAMA. 2012;308:890–6.
6. Barbier CE, Nylander R, Themudo R, Ahlström H, Lind L, Larsson EM, et al. Prevalence of unrecognized myocardial infarction detected with magnetic resonance imaging and its relationship to cerebral ischemic lesions in both sexes. J Am Coll Cardiol. 2011;58:1372–7.
7. Barbier CE, Bjerner T, Johansson L, Lind L, Ahlström H. Myocardial scars more frequent than expected: magnetic resonance imaging detects potential risk group. J Am Coll Cardiol. 2006;48:765–71.
8. Kim HW, Klem I, Shah DJ, Wu E, Meyers SN, Parker MA, et al. Unrecognized non-Q-wave myocardial infarction: prevalence and prognostic significance in patients with suspected coronary disease. PLoS Med. 2009;6:e1000057.
9. Cerqueira MD, Weissman NJ, Dilsizian V, Jacobs AK, Kaul S, Laskey WK, et al. American Heart Association Writing Group on Myocardial Segmentation and Registration for Cardiac Imaging. Standardized myocardial segmentation and nomenclature for tomographic imaging of the heart. A statement for healthcare professionals from the Cardiac Imaging Committee of the Council on Clinical Cardiology of the American Heart Association. Circulation. 2002;105:539–42.
10. Hunold P, Schlosser T, Vogt FM, Eggebrecht H, Schmermund A, Bruder O, et al. Myocardial late enhancement in contrast-enhanced cardiac MRI: distinction between infarction scar and non-infarction-related disease. AJR Am J Roentgenol. 2005;184:1420–6.
11. Austen WG, Edwards JE, Frye RL, Gensini GG, Gott VL, Griffith LS, et al. A reporting system on patients evaluated for coronary artery disease. Report of the Ad Hoc Committee for Grading of Coronary Artery Disease, Council on Cardiovascular Surgery, American Heart Association. Circulation. 1975;51:5–40.
12. Velders MA, James SK, Libungan B, Sarno G, Fröbert O, Carlsson J, et al. Prognosis of elderly patients with ST-elevation myocardial infarction treated with primary percutaneous coronary intervention in 2001 to 2011: A report from the Swedish Coronary Angiography and Angioplasty Registry (SCAAR) registry. Am Heart J. 2014;167:666–73.
13. Pereztol-Valdés O, Candell-Riera J, Santana-Boado C, Angel J, Aguadé-Bruix S, Castell-Conesa J, et al. Correspondence between left ventricular 17 myocardial segments and coronary arteries. Eur Heart J. 2005;26:2637–43.
14. Ortiz-Pérez JT, Rodríguez J, Meyers SN, Lee DC, Davidson C, Wu E. Correspondence between the 17-segment model and coronary arterial anatomy using contrast-enhanced cardiac magnetic resonance imaging. JACC Cardiovasc Imaging. 2008;1:282–93.
15. Zeger SL, Liang KY. Longitudinal data analysis for discrete and continuous outcomes. Biometrics. 1986;42:121–30.
16. Kwong RY, Sattar H, Wu H, Vorobiof G, Gandla V, Steel K, et al. Incidence and prognostic implication of unrecognized myocardial scar characterized by cardiac magnetic resonance in diabetic patients without clinical evidence of myocardial infarction. Circulation. 2008;118:1011–20.
17. Geske JB, Edwards WD, MacDonald RJ, Holmes Jr DR. Location of coronary culprit lesions at autopsy in 41 nondiabetic patients with acute myocardial infarction. Am J Forensic Med Pathol. 2010;31:213–7.
18. Choi JH, Chang SA, Choi JO, Song YB, Hahn JY, Choi SH, et al. Frequency of myocardial infarction and its relationship to angiographic collateral flow in territories supplied by chronically occluded coronary arteries. Circulation. 2013;127:703–9.
19. Niccoli G, Stefanini GG, Capodanno D, Crea F, Ambrose JA, Berg R. Are culprit lesions severely stenotic? JACC Cardiovasc Imaging. 2013;6:1108–14.
20. De Bruyne B, Fearon WF, Pijls NHJ, Barbato E, Tonino P, Piroth Z, et al. Fractional flow reserve-guided PCI for stable coronary artery disease. N Engl J Med. 2014;371:1208–17.
21. Thygesen K, Alpert JS, Jaffe AS, Simoons ML, Chaitman BR, White HD. Third universal definition of myocardial infarction. Eur Heart J. 2012;33:2551–67.
22. Paiva L, Providência R, Barra S, Dinis P, Faustino AC, Gonçalves L. Universal definition of myocardial infarction: clinical insights. Cardiology. 2015;131:13–21.
23. Fischer JJ, Samady H, McPherson JA, Sarembock IJ, Powers ER, Gimple LW, et al. Comparison between visual assessment and quantitative angiography versus fractional flow reserve for native coronary narrowings of moderate severity. Am J Cardiol. 2002;90:210–5.
24. Sianos G, Morel MA, Kappetein AP, Morice MC, Colombo A, Dawkins K, et al. The SYNTAX Score: an angiographic tool grading the complexity of coronary artery disease. EuroIntervention. 2005;1:219–27.
25. Herrman J, Kaski JC, Lerman A. Coronary microvascular dysfunction in the clinical setting: from mystery to reality. Eur Heart J. 2012;33:2771–81.

6

Role of cardiovascular magnetic resonance in the guidelines of the European Society of Cardiology

Florian von Knobelsdorff-Brenkenhoff* and Jeanette Schulz-Menger

Abstract

Background: Despite common enthusiasm for cardiovascular magnetic resonance (CMR), its application in Europe is quite diverse. Restrictions are attributed to a number of factors, like limited access, deficits in training, and incomplete reimbursement. Aim of this study is to perform a systematic summary of the representation of CMR in the guidelines of the European Society of Cardiology (ESC).

Methods: Twenty-nine ESC guidelines were screened for the terms "magnetic", "MRI", "CMR", "MR" and "imaging". As 3 topics were published twice (endocarditis, pulmonary hypertension, NSTEMI), 26 guidelines were finally included. MRI in the context of non-cardiovascular examinations was not recognized. The main CMR-related conclusions and, if available, the level of evidence and the class of recommendation were extracted.

Results: Fourteen of the 26 guidelines (53.8 %) contain specific recommendations regarding the use of CMR. Nine guidelines (34.6 %) mention CMR in the text, and 3 (11.5 %) do not mention CMR. The 14 guidelines with recommendations regarding the use of CMR contain 39 class-I recommendations, 12 class-IIa recommendations, 10 class-IIb recommendations and 2 class-III recommendations. Most of the recommendations have evidence level C (41/63; 65.1 %), followed by level B (16/63; 25.4 %) and level A (6/63; 9.5 %). The four guidelines, which absolutely contained most recommendations for CMR, were stable coronary artery disease ($n = 14$), aortic diseases ($n = 9$), HCM ($n = 7$) and myocardial revascularization ($n = 7$).

Conclusions: CMR is represented in the majority of the ESC guidelines. They contain many recommendations in favour of the use of CMR in specific scenarios. Issues regarding access, training and reimbursement have to be solved to offer CMR to patients in accordance with the ESC guidelines.

Keywords: Cardiovascular magnetic resonance, Guideline, Cardiology, Reimbursement

Background

Cardiovascular magnetic resonance (CMR) has been applied in a wide variety of indications in clinical cardiology. The most frequent indications are inflammatory and ischemic heart disease as well as cardiomyopathies. But also in rare diseases like amyloidosis, as well as in congenital heart disease, CMR has demonstrated its usefulness [1, 2]. CMR provides detailed information about cardiovascular anatomy and function by combining diverse techniques. In particular, the characterization of the myocardial tissue including the detection of oedema and the highly resolved determination of fibrosis is a unique feature of CMR [3]. Furthermore, with myocardial stress-perfusion imaging – free of ionizing radiation and with high diagnostic accuracy – the large patient group with (suspected) coronary artery disease is addressed [4]. Finally, the introduction of robust and fast imaging techniques as well as targeted examination protocols facilitated the clinical use [5].

Despite common enthusiasm for this modality, its use in Europe is quite diverse. This restriction is attributed to a number of factors, like missing skills

* Correspondence: florian.von-knobelsdorff@charite.de
Working Group Cardiovascular Magnetic Resonance, Experimental and Clinical Research Center, a joint cooperation between the Charité Medical Faculty and the Max-Delbrueck Center for Molecular Medicine; and HELIOS Klinikum Berlin Buch, Department of Cardiology and Nephrology, Berlin, Germany

both to run a CMR examination and to interpret the images under integration of profound cardiologic knowledge; relatively high costs and incomplete reimbursement; and limited access to scanners with cardiac dedication.

Aim of this study is to perform a systematic summary of the representation of CMR in the guidelines of the European Society of Cardiology (ESC) in order to stimulate the discussion about future plans for training, distribution and reimbursement of CMR in Europe.

Methods

All ESC guidelines, which are listed on the ESC website (http://www.escardio.org/Guidelines-&-Education/Clinical-Practice-Guidelines/ESC-Clinical-Practice-Guidelines-list/listing) were collected (Table 1). If more than one guideline for the same topic has been published in this period, both were analysed for changes, but only the most recent was included in the final analysis. The documents were screened for the terms "magnetic", "MRI", "CMR", "MR" and "imaging". MRI in the context of non-cardiovascular examinations like brain MRI was not recognized. The main

Table 1 List of ESC guidelines used for this summary. 1 = guideline contains specific recommendations regarding the use of CMR; 2 = guideline mentions scenarios in which CMR may be used, but without giving any specific recommendation; 3 = guideline does not mention CMR at all

Nr.	Title	Year	Role of CMR
1	ESC Guidelines for the management of patients with ventricular arrhythmias and the prevention of sudden cardiac death [6]	2015	1
2	ESC/ERS Guidelines for the diagnosis and treatment of pulmonary hypertension [7]	2015	2
3	ESC guidelines for the management of acute coronary syndromes in patients presenting without persistent ST-segment elevation [9]	2015	1
4	ESC Guidelines for the diagnosis and management of pericardial diseases [11]	2015	1
5	ESC Guidelines for the management of infective endocarditis [12]	2015	1
6	ESC Guidelines on diagnosis and management of hypertrophic cardiomyopathy [14]	2014	1
7	ESC Guidelines on the diagnosis and treatment of aortic diseases [15]	2014	1
8	ESC/EACTS Guidelines on myocardial revascularization [16]	2014	1
9	ESC Guidelines on the diagnosis and management of acute pulmonary embolism [17]	2014	1
10	ESC/ESA Guidelines on non-cardiac surgery: cardiovascular assessment and management [18]	2014	1
11	ESC Guidelines on diabetes, pre-diabetes, and cardiovascular diseases developed in collaboration with the EASD [19]	2013	2
12	ESC guidelines on the management of stable coronary artery disease [20]	2013	1
13	ESC Guidelines on cardiac pacing and cardiac resynchronization therapy [21]	2013	2
14	ESH/ESC Guidelines for the management of arterial hypertension [22]	2013	1
15	ESC/EACTS Guidelines on the management of valvular heart disease [23]	2012	2
16	Focused update of the ESC Guidelines for the management of atrial fibrillation [24]	2012	3
17	ESC/ACCF/AHA/WHF Third universal definition of myocardial Infarction [25]	2012	2
18	ESC Guidelines for the management of acute myocardial infarction in patients presenting with ST-segment elevation [26]	2012	1
19	ESC Guidelines for the diagnosis and treatment of acute and chronic heart failure [27]	2012	1
20	European Guidelines on cardiovascular disease prevention in clinical practice [28]	2012	2
21	ESC/EAS Guidelines for the management of dyslipidaemias [29]	2011	3
22	ESC Guidelines for the management of acute coronary syndromes in patients presenting without persistent ST-segment elevation [10]	2011	(new guideline 2015)
23	ESC Guidelines on the management of cardiovascular diseases during pregnancy [30]	2011	1
24	ESC Guidelines on the diagnosis and treatment of peripheral artery diseases [31]	2011	1
25	ESC Guidelines for the management of grown-up congenital heart disease [32]	2010	2
26	Focused Update of ESC Guidelines on device therapy in heart failure [34]	2010	3
27	Guidelines on the prevention, diagnosis, and treatment of infective endocarditis [23]	2009	(new guideline 2015)
28	Guidelines for the diagnosis and management of syncope [35]	2009	2
29	Guidelines for the diagnosis and treatment of pulmonary hypertension [8]	2009	(new guideline 2015)

conclusions were extracted and if available, the level of evidence and the class of recommendation were given (Tables 2 and 3). The number in parenthesis behind the citation provides the page of the fulltext guideline. If a recommendation refers to "imaging" in general, it was registered if the context included CMR. This process was done twice for every guideline to reassure that no relevant information was missed. The absolute number of recommendations is finally summarized, whereby equal recommendations that appeared in more than one guideline were only counted once. The order of the guidelines is chronologic beginning with the most recent. Guidelines other than by the ESC as well as ESC position statements were not included to guarantee one common level of guideline.

Results

Of the 29 ESC guidelines we screened, three topics were covered twice (endocarditis 2015 and 2009, pulmonary hypertension 2015 and 2009, NSTEMI 2015 and 2011). Of the remaining 26 ESC guidelines, 14 (53.8 %) contain specific recommendations regarding the use of CMR (Fig. 1, Table 1). Nine guidelines (34.6 %; endocarditis, pulmonary hypertension, diabetes, pacing, heart valve disease, definition of infarction, prevention, congenital heart disease, syncope) principally mention scenarios in which CMR may be used, but without giving any specific recommendation. Three guidelines (11.5 %; atrial fibrillation, dyslipidaemias, device therapy in heart failure) do not mention CMR at all. The 14 guidelines with recommendations regarding the use of CMR contain 39 class-I recommendations, 12 class-IIa recommendations, 10 class-IIb recommendations and 2 class-III recommendations (Fig. 2). (The diverse recommendations for myocardial revascularization in dependency of the evidence of ischemia were only counted once as IA). Most of the recommendations have evidence level C (41/63; 65.1 %), followed by level B (16/63; 25.4 %) and level A (6/63; 9.5 %). The two class-III recommendations in the context of CMR are: i) In the guideline for pulmonary embolism, MR angiography should not be used to rule out pulmonary embolism. ii) In the guideline about assessment before

Table 3 Level of evidence

Level of evidence A	Data derived from multiple randomized clinical trials or meta-analyses.
Level of evidence B	Data derived from a single randomized clinical trial or large non-randomized studies.
Level of evidence C	Consensus of opinion of the experts and/or small studies, retrospective studies, registries.

non-cardiac surgery, imaging stress testing in general is not recommended before low-risk surgery. The four guidelines, which absolutely contained most recommendations with referral to CMR, were stable coronary artery disease from 2013 ($n = 14$), aortic diseases ($n = 9$), HCM ($n = 7$) as well as myocardial revascularization ($n = 7$) from 2014. Twenty-eight recommendations refer to stress-imaging, 17 recommendations refer to the vasculature, 7 to cardiomyopathies, 5 to left- and right-ventricular function assessment (in part including fibrosis imaging), 4 to the pericardium and 2 to myocarditis. A summary of clinical scenarios/diagnoses, where the ESC made recommendations regarding CMR, is provided in the appendix of this paper.

2015 ESC guidelines for the management of patients with ventricular arrhythmias and the prevention of sudden cardiac death [6]

Table 4 summarizes the recommendations for CMR in the context of patients with ventricular arrhythmias and the prevention of sudden cardiac death.

For family members of sudden unexplained death syndrome or sudden arrhythmic death syndrome victims, echocardiography and/or CMR is recommended (Appendix on page 11 of the guideline). In patients with sustained ventricular tachycardia or ventricular fibrillation, the recommended algorithm for further patient assessment includes CMR (Fig. 1 on page 14). For instance myocarditis should also be suspected and a CMR scan may reveal abnormal fibrotic myocardial tissue (page 54). In patients with non-ischaemic cardiomyopathy, CMR fibrosis imaging (using late gadolinium enhancement, LGE) is associated with increased risk of all-cause mortality, heart failure hospitalization and sudden

Table 2 Class of recommendations

Class of recommendation	Definition	Suggested wording to use
Class I	Evidence and/or general agreement that a given treatment or procedure is beneficial, useful, effective.	Is recommended/is indicated
Class II	Conflicting evidence and/or a divergence of opinion about the usefulness/efficacy of the given treatment or procedure.	
Class IIa	Weight of evidence/opinion is in favour of usefulness/efficacy.	Should be considered
Class IIb	Usefulness/efficacy is less well established by evidence/opinion.	May be considered
Class III	Evidence or general agreement that the given treatment or procedure is not useful/effective, and in some cases may be harmful.	Is not recommended

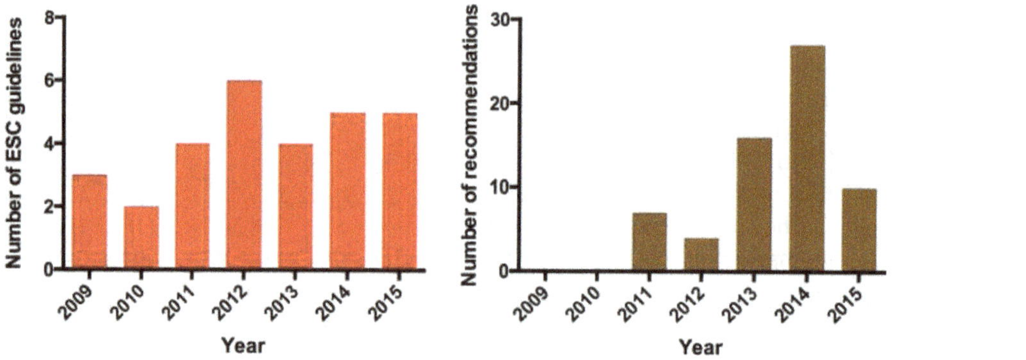

Fig. 1 *Left:* Number of ESC guidelines screened for this analysis per year. *Right:* Number of specific recommendations regarding CMR per year

cardiac death. The incremental value of LGE over other prognostic markers needs to be determined (page 36). Standardized evaluation of patients with HCM should include CMR in the case of inadequate echo window (page 39). LGE has been suggested to be used to guide ICD therapy in individuals with HCM with intermediate risk, however with few supportive data (page 38). Similarly, LGE on CMR of the right and left ventricle has been reported as risk factors for sudden cardiac death or appropriate ICD discharge in ARVC (page 40). In particular in ARVC, CMR provides excellent assessment of right ventricular size, function and regional wall motion. In paediatric patients with frequent premature ventricular complexes, cardiac evaluation including CMR is recommended (page 46). Non-invasive imaging of cardiac structure, best done by CMR, can be used to plan and guide ablation procedures for ventricular tachycardia (page 22).

2015 ESC/ERS guidelines for the diagnosis and treatment of pulmonary hypertension [7]

CMR is listed among the tests to contribute to the diagnosis of pulmonary hypertension, being accurate and reproducible in the assessment of right ventricular size, morphology and function and of blood flow, stroke volume, cardiac output, pulmonary arterial distensibility and right ventricular mass. The presence of LGE, reduced pulmonary arterial distensibility and retrograde flow have high predictive value for the identification of pulmonary hypertension. In patients with pulmonary hypertension, CMR may also be useful in cases of suspected congenital heart disease if echocardiography is not conclusive. MR angiography has a potential in patients with suspected chronic thromboembolic pulmonary hypertension. CMR provides useful prognostic information in patients with pulmonary artery hypertension (page 12).

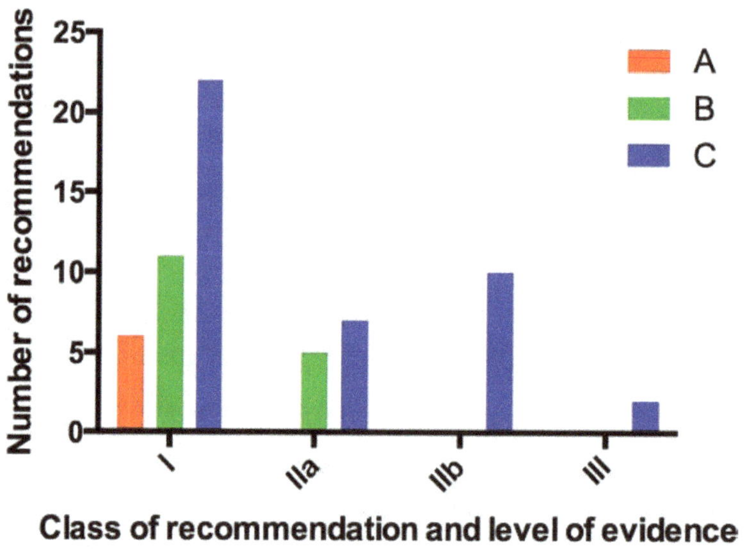

Fig. 2 Class and level of the recommendations for CMR in the ESC guidelines

Table 4 Recommendations for CMR in patients with ventricular arrhythmias and for the prevention of sudden cardiac death

Non-invasive evaluation of patients with suspected or known ventricular arrhythmias	Class[a]	Level[b]	Page
Pharmacological stress testing plus imaging modality is recommended to detect silent ischaemia in patients with ventricular arrhythmias who have an intermediate probability of having coronary artery disease by age or symptoms and are physically unable to perform a symptom-limited exercise test.	I	B	12
CMR or CT should be considered in patients with ventricular arrhythmias when echocardiography does not provide accurate assessment of LV and RV function and/or evaluation of structural changes.	IIa	B	12
Management of ventricular arrhythmias in inflammatory heart disease	**Class[a]**	**Level[b]**	**Page**
Demonstration of persistent myocardial inflammatory infiltrates by immunohistological evidence and/or abnormal localized fibrosis by CMR after acute myocarditis may be considered as an additional indicator of increased risk of SCD in inflammatory heart disease.	IIb	C	53
Prevention of sudden cardiac death in athletes	**Class[a]**	**Level[b]**	**Page**
Upon identification of ECG abnormalities suggestive of structural heart disease, echocardiography and/or CMR imaging is recommended.	I	C	62

[a] Class of recommendation
[b] Level of evidence

Specifically, right atrial size and the presence of pericardial effusion as assessed by CMR are used for risk assessment in pulmonary arterial hypertension (table 13 of the guideline). There is no specific recommendation regarding CMR and no significant change regarding the role of CMR in pulmonary hypertension between the present guideline and the 2009 version [8].

2015 ESC guidelines for the management of acute coronary syndromes in patients presenting without persistent ST-segment elevation [9]

CMR can assess both perfusion and wall motion abnormalities, and patients presenting with acute chest pain with a normal stress CMR have an excellent short- and midterm prognosis. CMR also permits detection of scar tissue and can differentiate this from recent infarction. CMR can facilitate the differential diagnosis between infarction and myocarditis or Tako-Tsubo cardiomyopathy (page 11). In subjects with no criteria for early invasive strategy, a non-invasive imaging stress test is recommended. No specific test is mentioned (Table 5). There is no significant change of the role of CMR compared to the 2011 NSTEMI guideline [10].

2015 ESC guidelines for the diagnosis and management of pericardial diseases [11]

CMR has shifted towards a comprehensive imaging modality, allowing visualization and tissue characterization of the pericardium (and heart) in patients with pericardial disease and appraisal of the consequences of pericardial abnormalities on cardiac function and filling patterns (page 20). Table 12 of the guideline summarizes the contribution of different imaging modalities in various pericardial diseases and table 13 of the guideline compares non-invasive imaging modalities to study the pericardium. Thereby, CMR is predominantly ranked as good ("++") or excellent ("+++"). Under the headline "what is new", CMR is recommended for the detection of pericardial inflammation to identify forms of initial reversible constrictive pericarditis, allowing a trial of medical anti-inflammatory therapy (page 5). The evidence of pericardial inflammation by CMR is also mentioned as one diagnostic criterion for acute pericarditis (table 4 of the guideline). In patients with myocarditis, CMR is recommended for the confirmation of myocardial involvement (page 13). CMR may be helpful to detect loculated pericardial effusion and pericardial thickening and masses, as well as associated chest abnormalities. CMR can contribute to the differentiation of constrictive pericarditis and restrictive cardiomyopathy (table 10 of the guideline), e.g. by assessment of ventricular coupling with real-time cine magnetic resonance during free breathing (page 19). In some cases of pericardial cysts, CMR may be helpful (page 35). The recommendations made for CMR in pericardial diseases are summarized in Table 6.

Table 5 Recommendations for imaging in patients with suspected non-ST-elevation acute coronary syndromes

Recommendations for imaging in patients with suspected non-ST-elevation acute coronary syndromes	Class[a]	Level[b]	Page
In patients with no recurrence of chest pain, normal ECG findings and normal levels of cardiac troponin (preferably high-sensitivity), but suspected acute coronary syndrome, a non-invasive stress test (preferably with imaging) for inducible ischaemia is recommended before deciding on an invasive strategy.	I	A	15

[a] Class of recommendation
[b] Level of evidence

Table 6 Recommendations for CMR in pericardial diseases

Recommendation for diagnostic work-up of pericardial diseases	Class[a]	Level[b]	Page
CT and/or CMR are second-level testing for diagnostic workup in pericarditis	I	C	38
Recommendations for the diagnosis and management of pericarditis associated with myocarditis	**Class[a]**	**Level[b]**	**Page**
CMR is recommended for the confirmation of myocardial involvement	I	C	13
Recommendations for the diagnosis of pericardial effusion	**Class[a]**	**Level[b]**	**Page**
CT or CMR should be considered in suspected cases of loculated pericardial effusion, pericardial thickening and masses, as well as associated chest abnormalities	IIa	C	14
Recommendations for the diagnosis of constrictive pericarditis	**Class[a]**	**Level[b]**	**Page**
CT and/or CMR are indicated as second-level imaging techniques to assess calcifications (CT), pericardial thickness, degree and extension of pericardial involvement	I	C	17
Recommendations for therapy of constrictive pericarditis	**Class[a]**	**Level[b]**	**Page**
Empiric anti-inflammatory therapy may be considered in cases with transient or new diagnosis of constriction with concomitant evidence of pericardial inflammation (i.e. CRP elevation or pericardial enhancement on CT/CMR)	IIb	C	19

[a] Class of recommendation
[b] Level of evidence

2015 ESC guidelines for the management of infective endocarditis [12]

Within the subchapter about 'complications of infective endocarditis' dealing with 'myocarditis and pericarditis', CMR is mentioned (next to echocardiography) to assess myocardial involvement during infective endocarditis (page 30). This CMR indication is new compared to the 2009 guideline [13].

2014 ESC guidelines on diagnosis and management of hypertrophic cardiomyopathy [14]

HCM in adults is defined by a wall thickness ≥15 mm and in first-degree relatives ≥13 mm in one or more LV myocardial segments - as measured by any imaging technique, including CMR (page 7, 8). Some patients with apical or distal hypertrophy develop small apical aneurysms, sometimes associated with myocardial scarring. These may only be detectable on CMR, ventriculography or contrast echo (page 9). The prevalence of non-sustained ventricular tachycardia increases with age and correlates with LV wall thickness and the presence of LGE on CMR (page 36). However, even though the extent of LGE on CMR has some utility in predicting cardiovascular mortality, current data do not support the use of LGE in prediction of sudden cardiac death risk (page 14). LGE at the right ventricular insertion points or localized to segments of maximum LV thickening on CMR assists for differentiating the diagnosis of hypertensive heart disease and HCM (table 9 of the guideline). The specific recommendations made for CMR in HCM are summarized in Table 7.

2014 ESC guidelines on the diagnosis and treatment of aortic diseases [15]

CMR is regarded as a valuable tool to image the aorta. On a scale from "+" to "+++", the ease of use is graded as "++", diagnostic reliability as "+++", serial examinations as "+++", and aortic wall visualization as "+++" (page 11). CMR is considered the leading technique for diagnosis of aortic dissection, with a reported sensitivity and specificity of 98 %. However, several methodological and practical limitations preclude the use of this modality in the majority of cases and in unstable patients (page 21). Recommendations for the use of CMR in patients with aortic diseases are given Table 8.

2014 ESC/EACTS guidelines on myocardial revascularization [16]

This guideline contains recommendations for CMR both for determining myocardial ischemia and for follow-up patients after myocardial revascularization, as well as for preparation before surgical myocardial revascularization. Table 9 shows the specific recommendations. There is no clear recommendation for CMR viability testing. Even though CMR has a high diagnostic accuracy for assessing the transmural extent of myocardial scar tissue and contractile reserve, its ability to detect viability and predict recovery of wall motion is no better than other imaging techniques (page 15).

2014 ESC guidelines on the diagnosis and management of acute pulmonary embolism [17]

MR angiography, although promising, is not yet ready for clinical practice due to its low sensitivity, high proportion of inconclusive MR angiography scans, and low availability in most emergency settings (Table 10).

Table 7 Recommendations for CMR in patients with HCM

Recommendations for CMR in patients with HCM	Class[a]	Level[b]	Page
It is recommended that CMR studies be performed and interpreted by teams experienced in cardiac imaging and in the evaluation of heart muscle disease	I	B	14
In the absence of contraindications, CMR with LGE is recommended in patients with suspected HCM who have inadequate echocardiographic windows, in order to confirm the diagnosis.	I	C	14
In the absence of contraindications, CMR with LGE should be considered in patients fulfilling diagnostic criteria for HCM, to assess cardiac anatomy, ventricular function, and the presence and extent of myocardial fibrosis.	IIa	B	14
CMR with LGE imaging should be considered in patients with suspected apical hypertrophy or aneurysm.	IIa	C	14
CMR with LGE imaging should be considered in patients with suspected cardiac amyloidosis.	IIa	C	14
CMR with LGE may be considered before septal alcohol ablation or myectomy, to assess the extent and distribution of hypertrophy and myocardial fibrosis.	IIb	C	14
CMR may be considered every 5 years in clinically stable patients, or every 2–3 years in patients with progressive disease.	IIb	C	37

[a] Class of recommendation
[b] Level of evidence

2014 ESC/ESA guidelines on non-cardiac surgery: cardiovascular assessment and management [18]

Resting LV function can be evaluated before non-cardiac surgery in high-risk surgery (IIb, C). Following the guidelines, this can be done by radionuclide ventriculography, gated single photon emission computed tomography, echocardiography, CMR or multislice CT all with similar accuracy. The recommendations for non-invasive stress testing of ischemic heart disease are given in Table 11. As nuclear myocardial perfusion imaging and stress echocardiography were mainly used in clinical studies about preoperative ischemic testing, these modalities are pronounced. CMR (both perfusion and wall motion analysis) is mentioned as an accurate alternative method.

2013 ESC guidelines on diabetes, pre-diabetes, and cardiovascular diseases developed in collaboration with the EASD [19]

Patients with glucose perturbations are in need of early risk assessment to identify co-morbidities and factors that increase cardiovascular risk. This includes among other the evaluation of myocardial viability and LV function by means of echo-Doppler and/or CMR (page 28), and Duplex ultrasonography, computed tomography angiography and CMR to evaluate carotid artery stenosis (page 45). To evaluate inducible ischaemia, only exercise testing, stress echocardiography, or myocardial scintigraphy are mentioned (page 28).

Table 8 Recommendations for CMR in aortic diseases

Recommendations on diagnostic work-up of acute aortic syndrome	Class[a]	Level[b]	Page
In stable patients with a suspicion of acute aortic syndrome, CMR is recommended (or should be considered) according to local availability and expertise	I	C	22
In case of initially negative imaging with persistence of suspicion of acute aortic syndrome, repetitive imaging (CT or CMR) is recommended.	I	C	22
In case of uncomplicated Type B aortic dissection treated medically, repeated imaging (CT or CMR) during the first days is recommended.	I	C	22
In uncomplicated Type B intramural hematoma, repetitive imaging (CMR or CT) is indicated.	I	C	26
In uncomplicated Type B penetrating aortic ulcer, repetitive imaging (CMR or CT) is indicated.	I	C	27
Recommendations for the management of aortic root dilation in patients with bicuspid aortic valve	**Class[a]**	**Level[b]**	**Page**
CMR or CT is indicated in patients with bicuspid aortic valve when the morphology of the aortic root and the ascending aorta cannot be accurately assessed by TTE.	I	C	42
In the case of aortic diameter >50 mm or an increase >3 mm/year measured by echocardiography, confirmation of the measurement is indicated, using another imaging modality (CT or CMR).	I	C	42
Recommendations for follow-up and management in chronic aortic diseases	**Class[a]**	**Level[b]**	**Page**
Contrast CT or CMR is recommended to confirm the diagnosis of chronic aortic dissection.	I	C	48
For follow-up after (T)EVAR in young patients, CMR should be preferred to CT for magnetic resonance-compatible stent grafts, to reduce radiation exposure.	IIa	C	48

[a] Class of recommendation
[b] Level of evidence

Table 9 Recommendations for CMR in the context of myocardial revascularization

Recommendations for imaging to determine ischemia to plan revascularization	Class[a]	Level[b]	Page
Stress CMR, stress-echo, SPECT or PET are recommended in subjects with intermediate pretest probability for suspected coronary artery disease and stable symptoms	I	A	14
To achieve a prognostic benefit by revascularization in patients with coronary artery disease, ischemia has to be documented by non-invasive imaging			
Left main disease with stenosis >50 %	I	A	18
Any proximal LAD stenosis >50 %	I	A	18
Two-vessel or three-vessel disease with stenosis > 50 % with impaired LV function (LVEF < 40 %)a	I	A	18
Large area of ischaemia (>10 % LV)	I	B	18
Single remaining patent coronary artery with stenosis >50 %	I	C	18
Recommendations for follow-up and management after myocardial revascularization for asymptomatic patients	**Class[a]**	**Level[b]**	**Page**
Early imaging testing should be considered in specific patient subsets.	IIa	C	72
Routine stress testing may be considered >2 years after PCI and >5 years after CABG.	IIa	B	72
Recommendations for follow-up and management after myocardial revascularization for symptomatic patients	**Class[a]**	**Level[b]**	**Page**
It is recommended to reinforce medical therapy and lifestyle changes in patients with low-risk findings at stress testing.	I	C	72
With intermediate- to high-risk findings at stress testing, coronary angiography is recommended.	I	C	72
Recommendation for carotid artery screening before CABG	**Class[a]**	**Level[b]**	**Page**
CMR, CT, or digital subtraction angiography may be considered if carotid artery stenosis by ultrasound is >70 % and myocardial revascularization is contemplated.	IIb	C	39

[a] Class of recommendation
[b] Level of evidence

2013 ESC guidelines on the management of stable coronary artery disease [20]

Table 12 summarizes the corresponding recommendations for CMR in the context of stable coronary artery disease. CMR may be used to define structural cardiac abnormalities and evaluate ventricular function. Use of CMR is recommended in patients, in whom, despite the use of echo contrast agents, transthoracic echocardiography is unable to answer the clinical question (usually because of a restricted acoustic window) and who have no contra-indications for CMR (page 13). In patients with suspected coronary artery disease and intermediate pretest probability, non-invasive testing is recommended. Among the modalities to perform stress imaging, CMR is mentioned on the same level as stress echocardiography, SPECT and PET. To stratify the risk for events, high risk is assumed in stress CMR if there are ≥2/16 segments with new perfusion defects or ≥3 dobutamine-induced dysfunctional segments (page 20). CMR coronary arteriography must still be regarded primarily as a research tool and is not recommended for routine clinical practice in the diagnostic evaluation of suspected coronary artery disease (page 19).

2013 ESC guidelines on cardiac pacing and cardiac resynchronization therapy [21]

Regarding patient selection for cardiac resynchronization therapy, it is mentioned that CMR and other imaging techniques were evaluated. However, the real value of these novel technologies remains to be determined in randomized trials (page 23). Furthermore, general safety-based recommendations for MR imaging in patients with implanted cardiac devices are given, according to conventional or MR-conditional devices (page 44).

2013 ESH/ESC guidelines for the management of arterial hypertension [22]

When searching for asymptomatic organ damage in patients with arterial hypertension, CMR should be considered for assessment of LV size and mass when echocardiography is

Table 10 Recommendation for CMR in pulmonary embolism

Recommendations for CMR in pulmonary embolism	Class[a]	Level[b]	Page
MR angiography should not be used to rule out pulmonary embolism.	III	C	11

[a] Class of recommendation
[b] Level of evidence

Table 11 Recommendations for CMR in the context of non-cardiac surgery

Recommendations for non-invasive stress testing of ischemic heart disease	Class[a]	Level[b]	Page
Imaging stress testing is recommended before high-risk surgery in patients with more than two clinical risk factors and poor functional capacity (<4 METs).	I	C	12
Imaging stress testing may be considered before high- or intermediate-risk surgery in patients with one or two clinical risk factors and poor functional capacity (<4 METs).	IIb	C	12
Imaging stress testing is not recommended before low-risk surgery, regardless of the patient's clinical risk.	III	C	12

[a] Class of recommendation
[b] Level of evidence

technically not feasible and when LGE imaging would have therapeutic consequences (page 17). On a scale from "+" to "++++", CMR was graded with "++" regarding cardiovascular predictive value, "+" regarding availability, "+++" regarding reproducibility" and "++" regarding cost-effectiveness (page 20). CMR is rated as highly sensitive to detect changes of LV hypertrophy, superior to echocardiography and ECG (page 51). Concerning renal artery stenosis as cause of secondary hypertension, CMR is named as additional/confirmatory test after renal ultrasonography (page 22). The recommendation for CMR in suspected ischemic heart disease in the context of hypertension-induced organ damage is given in Table 13.

Table 12 Recommendations for CMR in stable coronary artery disease

Recommendations for non-invasive testing for ischemic heart disease	Class[a]	Level[b]	Page
In patients with suspected stable coronary artery disease and intermediate pretest probability of 15 % - 65 % and LVEF ≥50 %, stress imaging is preferred as the initial test option if local expertise and availability permit.	I	B	17
An imaging stress test is recommended as the initial test for diagnosing stable coronary artery disease if the pretest probability is between 66-85 % or if LVEF is <50 % in patients without typical angina.	I	B	17
An imaging stress test is recommended in patients with resting ECG abnormalities, which prevent accurate interpretation of ECG changes during stress.	I	B	17
An imaging stress test should be considered in symptomatic patients with prior revascularization (PCI or CABG).	IIa	B	17
An imaging stress test should be considered to assess the functional severity of intermediate lesions on coronary arteriography.	IIa	B	17
Recommendations for risk stratification using ischemia testing	**Class[a]**	**Level[b]**	**Page**
Risk stratification is recommended based on clinical assessment and the results of the stress test initially employed for making a diagnosis of stable coronary artery disease	I	B	22
Stress imaging for risk stratification is recommended in patients with a non-conclusive exercise ECG	I	B	22
Risk stratification using stress ECG (unless they cannot exercise or display ECG changes which make the ECG non evaluable) or preferably stress imaging if local expertise and availability permit is recommended in patients with stable coronary disease after a significant change in symptom level	I	B	22
Stress imaging is recommended for risk stratification in patients with known stable coronary artery disease and a deterioration in symptoms if the site and extent of ischemia would influence clinical decision making	I	B	22
In asymptomatic adults with diabetes or asymptomatic adults with a strong family history of coronary artery disease or when previous risk assessment testing suggests high risk of coronary artery disease, such as a coronary artery calcium score of 400 or greater stress imaging tests (MPI, stress echocardiography, perfusion CMR) may be considered for advanced cardiovascular risk assessment.	IIb	C	24
Recommendation for re-assessment in patients with stable coronary artery disease	**Class[a]**	**Level[b]**	**Page**
An exercise ECG or stress imaging if appropriate is recommended in the presence of recurrent or new symptoms once instability has been ruled out.	I	C	25
Reassessment of the prognosis using stress testing may be considered in asymptomatic patients after the expiration of the period for which the previous test was felt to be valid ("warranty period")	IIb	C	25
In symptomatic patients with revascularized stable coronary artery disease, stress imaging (stress echocardiography, CMR or MPS) is indicated rather than stress ECG.	I	C	47
Late (6 months) stress imaging test after revascularization may be considered to detect patients with restenosis after stenting or graft occlusion irrespective of symptoms.	IIb	C	47

[a] Class of recommendation
[b] Level of evidence

Table 13 Recommendation for CMR in the management of arterial hypertension

Recommendations for stress-testing in arterial hypertension	Class[a]	Level[b]	Page
Whenever history suggests myocardial ischaemia, a stress ECG test is recommended, and, if positive or ambiguous, an imaging stress test (stress echocardiography, stress CMR or nuclear scintigraphy) is recommended.	I	C	21

[a] Class of recommendation
[b] Level of evidence

2012 guidelines on the management of valvular heart disease [23]
In patients with inadequate echocardiographic quality or discrepant results, CMR should be used to assess the severity of valvular lesions - particularly regurgitant lesions - and to assess ventricular volumes and systolic function, as CMR assesses these parameters with higher reproducibility than echocardiography. CMR is the reference method for the evaluation of right ventricular volumes and function and is therefore useful to evaluate the consequences of tricuspid regurgitation. In practice, the routine use of CMR is limited because of its limited availability, compared with echocardiography (page 7).

In *aortic regurgitation*, CMR (or CT) is recommended for the evaluation of the aorta in patients with Marfan syndrome, or if an enlarged aorta is detected by echocardiography, particularly in patients with bicuspid aortic valves (page 10). Furthermore, CT or preferably CMR are advisable when the distal ascending aorta is not well visualized and/or when the surgical indication may be based on aortic enlargement, rather than LV size or function.

In *aortic stenosis* with paradoxical low flow, the diagnosis of severe AS requires careful exclusion of diverse reasons for the echo constellation before making the decision to intervene. In addition to more detailed echocardiographic measurements, this may require CMR and catheterization (page 14). (CT and) CMR provide additional information on the assessment of the ascending aorta when it is enlarged (page 14). Furthermore, CMR may also be useful for the detection and quantification of myocardial fibrosis, providing additional prognostic information in symptomatic patients without coronary artery disease (page 14).

In secondary mitral regurgitation and low LVEF, it is also mandatory to assess the absence, or presence and extent, of myocardial viability by one of the available imaging techniques (dobutamine echocardiography, SPECT, PET or CMR) (page 23). There are no specific recommendations for CMR in this guideline.

2012 focused update of the ESC Guidelines for the management of atrial fibrillation [24]
CMR is not mentioned in this guideline.

2012 third universal definition of myocardial infarction [25]
Imaging evidence of new loss of viable myocardium or new regional wall motion abnormality is listed among the criteria for acute myocardial infarction. Among the criteria for prior myocardial infarction, imaging evidence of a region of loss of viable myocardium that is thinned and fails to contract, in the absence of a non-ischaemic cause, is listed (page 3). CMR is mentioned next to other imaging tests (page 9) for assessing myocardial viability, perfusion, and function. Furthermore, its value in detecting myocardial disease states that can mimic myocardial infarct, such as myocarditis, is emphasized (page 10). There are no specific recommendations for CMR in this guideline.

2012 ESC guidelines for the management of acute myocardial infarction in patients presenting with ST-segment elevation [26]
Contrast-enhanced CMR is mentioned as one of several techniques to make the diagnosis of no-reflow. If, in spite of the angiography performed in the acute phase, there are concerns about inducible ischaemia, an outpatient exercise-testing or stress-imaging test (using scintigraphy, echocardiography or CMR) is appropriate. Regarding the assessment of viability, the same statement as within the revascularization guidelines from 2014 is given: CMR has a high diagnostic accuracy for assessing transmural extent of myocardial scar tissue, but its ability to detect viability and predict recovery of wall motion is not superior to other imaging techniques

Table 14 Recommendations for CMR in patients with STEMI

Recommendations for imaging during hospitalization and at discharge in patients with STEMI	Class[a]	Level[b]	Page
If echocardiography is not feasible, CMR may be used as an alternative for assessment of infarct size and resting LV function.	IIb	C	26
For patients with multivessel disease, or in whom revascularization of other vessels is considered, stress testing or imaging (e.g. using stress myocardial perfusion scintigraphy, stress echocardiography, positron emission tomography or CMR) for ischaemia and viability is indicated before or after discharge.	I	A	26

[a] Class of recommendation
[b] Level of evidence

Table 15 Recommendations for CMR in acute and chronic heart failure

Recommendations for CMR in ambulatory patients suspected of having heart failure	Class[a]	Level[b]	Page
CMR imaging is recommended to evaluate cardiac structure and function, to measure LVEF, and to characterize cardiac tissue, especially in subjects with inadequate echocardiographic images or where the echocardiographic findings are inconclusive or incomplete (but taking account of cautions/contraindications to CMR).	I	C	10
Myocardial perfusion/ischaemia imaging (echocardiography, CMR, SPECT, or PET) should be considered in patients thought to have coronary artery disease, and who are considered suitable for coronary revascularization, to determine whether there is reversible myocardial ischaemia and viable myocardium.	IIa	C	10

[a] Class of recommendation
[b] Level of evidence

(page 27). Table 14 shows the recommendations for CMR in patients with STEMI.

2012 ESC guidelines for the diagnosis and treatment of acute and chronic heart failure [27]

CMR is particularly valuable in identifying inflammatory and infiltrative conditions as well as in the work-up of patients with suspected cardiomyopathy, arrhythmias, suspected cardiac tumours, or pericardial diseases, and is the imaging method of choice in patients with complex congenital heart disease (pages 16–17). Table 7 of the guideline summarizes possible applications of various imaging techniques in the diagnosis of heart failure. Thereby, the value of CMR is rated - on a scale from "+" to "+++" - with "+++" regarding coronary artery disease, myocarditis, sarcoidosis, amyloidosis, eosinophilic syndromes, iron overload, arrhythmogenic right ventricular cardiomyopathy, endomyocardial fibrosis; with "++" regarding valvular regurgitation, HCM, pericarditis, Takotsubo-cardiomyopathy, and with "+" regarding valvular stenosis and Anderson-Fabry-Disease. In patients presenting with heart failure and ECG signs of LV hypertrophy or low QRS voltage, CMR is recommended for further work-up. Table 15 provides recommendations for CMR in ambulatory patients suspected of having heart failure.

2012 European guidelines on cardiovascular disease prevention in clinical practice [28]

This guideline dedicates a chapter to the early detection of cardiovascular disease in asymptomatic subjects by CMR. It concludes that at present, CMR is a promising research tool, but its routine use remains limited and it is not yet appropriate for identifying patients at high risk for cardiovascular disease (page 23).

2011 ESC/EAS guidelines for the management of dyslipidaemias [29]

This guideline does not contain relevant paragraphs regarding CMR.

2011 ESC guidelines on the management of cardiovascular diseases during pregnancy [30]

CMR may be useful in diagnosing complex heart disease or pathology of the aorta. Limited data during organogenesis are available, but CMR is probably safe, especially after the first trimester. Gadolinium can be assumed to cross the fetal blood-placental barrier, but data are limited. The long-term risks of exposure of the developing fetus to free gadolinium ions are not known, and therefore gadolinium should be avoided (page 8). In bicuspid aortic valve disease, dilatation is often maximal in the distal part of the ascending aorta, which cannot be adequately visualized echocardiographically; therefore, CMR or CT should be performed before pre-pregnancy (page 21). Table 16 summarizes recommendations for CMR during pregnancy.

2011 ESC guidelines on the diagnosis and treatment of peripheral artery diseases [31]

MR angiography (MRA) is regarded as one of the main diagnostic modalities to assess peripheral artery disease. Table 17 summarizes the recommendations for MRA to assess peripheral artery disease.

Table 16 Recommendations for CMR during pregnancy ·

Recommendations	Class[a]	Level[b]	Page
CMR (without gadolinium) should be considered if echocardiography is insufficient for diagnosis.	IIa	C	14
Imaging of the entire aorta (CT/CMR) should be performed before pregnancy in patients with Marfan syndrome or other known aortic disease.	I	C	22
For imaging of pregnant women with dilatation of the distal ascending aorta, aortic arch or descending aorta, CMR (without gadolinium) is recommended.	I	C	22

[a] Class of recommendation
[b] Level of evidence

Table 17 Recommendations for MRA to assess peripheral artery disease

Recommendations for evaluation of carotid artery stenosis	Class[a]	Level[b]	Page
Duplex ultrasound, CT-angiography, and/or MRA are indicated to evaluate carotid artery stenosis.	I	A	11
Recommendations for diagnosis of symptomatic chronic mesenteric ischaemia	**Class[a]**	**Level[b]**	**Page**
When Duplex ultrasound is inconclusive, CT-angiography or gadolinium-enhanced MRA are indicated.	I	B	19
Recommendations for diagnostic strategies for renal artery stenosis	**Class[a]**	**Level[b]**	**Page**
MRA (in patients with creatinine clearance >30 mL/min) is recommended to establish the diagnosis of renal artery stenosis.	I	B	21
Recommendations for diagnostic tests in patients with lower extremity artery disease	**Class[a]**	**Level[b]**	**Page**
Duplex ultrasound and/or CT-angiography and/or MRA are indicated to localize lower extremity artery disease lesions and consider revascularization options.	I	A	26

[a] Class of recommendation
[b] Level of evidence

2010 ESC guidelines for the management of grown-up congenital heart disease [32]

CMR has become increasingly important in grown-up with congenital heart disease (GUCH) and is an essential facility in the specialist unit. ESC recommendations for the use of CMR in GUCH patients have been published separately [33]. There are several groups of indications for CMR when assessing adult congenital heart disease in clinical practice:

1. CMR as an alternative to echocardiography, when both techniques can provide similar information but echocardiography cannot be obtained with sufficient quality.
2. CMR as a second method when echocardiography measurements are borderline or ambiguous.
3. Indications where CMR is considered superior to echocardiography and should be regularly used when the information is essential for patient management. These indications include the quantification of right ventricular (RV) volumes and ejection fraction, RV and LV mass, evaluation of RV outflow tract and conduits, quantification of pulmonary regurgitation, evaluation of pulmonary arteries, aorta, systemic and pulmonary veins, collaterals and arteriovenous malformations, coronary anomalies and coronary artery disease, evaluation of intra- and extracardiac masses, and myocardial tissue characterization (fibrosis, fat, iron).

2010 focused update of ESC Guidelines on device therapy in heart failure [34]

CMR is not mentioned in this guideline.

2009 guidelines for the diagnosis and management of syncope [35]

In the diagnostic work-up of syncope, CMR - along with other imaging modalities - may be performed in selected cases (e.g. aortic dissection and haematoma, pulmonary embolism, cardiac masses, pericardial and myocardial diseases, congenital anomalies of coronary arteries) (page 23).

Discussion

This is the first systematic summary of the representation of CMR in the ESC guidelines. It shows that CMR is mentioned in the majority of guidelines (89 %) and that more than 50 % of the guidelines contain specific recommendations, when and how to use CMR. Almost all recommendations are in favour of the use of CMR.

The majority of recommendations refer to stress imaging to assess coronary artery disease in general. Even though CMR is not listed as the only recommended modality, it is ranked equally to nuclear studies and stress-echocardiography. Recently, large and important studies like CE-Marc have promoted this favourable position of CMR [4]. Accordingly, the evaluation of suspected coronary artery disease or ischemia in known coronary artery disease makes up the largest indication group for CMR in the EuroCMR registry [2].

Interestingly, in the context of ischemic heart disease, the ESC guidelines are relatively conservative in the evaluation of CMR viability testing. They rate its ability to detect viability and predict recovery of wall motion no better than with other imaging techniques and do not word a specific recommendation [16]. By way of contrast, viability testing makes up the third largest indication group in the EuroCMR registry [2].

The use of CMR in HCM is also well represented in the corresponding guideline. Thereby, CMR is mainly recommended to describe the phenotype and make the diagnosis, while its value for risk stratification for sudden cardiac death is still under debate [36]. Other cardiomyopathies (e.g. DCM, ARVC) and myocarditis are less well expressed in specific ESC recommendations. This can be attributed to the lack of large-scale data, as well as the absence of specific ESC-guidelines dedicated to cardiomyopathies (other than HCM) or inflammatory heart disease. The significance of CMR in these indication groups is underlined by several ESC position statements: A recent document about myocarditis stated that CMR may be considered in clinically stable patients with myocarditis [37]. A recent document about cardiomyopathies stated that the incremental contribution of CMR to the diagnosis of cardiomyopathies derives from accurate assessment of the morphology and function of the heart and tissue characterization [38]. Finally, a document about the role of endomyocardial biopsy in the management of cardiovascular disease mentions CMR repeatedly as a valuable tool in patients scheduled for biopsy either to assist or to replace biopsy [39]. In those centers taking part in the EuroCMR registry, cardiomyopathies and myocarditis make up the second largest CMR indication group [2].

Other well-established indications for CMR are completely unmentioned in the ESC guidelines, like CMR in the context of sarcoid disease. A recent consensus statement by the Heart Rhythm Society from 2014 on the diagnosis and management of arrhythmias associated with cardiac sarcoid defined the presence of LGE on CMR as one criteria for the diagnosis of cardiac sarcoid [40]. Screening for cardiac involvement in patients with biopsy-proven extracardiac sarcoidosis should include advanced cardiac imaging like CMR under certain circumstances. Planning the ablation procedure based on the predominant location of scarring as detected by LGE-CMR may be helpful and CMR may support sudden death risk stratification. Nevertheless, for the present analysis we decided to stick only to the ESC guidelines to warrant a consistent level of guideline standard.

Regarding valvular and congenital heart disease, the ESC guidelines contain extensive text passages about the value of CMR, reflecting current practice, where these indications make up a substantial part of all examinations [2]. In future guideline versions, the translation of these paragraphs into specific recommendations is needed to clarify the position of CMR.

This study touches several aspects: First, the frequent representation of CMR in the ESC guidelines demonstrates that the cardiology society has accepted CMR as an integral part of the armamentarium of cardiovascular diagnostic modalities (e.g. stress testing). As a next step, studies are needed that analyse the adherence to the ESC guidelines and how it impacts patients' management [41]. Second, there are several clinical scenarios, where CMR is already used at dedicated centres, but which are not well represented in the ESC guidelines (e.g. myocarditis). Here, further studies are needed to provide the required evidence. Third, CMR has not yet arrived in the clinical reality in many regions of Europe. Hence, not everywhere in Europe can the patients be managed according to the ESC guidelines. The reasons are certainly multifactorial, with economic issues playing a central role: i) in some diseases alternative techniques are often readily available that provide similar information as CMR does. This is especially true for testing for myocardial ischemia, where SPECT and stress echocardiography are still the dominant modalities. ii) CMR is recognized as expensive and reimbursement not aspired by the medical insurances in many countries. iii) knowledge both to run a CMR examination and to interpret the images with profound cardiologic knowledge is often limited and structures for systematic training are needed, including the establishment of cooperation between radiologists and cardiologists.

Already now, there are attempts how to overcome the latter obstacles and to enable the use of CMR in accordance with the guidelines: Recent large-scale studies demonstrated the diagnostic accuracy of CMR and its superiority in some indications [4]; prognostic data are available that demonstrate the benefit of CMR [42]; there are studies that demonstrate the potential for saving resources by using CMR [43]; structures for acquiring CMR skills including e-based learning are evolving [44]; and CMR imaging became faster and the user interfaces easier to handle.

Limitations of the study

This summary is not intended to provide a balanced comparison of the various imaging modalities in the ESC guidelines, but aimed at describing only the role of CMR.

Conclusions

CMR is represented in the majority of the ESC guidelines. They contain many recommendations in favour of the use of CMR in specific scenarios. Issues regarding training, costs and reimbursement have to be solved to provide CMR to the patients in accordance with the ESC recommendations.

Appendix: Summary of clinical scenarios/diagnoses, where the ESC made recommendations regarding CMR

Suspected/stable coronary artery disease	Class[a]	Level[b]	Guideline
Whenever history suggests myocardial ischaemia, a stress ECG test is recommended, and, if positive or ambiguous, an imaging stress test (stress echocardiography, stress CMR or nuclear scintigraphy) is recommended.	I	C	[22]
In subjects with intermediate pretest probability for suspected coronary artery disease and stable symptoms, stress CMR, stress-echo, SPECT or PET are recommended	I	A	[16]
In patients with suspected stable coronary artery disease and intermediate pretest probability of 15 % - 65 % and LVEF =50 %, stress imaging is preferred as the initial test option if local expertise and availability permit.	I	B	[20]
An imaging stress test is recommended as the initial test for diagnosing stable coronary artery disease if the pretest probability is between 66-85 % or if LVEF is <50 % in patients without typical angina.	I	B	[20]
An imaging stress test is recommended in patients with resting ECG abnormalities, which prevent accurate interpretation of ECG changes during stress.	I	B	[20]
Stress imaging for risk stratification is recommended in patients with a non-conclusive exercise ECG	I	B	[20]
Risk stratification is recommended based on clinical assessment and the results of the stress test initially employed for making a diagnosis of stable coronary artery disease	I	B	[20]
In asymptomatic adults with diabetes or asymptomatic adults with a strong family history of coronary artery disease or when previous risk assessment testing suggests high risk of coronary artery disease, such as a coronary artery calcium score of 400 or greater stress imaging tests (MPI, stress echocardiography, perfusion CMR) may be considered for advanced cardiovascular risk assessment.	IIb	C	[20]
In patients with stable coronary disease after a significant change in symptom level, risk stratification using stress ECG (unless they cannot exercise or display ECG changes which make the ECG non evaluable) or preferably stress imaging if local expertise and availability permit is recommended	I	B	[20]
In patients with known stable coronary artery disease and a deterioration in symptoms, stress imaging is recommended for risk stratification if the site and extent of ischemia would influence clinical decision making	I	B	[20]
An exercise ECG or stress imaging if appropriate is recommended in the presence of recurrent or new symptoms once instability has been ruled out.	I	C	[20]
Reassessment of the prognosis using stress testing may be considered in asymptomatic patients after the expiration of the period for which the previous test was felt to be valid ("warranty period")	IIb	C	[20]
Risk stratification before non-cardiac surgery	**Class[a]**	**Level[b]**	**Guideline**
Imaging stress testing is recommended before high-risk surgery in patients with more than two clinical risk factors and poor functional capacity (<4 METs).	I	C	[18]
Imaging stress testing may be considered before high- or intermediate-risk surgery in patients with one or two clinical risk factors and poor functional capacity (<4 METs).c	IIb	C	[18]
Imaging stress testing is not recommended before low-risk surgery, regardless of the patient's clinical risk.	III	C	[18]
Acute coronary syndrome	**Class[a]**	**Level[b]**	**Guideline**
In patients with no recurrence of chest pain, normal ECG findings and normal levels of cardiac troponin (preferably high-sensitivity), but suspected acute coronary syndrome, a non-invasive stress test (preferably with imaging) for inducible ischaemia is recommended before deciding on an invasive strategy.	I	A	[9]
If echocardiography is not feasible, CMR may be used as an alternative for assessment of infarct size and resting LV function after STEMI.	IIb	C	[26]
For patients with multivessel disease, or in whom revascularization of other vessels is considered, stress testing or imaging (e.g. using stress myocardial perfusion scintigraphy, stress echocardiography, positron emission tomography or CMR) for ischaemia and viability is indicated after STEMI before or after discharge.	I	A	[26]
Before coronary revascularization	**Class[a]**	**Level[b]**	**Guideline**
An imaging stress test should be considered to assess the functional severity of intermediate lesions on coronary arteriography.	IIa	B	[20]
To achieve a prognostic benefit by revascularization in patients with coronary artery disease, ischemia has to be documented by non-invasive imaging	I	A-C	[16]
After coronary revascularization	**Class[a]**	**Level[b]**	**Guideline**
In asymptomatic patients after revascularisation, early imaging testing should be considered in specific patient subsets.	IIa	C	[16]
Late (6 months) stress imaging test after revascularization may be considered to detect patients with restenosis after stenting or graft occlusion irrespective of symptoms.	IIb	C	[20]
In asymptomatic patients, routine stress testing may be considered >2 years after PCI and >5 years after CABG.	IIa	B	[16]

(Continued)

In symptomatic patients with revascularized stable coronary artery disease, stress imaging (stress echocardiography, CMR or MPS) is indicated rather than stress ECG.	I	C	[20]
In symptomatic patients with prior revascularization (PCI or CABG), an imaging stress test should be considered	IIa	B	[20]
In symptomatic patients after revascularization with low-risk findings at stress testing, it is recommended to reinforce medical therapy and lifestyle changes.	I	C	[16]
In symptomatic patients after revascularization with intermediate- to high-risk findings at stress testing, coronary angiography is recommended.	I	C	[16]
Heart failure	Class[a]	Level[b]	Guideline
CMR imaging is recommended to evaluate cardiac structure and function, to measure LVEF, and to characterize cardiac tissue, especially in subjects with inadequate echocardiographic images or where the echocardiographic findings are inconclusive or incomplete (but taking account of cautions/contraindications to CMR).	I	C	[27]
Myocardial perfusion/ischaemia imaging (echocardiography, CMR, SPECT, or PET) should be considered in patients thought to have coronary artery disease, and who are considered suitable for coronary revascularization, to determine whether there is reversible myocardial ischaemia and viable myocardium.	IIa	C	[27]
Ventricular arrhythmia	Class[a]	Level[b]	Guideline
Pharmacological stress testing plus imaging modality is recommended to detect silent ischaemia in patients with ventricular arrhythmias who have an intermediate probability of having coronary artery disease by age or symptoms and are physically unable to perform a symptom-limited exercise test.	I	B	[6]
CMR should be considered in patients with ventricular arrhythmias when echocardiography does not provide accurate assessment of LV and RV function and/or evaluation of structural changes.	IIa	B	[6]
Inflammatory heart disease	Class[a]	Level[b]	Guideline
Demonstration of persistent myocardial inflammatory infiltrates by immunohistological evidence and/or abnormal localized fibrosis by CMR after acute myocarditis may be considered as an additional indicator of increased risk of SCD in inflammatory heart disease.	IIb	C	[6]
CMR is recommended for the confirmation of myocardial involvement in pericarditis	I	C	[11]
Hypertrophic cardiomyopathy	Class[a]	Level[b]	Guideline
It is recommended that CMR studies in suspected HCM be performed and interpreted by teams experienced in cardiac imaging and in the evaluation of heart muscle disease	I	B	[14]
In the absence of contraindications, CMR with LGE is recommended in patients with suspected HCM who have inadequate echocardiographic windows, in order to confirm the diagnosis.	I	C	[14]
In the absence of contraindications, CMR with LGE should be considered in patients fulfilling diagnostic criteria for HCM, to assess cardiac anatomy, ventricular function, and the presence and extent of myocardial fibrosis.	IIa	B	[14]
CMR with LGE imaging should be considered in patients with suspected apical hypertrophy or aneurysm.	IIa	C	[14]
CMR with LGE may be considered before septal alcohol ablation or myectomy, to assess the extent and distribution of hypertrophy and myocardial fibrosis.	IIb	C	[14]
CMR may be considered every 5 years in clinically stable patients, or every 2–3 years in patients with progressive disease.	IIb	C	[14]
Athlete's heart	Class[a]	Level[b]	Guideline
For prevention of sudden cardiac death in athletes, upon identification of ECG abnormalities suggestive of structural heart disease, echocardiography and/or CMR imaging is recommended.	I	C	[6]
Storage disease	Class[a]	Level[b]	Guideline
CMR with LGE imaging should be considered in patients with suspected cardiac amyloidosis.	IIa	C	[14]
Pericardial diseases	Class[a]	Level[b]	Guideline
CMR is second-level testing for diagnostic workup in pericarditis	I	C	[11]
CMR should be considered in suspected cases of loculated pericardial effusion, pericardial thickening and masses, as well as associated chest abnormalities	IIa	C	[11]
CMR is indicated as second-level imaging technique to assess pericardial thickness, degree and extension of pericardial involvement for the diagnosis of constrictive pericarditis	I	C	[11]
Empiric anti-inflammatory therapy may be considered in cases with transient or new diagnosis of constrictive pericarditis with concomitant evidence of pericardial inflammation (i.e. pericardial enhancement on CMR)	IIb	C	[11]
Pregnancy	Class[a]	Level[b]	Guideline
CMR (without gadolinium) should be considered if echocardiography is insufficient for diagnosis.	IIa	C	[30]

(Continued)

Imaging of the entire aorta (CT/CMR) should be performed before pregnancy in patients with Marfan syndrome or other known aortic disease.	I	C	[30]
For imaging of pregnant women with dilatation of the distal ascending aorta, aortic arch or descending aorta, CMR (without gadolinium) is recommended.	I	C	[30]
Vessel disease	Class[a]	Level[b]	Guideline
In stable patients with a suspicion of acute aortic syndrome, CMR is recommended (or should be considered) according to local availability and expertise	I	C	[15]
In case of initially negative imaging with persistence of suspicion of acute aortic syndrome, repetitive imaging (CT or CMR) is recommended.	I	C	[15]
In case of uncomplicated Type B aortic dissection treated medically, repeated imaging (CT or CMR) during the first days is recommended.	I	C	[15]
In uncomplicated Type B intramural hematoma, repetitive imaging (CMR or CT) is indicated.	I	C	[15]
In uncomplicated Type B penetrating aortic ulcer, repetitive imaging (CMR or CT) is indicated.	I	C	[15]
CMR or CT is indicated in patients with bicuspid aortic valve when the morphology of the aortic root and the ascending aorta cannot be accurately assessed by TTE.	I	C	[15]
In the case of aortic diameter >50 mm or an increase >3 mm/year measured by echocardiography, confirmation of the measurement is indicated, using another imaging modality (CT or CMR).	I	C	[15]
Contrast CT or CMR is recommended to confirm the diagnosis of chronic aortic dissection.	I	C	[15]
For follow-up after (T)EVAR in young patients, CMR should be preferred to CT for magnetic resonance-compatible stent grafts, to reduce radiation exposure.	IIa	C	[15]
CMR, CT, or digital subtraction angiography may be considered if carotid artery stenosis by ultrasound is >70 % and myocardial revascularization is contemplated.	IIb	C	[16]
MR angiography should not be used to rule out pulmonary embolism.	III	C	[17]
Duplex ultrasound, CT-angiography, and/or MRA are indicated to evaluate carotid artery stenosis.	I	A	[31]
When Duplex ultrasound is inconclusive, CT-angiography or gadolinium-enhanced MRA are indicated to evaluate chronic mesenteric ischaemia.	I	B	[31]
MRA (in patients with creatinine clearance >30 mL/min) is recommended to establish the diagnosis of renal artery stenosis.	I	B	[31]
Duplex ultrasound and/or CT-angiography and/or MRA are indicated to localize lower extremity artery disease lesions and consider revascularization options.	I	A	[31]

[a] Class of recommendation
[b] Level of evidence

Abbreviations
CMR: cardiovascular magnetic resonance; CT: computed tomography; ECG: electrocardiography; ESC: European society for cardiology; LAD: left anterior descending coronary artery; LGE: late gadolinium enhancement; LV: left ventricle; MRA: magnetic resonance angiography; PET: positron emission tomography; RV: right ventricle; SPECT: single photon emission computed tomography; STEMI: ST elevation myocardial infarct; TTE: transthoracic echocardiography.

Competing interests
The authors declare that they have no competing interests.

Authors' contributions
FvKB was responsible for conception and design, acquisition of data, analysis and interpretation of data and drafted the manuscript. JSM revised the manuscript critically for important intellectual content and has given final approval of the version to be published. Both authors agree to be accountable for all aspects of the work in ensuring that questions related to the accuracy or integrity of any part of the work are appropriately investigated and resolved. All authors read and approved the final manuscript.

Acknowledgements
We thank Kai Philipp Hasemann for assisting during the analysis of the guideline fulltextes.

References
1. von Knobelsdorff-Brenkenhoff F, Bublak A, El-Mahmoud S, Wassmuth R, Opitz C, Schulz-Menger J. Single-centre survey of the application of cardiovascular magnetic resonance in clinical routine. Eur Heart J Cardiovasc Imaging. 2013;14:62–8.
2. Bruder O, Wagner A, Lombardi M, Schwitter J, van Rossum A, Pilz G, et al. European Cardiovascular Magnetic Resonance (EuroCMR) registry–multi national results from 57 centers in 15 countries. J Cardiovasc Magn Reson. 2013;15:9.
3. Friedrich MG. There is more than shape and function. J Am Coll Cardiol. 2008;52:1581–3.
4. Greenwood JP, Maredia N, Younger JF, Brown JM, Nixon J, Everett CC, et al. Cardiovascular magnetic resonance and single-photon emission computed tomography for diagnosis of coronary heart disease (CE-MARC): a prospective trial. Lancet. 2012;379:453–60.
5. Kramer CM, Barkhausen J, Flamm SD, Kim RJ, Nagel E. Society for Cardiovascular Magnetic Resonance Board of Trustees Task Force on Standardized P. Standardized cardiovascular magnetic resonance (CMR) protocols 2013 update. J Cardiovasc Magn Reson. 2013;15:91.
6. Authors/Task Force M, Priori SG, Blomstrom-Lundqvist C, Mazzanti A, Blom N, Borggrefe M et al. 2015 ESC Guidelines for the management of patients with ventricular arrhythmias and the prevention of sudden cardiac death: The Task Force for the Management of Patients with Ventricular Arrhythmias and the Prevention of Sudden Cardiac Death of the European Society of Cardiology (ESC) Endorsed by: Association for European Paediatric and Congenital Cardiology (AEPC). Eur Heart J. 2015. pii: ehv316. [Epub ahead of print]

7. Authors/Task Force M, Galie N, Humbert M, Vachiery JL, Gibbs S, Lang I, et al. 2015 ESC/ERS Guidelines for the diagnosis and treatment of pulmonary hypertension: The Joint Task Force for the Diagnosis and Treatment of Pulmonary Hypertension of the European Society of Cardiology (ESC) and the European Respiratory Society (ERS) Endorsed by: Association for European Paediatric and Congenital Cardiology (AEPC), International Society for Heart and Lung Transplantation (ISHLT). Eur Heart J. 2016;37:67–119.
8. Galie N, Hoeper MM, Humbert M, Torbicki A, Vachiery JL, Barbera JA, et al. Guidelines for the diagnosis and treatment of pulmonary hypertension: the Task Force for the Diagnosis and Treatment of Pulmonary Hypertension of the European Society of Cardiology (ESC) and the European Respiratory Society (ERS), endorsed by the International Society of Heart and Lung Transplantation (ISHLT). Eur Heart J. 2009;30:2493–537.
9. Authors/Task Force M, Roffi M, Patrono C, Collet JP, Mueller C, Valgimigli M et al. 2015 ESC Guidelines for the management of acute coronary syndromes in patients presenting without persistent ST-segment elevation: Task Force for the Management of Acute Coronary Syndromes in Patients Presenting without Persistent ST-Segment Elevation of the European Society of Cardiology (ESC). Eur Heart J. 2015 pii: ehv320. [Epub ahead of print].
10. Hamm CW, Bassand JP, Agewall S, Bax J, Boersma E, Bueno H, et al. ESC Guidelines for the management of acute coronary syndromes in patients presenting without persistent ST-segment elevation: The Task Force for the management of acute coronary syndromes (ACS) in patients presenting without persistent ST-segment elevation of the European Society of Cardiology (ESC). Eur Heart J. 2011;32:2999–3054.
11. Authors/Task Force M, Adler Y, Charron P, Imazio M, Badano L, Baron-Esquivias G, et al. 2015 ESC Guidelines for the diagnosis and management of pericardial diseases: The Task Force for the Diagnosis and Management of Pericardial Diseases of the European Society of Cardiology (ESC)Endorsed by: The European Association for Cardio-Thoracic Surgery (EACTS). Eur Heart J. 2015;36:2921–64.
12. Authors/Task Force M, Habib G, Lancellotti P, Antunes MJ, Bongiorni MG, Casalta JP, et al. 2015 ESC Guidelines for the management of infective endocarditis: The Task Force for the Management of Infective Endocarditis of the European Society of Cardiology (ESC)Endorsed by: European Association for Cardio-Thoracic Surgery (EACTS), the European Association of Nuclear Medicine (EANM). Eur Heart J. 2015;36:3075–128.
13. Habib G, Hoen B, Tornos P, Thuny F, Prendergast B, Vilacosta I, et al. Guidelines on the prevention, diagnosis, and treatment of infective endocarditis (new version 2009): the Task Force on the Prevention, Diagnosis, and Treatment of Infective Endocarditis of the European Society of Cardiology (ESC). Endorsed by the European Society of Clinical Microbiology and Infectious Diseases (ESCMID) and the International Society of Chemotherapy (ISC) for Infection and Cancer. Eur Heart J. 2009;30:2369–413.
14. Authors/Task Force M, Elliott PM, Anastasakis A, Borger MA, Borggrefe M, Cecchi F, et al. 2014 ESC Guidelines on diagnosis and management of hypertrophic cardiomyopathy: the Task Force for the Diagnosis and Management of Hypertrophic Cardiomyopathy of the European Society of Cardiology (ESC). Eur Heart J. 2014;35:2733–79.
15. Erbel R, Aboyans V, Boileau C, Bossone E, Bartolomeo RD, Eggebrecht H, et al. 2014 ESC Guidelines on the diagnosis and treatment of aortic diseases: Document covering acute and chronic aortic diseases of the thoracic and abdominal aorta of the adult. The Task Force for the Diagnosis and Treatment of Aortic Diseases of the European Society of Cardiology (ESC). Eur Heart J. 2014;35:2873–926.
16. Authors/Task Force m, Windecker S, Kolh P, Alfonso F, Collet JP, Cremer J, et al. 2014 ESC/EACTS Guidelines on myocardial revascularization: The Task Force on Myocardial Revascularization of the European Society of Cardiology (ESC) and the European Association for Cardio-Thoracic Surgery (EACTS) Developed with the special contribution of the European Association of Percutaneous Cardiovascular Interventions (EAPCI). Eur Heart J. 2014;35:2541–619.
17. Konstantinides SV, Torbicki A, Agnelli G, Danchin N, Fitzmaurice D, Galie N, et al. 2014 ESC guidelines on the diagnosis and management of acute pulmonary embolism. Eur Heart J. 2014;35:3033–69. 69a-69k.
18. Kristensen SD, Knuuti J, Saraste A, Anker S, Botker HE, Hert SD, et al. 2014 ESC/ESA Guidelines on non-cardiac surgery: cardiovascular assessment and management: The Joint Task Force on non-cardiac surgery: cardiovascular assessment and management of the European Society of Cardiology (ESC) and the European Society of Anaesthesiology (ESA). Eur Heart J. 2014;35:2383–431.
19. Authors/Task Force M, Ryden L, Grant PJ, Anker SD, Berne C, Cosentino F, et al. ESC Guidelines on diabetes, pre-diabetes, and cardiovascular diseases developed in collaboration with the EASD: the Task Force on diabetes, pre-diabetes, and cardiovascular diseases of the European Society of Cardiology (ESC) and developed in collaboration with the European Association for the Study of Diabetes (EASD). Eur Heart J. 2013;34:3035–87.
20. Task Force M, Montalescot G, Sechtem U, Achenbach S, Andreotti F, Arden C, et al. 2013 ESC guidelines on the management of stable coronary artery disease: the Task Force on the management of stable coronary artery disease of the European Society of Cardiology. Eur Heart J. 2013;34:2949–3003.
21. Brignole M, Auricchio A, Baron-Esquivias G, Bordachar P, Boriani G, Breithardt OA, et al. 2013 ESC Guidelines on cardiac pacing and cardiac resynchronization therapy: the Task Force on cardiac pacing and resynchronization therapy of the European Society of Cardiology (ESC). Developed in collaboration with the European Heart Rhythm Association (EHRA). Eur Heart J. 2013;34:2281–329.
22. Mancia G, Fagard R, Narkiewicz K, Redon J, Zanchetti A, Bohm M, et al. 2013 ESH/ESC guidelines for the management of arterial hypertension: the Task Force for the Management of Arterial Hypertension of the European Society of Hypertension (ESH) and of the European Society of Cardiology (ESC). Eur Heart J. 2013;34:2159–219.
23. Joint Task Force on the Management of Valvular Heart Disease of the European Society of C, European Association for Cardio-Thoracic S, Vahanian A, Alfieri O, Andreotti F, Antunes MJ, et al. Guidelines on the management of valvular heart disease (version 2012). Eur Heart J. 2012;33:2451–96.
24. Camm AJ, Lip GY, De Caterina R, Savelieva I, Atar D, Hohnloser SH, et al. 2012 focused update of the ESC Guidelines for the management of atrial fibrillation: an update of the 2010 ESC Guidelines for the management of atrial fibrillation. Developed with the special contribution of the European Heart Rhythm Association. Eur Heart J. 2012;33:2719–47.
25. Thygesen K, Alpert JS, Jaffe AS, Simoons ML, Chaitman BR, White HD, et al. Third universal definition of myocardial infarction. Eur Heart J. 2012;33:2551–67.
26. Task Force on the management of STseamiotESoC, Steg PG, James SK, Atar D, Badano LP, Blomstrom-Lundqvist C, et al. ESC Guidelines for the management of acute myocardial infarction in patients presenting with ST-segment elevation. Eur Heart J. 2012;33:2569–619.
27. McMurray JJ, Adamopoulos S, Anker SD, Auricchio A, Bohm M, Dickstein K, et al. ESC Guidelines for the diagnosis and treatment of acute and chronic heart failure 2012: The Task Force for the Diagnosis and Treatment of Acute and Chronic Heart Failure 2012 of the European Society of Cardiology. Developed in collaboration with the Heart Failure Association (HFA) of the ESC. Eur Heart J. 2012;33:1787–847.
28. Perk J, De Backer G, Gohlke H, Graham I, Reiner Z, Verschuren M, et al. European Guidelines on cardiovascular disease prevention in clinical practice (version 2012). The Fifth Joint Task Force of the European Society of Cardiology and Other Societies on Cardiovascular Disease Prevention in Clinical Practice (constituted by representatives of nine societies and by invited experts). Eur Heart J. 2012;33:1635–701.
29. European Association for Cardiovascular P, Rehabilitation, Reiner Z, Catapano AL, De Backer G, Graham I, et al. ESC/EAS Guidelines for the management of dyslipidaemias: the Task Force for the management of dyslipidaemias of the European Society of Cardiology (ESC) and the European Atherosclerosis Society (EAS). Eur Heart J. 2011;32:1769–818.
30. European Society of G, Association for European Paediatric C, German Society for Gender M, Regitz-Zagrosek V, Blomstrom Lundqvist C, Borghi C, et al. ESC Guidelines on the management of cardiovascular diseases during pregnancy: the Task Force on the Management of Cardiovascular Diseases during Pregnancy of the European Society of Cardiology (ESC). Eur Heart J. 2011;32:3147–97.
31. European Stroke O, Tendera M, Aboyans V, Bartelink ML, Baumgartner I, Clement D, et al. ESC Guidelines on the diagnosis and treatment of peripheral artery diseases: Document covering atherosclerotic disease of extracranial carotid and vertebral, mesenteric, renal, upper and lower extremity arteries: the Task Force on the Diagnosis and Treatment of Peripheral Artery Diseases of the European Society of Cardiology (ESC). Eur Heart J. 2011;32:2851–906.
32. Baumgartner H, Bonhoeffer P, De Groot NM, de Haan F, Deanfield JE, Galie N, et al. ESC Guidelines for the management of grown-up congenital heart disease (new version 2010). Eur Heart J. 2010;31:2915–57.
33. Kilner PJ, Geva T, Kaemmerer H, Trindade PT, Schwitter J, Webb GD. Recommendations for cardiovascular magnetic resonance in adults with

congenital heart disease from the respective working groups of the European Society of Cardiology. Eur Heart J. 2010;31:794–805.

34. Dickstein K, Vardas PE, Auricchio A, Daubert JC, Linde C, McMurray J, et al. 2010 Focused Update of ESC Guidelines on device therapy in heart failure: an update of the 2008 ESC Guidelines for the diagnosis and treatment of acute and chronic heart failure and the 2007 ESC guidelines for cardiac and resynchronization therapy. Developed with the special contribution of the Heart Failure Association and the European Heart Rhythm Association. Eur Heart J. 2010;31:2677–87.
35. Task Force for the D, Management of S, European Society of C, European Heart Rhythm A, Heart Failure A, Heart Rhythm S et al. Guidelines for the diagnosis and management of syncope (version 2009). Eur Heart J. 2009;30:2631–71.
36. Nicholls M. The 2014 ESC Guidelines on the Diagnosis and Management of Hypertrophic Cardiomyopathy have been published. Eur Heart J. 2014;35:2849–50.
37. Caforio AL, Pankuweit S, Arbustini E, Basso C, Gimeno-Blanes J, Felix SB, et al. Current state of knowledge on aetiology, diagnosis, management, and therapy of myocarditis: a position statement of the European Society of Cardiology Working Group on Myocardial and Pericardial Diseases. Eur Heart J. 2013;34:2636–48. 48a-48d.
38. Rapezzi C, Arbustini E, Caforio AL, Charron P, Gimeno-Blanes J, Helio T, et al. Diagnostic work-up in cardiomyopathies: bridging the gap between clinical phenotypes and final diagnosis. A position statement from the ESC Working Group on Myocardial and Pericardial Diseases. Eur Heart J. 2013;34:1448–58.
39. Cooper LT, Baughman KL, Feldman AM, Frustaci A, Jessup M, Kuhl U, et al. The role of endomyocardial biopsy in the management of cardiovascular disease: a scientific statement from the American Heart Association, the American College of Cardiology, and the European Society of Cardiology Endorsed by the Heart Failure Society of America and the Heart Failure Association of the European Society of Cardiology. Eur Heart J. 2007;28:3076–93.
40. Birnie DH, Sauer WH, Bogun F, Cooper JM, Culver DA, Duvernoy CS, et al. HRS expert consensus statement on the diagnosis and management of arrhythmias associated with cardiac sarcoidosis. Heart Rhythm. 2014;11:1305–23.
41. Maggioni AP, Anker SD, Dahlstrom U, Filippatos G, Ponikowski P, Zannad F, et al. Are hospitalized or ambulatory patients with heart failure treated in accordance with European Society of Cardiology guidelines? Evidence from 12,440 patients of the ESC Heart Failure Long-Term Registry. Eur J Heart Fail. 2013;15:1173–84.
42. Anderson LJ, Holden S, Davis B, Prescott E, Charrier CC, Bunce NH, et al. Cardiovascular T2-star (T2*) magnetic resonance for the early diagnosis of myocardial iron overload. Eur Heart J. 2001;22:2171–9.
43. Pilz G, Patel PA, Fell U, Ladapo JA, Rizzo JA, Fang H, et al. Adenosine-stress cardiac magnetic resonance imaging in suspected coronary artery disease: a net cost analysis and reimbursement implications. Int J Cardiovasc Imaging. 2010;27:113–21.
44. Muehlberg F, Neumann D, von Knobelsdorff-Brenkenhoff F, Traber J, Alwardt N, Schulz-Menger J. A Multicenter Cardiovascular MR Network for Tele-Training and Beyond: Setup and Initial Experiences. J Am Coll Radiol. 2015;12:876–83.

7

Blood correction reduces variability and gender differences in native myocardial T1 values at 1.5 T cardiovascular magnetic resonance – a derivation/validation approach

Jannike Nickander[1], Magnus Lundin[1], Goran Abdula[1], Peder Sörensson[2], Stefania Rosmini[3], James C. Moon[3], Peter Kellman[4], Andreas Sigfridsson[1] and Martin Ugander[1*]

Abstract

Background: Myocardial native T1 measurements are likely influenced by intramyocardial blood. Since blood T1 is both variable and longer compared to myocardial T1, this will degrade the precision of myocardial T1 measurements. Precision could be improved by correction, but the amount of correction and the optimal blood T1 variables to correct with are unknown. We hypothesized that an appropriate correction would reduce the standard deviation (SD) of native myocardial T1.

Methods: Consecutive patients ($n = 400$) referred for CMR with known or suspected heart disease were split into a derivation cohort for model construction ($n = 200$, age 51 ± 18 years, 50% male) and a validation cohort for assessing model performance ($n = 200$, age 48 ± 17 years, 50% male). Exclusion criteria included focal septal abnormalities. A Modified Look-Locker inversion recovery sequence (MOLLI, 1.5 T Siemens Aera) was used to acquire T1 and T1* maps. T1 and T1* maps were used to measure native myocardial T1, and blood T1 and T1*. A multivariate linear regression correction model was implemented using blood measurement of R1 (1/T1), R1* (1/T1*) or hematocrit. The correction model from the derivation cohort was applied to the validation cohort, and assessed for reduction in variability with the F-test.

Results: Blood [LV + RV] mean R1, mean R1* and hematocrit correlated with myocardial T1 (Pearson's r, range 0.37 to 0.45, $p < 0.05$ for all) in both the derivation and validation cohorts respectively, suggesting that myocardial T1 measurements are influenced by intramyocardial blood. Mean myocardial native T1 did not differ between the derivation and validation cohorts (1030 ± 42.6 ms and 1023 ± 45.2 ms respectively, $p = 0.07$). In the derivation cohort, correction using blood mean R1 and mean R1* yielded a decrease in myocardial T1 SD (45.2 ms to 36.6 ms, $p = 0.03$). When the model from the derivation cohort was applied to the validation cohort, the SD reduction was maintained (39.3 ms, $p = 0.049$). This 13% reduction in measurement variability leads to a 23% reduction in sample size to detect a 50 ms difference in native myocardial T1.

Conclusions: Correcting native myocardial T1 for R1 and R1* of blood improves the precision of myocardial T1 measurement by ~13%, and could consequently improve disease detection and reduce sample size needs for clinical research.

Keywords: Native T1, T1 Mapping, Post-processing, Quantification, Precision

* Correspondence: martin.ugander@gmail.com
[1]Department of Clinical Physiology, Karolinska Institutet and Karolinska University Hospital, Stockholm, Sweden
Full list of author information is available at the end of the article

Background

Parametric pixel-wise mapping has been developed to quantitatively measure and image the longitudinal magnetic relaxation time (T1) [1]. Native myocardial T1 mapping has shown diagnostic promise for differentiating healthy myocardium from various pathologies including acute myocardial infarction [2], myocarditis [3, 4], amyloidosis [5], edema [6], Anderson-Fabry disease [7] and other non-ischemic diseases [8, 9]. Reference values for native myocardial T1 in ischemic and several non-ischemic heart diseases have been reported, with cutoff values for age, and sex [10], which suggests that native myocardial T1 mapping is a robust diagnostic tool for myocardial tissue characterization in clinical use [5, 11, 12].

However, the normal myocardial blood volume (MBV) averages approximately 6% of the myocardium [13, 14]. The T1 value of blood is higher than the T1 value of the myocardium, thus the T1 value of the myocardium is expected to be influenced by both the T1 value, and the amount of blood in the myocardium. The partial volume effect describes the concept that a single voxel may contain tissue of different characteristics, whereas the pixel value for that voxel will represent a combination of these contents [15]. Furthermore, the myocardial T1 values reflect a volume of tissue consisting of myocytes, extracellular connective tissue, nerves, blood vessels and the blood therein [16, 17]. Therefore, myocardial T1 values should relate to the summed composition of the tissue, including the microcirculation. The T1 values of blood have been shown to vary due to a number of factors like hematocrit [18], sex [10], age [19], and oxygen pressure [18, 20] and variations in these factors may influence the interpretation of myocardial T1 values, and obscure the true T1 value of the myocardium.

Approaches for correcting for myocardial blood volume have been reported [21, 22]. Reiter et al. showed that myocardial T1 differences by age and sex were eliminated when corrected for T1 measured in the blood pool of the left ventricle (LV) [22]. This correction could therefore decrease the variability of native myocardial T1 between patients, thus improving the clinical accuracy. Therefore, the purpose of this study was to identify a blood correction model, with cardiovascular magnetic resonance (CMR) available measurements, which in a future implementation could allow automated inline blood-corrected T1 maps, and validate this model in a separate clinical cohort. A technical aspect of an automated method for blood correction is blood segmentation. Therefore, the mean blood T1 values of both ventricles (LV and right ventricle (RV)) were acquired. Blood T1* measurements were also investigated. Since there is no reference method for measuring myocardial T1 values, we hypothesized that blood correction could reduce the variability in native myocardial T1 values in a clinical population, measured as a decrease in standard deviation (SD).

Methods

Study population

Consecutive patients referred for diagnostic CMR for known or suspected heart disease at Karolinska University Hospital, Stockholm, Sweden, were retrospectively enrolled between 2014-01-02 and 2015-08-07. Inclusion was terminated when a total of 200 males and 200 females were included, respectively. A total of 543 patients were assessed for eligibility. Exclusion criteria included focal septal myocardial pathologies, cardiac shunts, poor image quality or presence of cardiac tumors, see Fig. 1. Included patients were randomly assigned to either the derivation or the validation cohort. Hematocrit was determined by venous blood sampling prior to CMR, as a part of the clinical routine. Venous blood was drawn with a syringe from an intravenous access cannula, and analyzed by an iSTAT Handheld Blood Analyzer®, using a CHEM8+ cartridge (Abbot Point of Care, Princeton, USA). The study was approved by the local research ethics committee, and all patients provided written informed consent.

Healthy volunteers ($n = 77$, mean age 49 ± 14 years, 49% males) were prospectively recruited between April 2014 and July 2015 through local advertising. None of the volunteers had any cardiovascular disease or diabetes. Five were on statins and one was on aspirin for primary prevention. All volunteers had a normal 12-lead ECG and all scans were reported as normal by experienced Level 3 CMR cardiologists. Imaging was performed on a 1.5 T MR scanner (Magnetom Avanto, Siemens, Erlangen, Germany) and a 32-channel cardiac phased array receiver coil was used. The imaging protocol included cines, native T1 mapping, T2 mapping, Late Gadolinium Enhancement

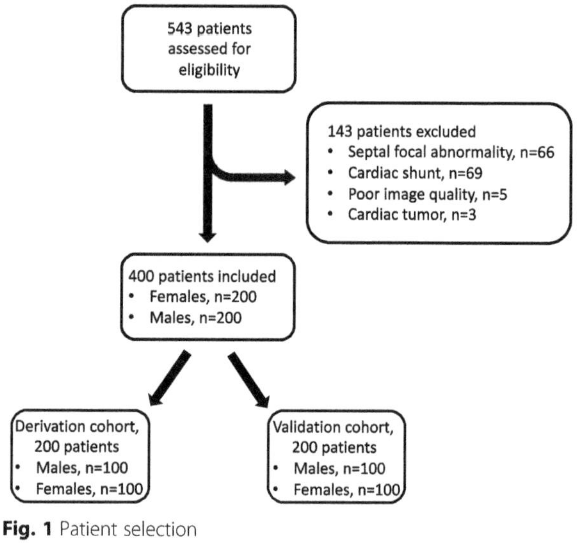

Fig. 1 Patient selection

(LGE) and post-contrast T1 mapping. For this study, only the native T1 and T1* maps were analysed. Whole blood for venous hematocrit was drawn in all subjects by venipuncture and analyzed as routine clinical samples using a Sysmex XE-2100 hematology analyzer (Sysmex, Kobe, Japan) [23].

Image acquisition

All patient CMR scans were conducted on a 1.5 T scanner (Siemens Aera, Erlangen, Germany) with a phased-array 18-channel body matrix coil together with a spine matrix coil. All patients were examined in the supine position. CMR scans assessing LV function used retrospectively electrocardiographically gated balanced steady-state free precession (bSSFP) cine imaging covering the entire LV. Typical imaging parameters included flip angle = 61°, voxel size = 2.0x2.0x8.0 mm^3, TR/TE = 37.05/1.19 ms, matrix size = 143x256 and field of view (FoV) 303x360 mm^2.

T1 maps were acquired using an electrocardiographically gated Modified Look-Locker inversion recovery (MOLLI) sequence [24] with a 5(3)3 sampling scheme (Siemens WIP 1041). T1 maps were reconstructed using inline motion correction [25], and reconstruction output included a T1 error map, a T1* map and a T1 map. Typical image acquisition parameters were: steady-state free precession single-shot read out with a trigger delay to coincide with end-diastole, flip angle = 35°, matrix size = 144x256, TE = 2.6 ms, TR = 278 ms, FoV = 270x360 mm^2, parallel acquisition technique (PAT) factor 2, number of inversion 2, data window duration 163 ms. Operators were allowed to perform standard cardiac planning adjusting for patient size, rendering a range of phase encoding lines 136–158, and FoV 241–384 x 300–410 mm^2.

The healthy volunteers were imaged using a 5s(3s)3s MOLLI protocol. The acquisition parameters were: pixel bandwidth 977 Hz/pixel; echo time = 1.1 ms; flip angle = 35°; matrix size = 256x144; slice thickness = 6 mm. Motion correction and a non-linear least-square curve fitting were performed with the set of images acquired at different inversion times to generate a pixel-wise T1 map and T1* map.

Image analysis

LV volumes, ejection fraction (EF) and myocardial mass were quantified using the SyngoVia Software, VA30 (Siemens, Erlangen, Germany). Body surface area (BSA) was calculated with the Du Bois formula [26]. Volumetric measurements and myocardial mass were indexed to BSA. Native myocardial T1 values were measured by one observer by manually delineating a region of interest (ROI), conservatively placed, to avoid partial volume effects, in the mid-mural third of the septum of a mid-ventricular short-axis T1 map using a clinical work station (IDS7, Sectra, Linköping, Sweden). Blood T1 and T1* values were measured in the blood pool of both ventricles as the mean value of two manually delineated ROIs in the corresponding mid-ventricular short-axis T1 and T1* maps. The ROIs were delineated as large as possible without including papillary muscle and trabeculae, see Fig. 2. Myocardial wall thickness was measured in the septum in the corresponding bSSFP cine short-axis slice, in end-diastole. Mean blood T1 and T1* values were calculated as the average of blood T1 and T1* from the RV and the LV, and converted to the T1 relaxation rate (R1 = 1/T1). This yielded mean blood R1 and mean blood R1*. R1, as opposed to T1, is linearly related to the concentration of differing T1 species such as contrast agent or blood in the setting of the current study.

A linear correlation between septal myocardial T1 and blood measurements was assumed. T1 was corrected using the equation, Equation 1:

$$T1_{corrected} = T1_{uncorrected} + constant \cdot \left(X_{mean} - X_{patient}\right)$$

where X is the blood measurement of mean R1, mean

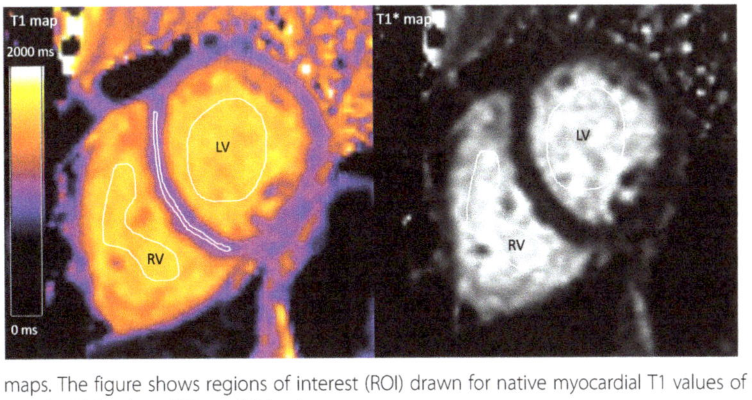

Fig. 2 Short-axis T1 and T1* maps. The figure shows regions of interest (ROI) drawn for native myocardial T1 values of the mid-mural septum, LV blood pool T1 and T1* values, and RV blood pool T1 and T1* values

R1* or hematocrit, mean is the mean for the patient cohort, and the constant was calculated as the slopes of linear regression between myocardial T1 and the blood measurements.

The T1 maps from the healthy volunteers were analysed using CVI42 software (Circle Cardiovascular Imaging Inc.,Version 5.1.2 [303], Calgary, Canada) by one observer. Global myocardial T1 values were acquired by carefully delineating the endo- and epicardial borders and eroding 10% to acquire the middle 80% of the myocardium. ROIs were drawn in the LV and RV blood pools of the mid-ventricular short-axis slice of the native T1 and T1* maps, and care was taken to avoid papillary muscles.

Statistical analysis

Continuous variables were reported as mean and SD. Statistical analysis was performed using Microsoft Excel (Microsoft, Redmond, Washington, USA), and statistical testing was performed using Statistical Product and Service Solutions® (IBM SPSS Statistics 23, IBM, New York, USA). Statistical significance was defined as $p < 0.05$.

Multivariate linear regression was performed for slopes used for correction of native myocardial T1 for combinations of blood characteristics in the derivation cohort. The blood correction model from the derivation cohort was applied to the validation cohort, and the healthy volunteers respectively. The relationships between corrected and uncorrected native myocardial T1 values were investigated by the SD of the mean native myocardial T1, and evaluated for differences with the F-test. Mean values were compared by using the paired or unpaired *t*-test as appropriate in normally distributed data, and Mann–Whitney *U*-test in data with non-normal distribution. Sample size calculations were performed using Microsoft Excel.

Results

Study population

Baseline characteristics of the derivation and validation cohorts are shown in Table 1. Mean uncorrected native myocardial T1 was 1030 ± 42.6 ms in the derivation cohort, 1023 ± 45.2 ms, ($p = 0.07$) in the validation cohort, and 1027 ± 37.5 ms in the healthy volunteers. Hematocrit range for all 400 patients was 25 to 57%. There was no difference in characteristics between the derivation and validation cohorts, except for LV stroke volume (SV) and indexed LVSV (LVSVI), which was lower in the derivation cohort, albeit with a small magnitude of difference. There was no difference in characteristics between the females in

Table 1 Baseline characteristics of the derivation and validation cohorts

Characteristic	Derivation cohort ($n = 200$)[a]	Validation cohort ($n = 200$)[a]	*p*-value
Age (years)	51 ± 18	48 ± 17	0.14
Female sex, n (%)	100 (50%)	100 (50%)	1.0
Height (cm)	173 ± 14	174 ± 10	0.44
Weight (kg)	77 ± 16	78 ± 18	0.79
BSA (m^2)	1.9 ± 0.3	1.9 ± 0.2	0.95
LVEDV (ml)	180 ± 63	183 ± 63	0.56
LVEDVI (ml/m^2)	94 ± 29	95 ± 32	0.61
LVESV (ml)	91 ± 57	88 ± 57	0.81
LVESVI (ml/m^2)	47 ± 28	46 ± 29	0.95
LVSV (ml)	89 ± 27	95 ± 25	0.02*
LVSVI (ml/m^2)	47 ± 14	50 ± 11	0.01*
LVEF (%)	52 ± 12	54 ± 11	0.06
LVM (g)	138 ± 46	137 ± 53	0.75
LVMI (g/m^2)	71 ± 19	72 ± 23	0.95
ECV (%)	28 ± 4	28 ± 4	0.51
Hematocrit (%)	40 ± 4	40 ± 5	0.71
Septal wall thickness (mm)	10 ± 2	10 ± 2	0.45
Myocardial T1 (ms)	1030 ± 43	1023 ± 45	0.07
Mean blood R1 (ms^{-1})	0.00064 ± 0.00004	0.00064 ± 0.00004	0.49
Mean blood R1* (ms^{-1})	0.00061 ± 0.00005	0.00061 ± 0.00005	0.98

Characteristics are given as means ± standard deviations, or percentages as appropriate. *p*-values refer to comparison of mean values between derivation and validation cohort. *marks significant result. [a]Data missing for LV volumes, EF and mass ($n = 2$), and ECV ($n = 4$) in the derivation cohort. Data missing for ECV ($n = 2$) in the validation cohort the validation and derivation cohorts shown in Table 2. There was no difference between the males in the derivation and validation cohorts, except for LVSV and LVSVI, Table 3.

Myocardial T1 correlation

All the blood measurements correlated with uncorrected native myocardial T1 in both the derivation and validation cohorts, see Table 4. Myocardial wall thickness was not correlated with native myocardial T1, and was therefore not included in the multivariate analysis. Hematocrit had the weakest correlation in both the derivation and validation cohort, respectively. Mean R1 and mean R1* had the same correlation in the derivation cohort, whereas mean R1 alone had the best correlation in the validation cohort.

Myocardial T1 blood correction

Multivariate linear regression in the derivation cohort showed that the best correction model was a combination of mean R1 and mean R1* (R^2 0.26, $p < 0.001$), see Table 4. The constants from the regression model were used to correct native myocardial T1 values according to Equation 1. The blood correction model for mean R1 and mean R1* decreased the SD of myocardial T1 to 36.6 ms ($p = 0.03$) in the derivation cohort, see Fig. 3. The model also decreased the SD of myocardial T1 values in the validation cohort to 39.3 ms ($p = 0.049$), see Fig. 3. Mean uncorrected myocardial T1 in the derivation cohort was 1015 ± 38.6 ms for males and 1046 ± 41.1 ms for females ($p < 0.001$). The difference in mean myocardial T1 between males and females was eliminated by blood correction in the derivation cohort (1025 ± 33.3 ms vs 1035 ± 39.2 ms, $p = 0.09$), see Fig. 4. In the validation cohort, the mean uncorrected myocardial T1 was 1005 ± 38.6 ms for males and 1040 ± 37.0 ms for females ($p < 0.001$). The difference in mean myocardial T1 between males and females was reduced, but remained significant following blood correction, albeit by a small magnitude (1015 ± 40 ms vs 1028 ± 37.6 ms, $p = 0.02$), see Fig. 5. The range in myocardial T1 values in the derivation cohort decreased with 25% following blood correction (908–1183 ms vs 941–1146 ms).

Myocardial blood correction in healthy volunteers

The SD of uncorrected myocardial T1 measurements of the healthy volunteers was 37.5 ms. The blood correction model for mean R1 and mean R1* did not decrease the SD (36.7 ms, $p = 0.85$). The mean uncorrected myocardial T1 in the healthy volunteers was 1012 ± 30.4 ms for males and 1042 ± 38.0 ms for females ($p < 0.001$). The difference in mean myocardial T1 between males

Table 2 Baseline characteristics of the females in the derivation and validation cohorts

Characteristic, females ($n = 200$)	Derivation cohort ($n = 100$)[a]	Validation cohort ($n = 100$)[a]	p-value
Age (years)	52 ± 18	49 ± 17	0.21
Female sex, n (%)	100 (100%)	100 (100%)	1.0
Height (cm)	165 ± 8	167 ± 7	0.17
Weight (kg)	69 ± 14	70 ± 16	0.89
BSA (m^2)	1.8 ± 0.2	1.8 ± 0.2	0.77
LVEDV (ml)	157 ± 52	159 ± 49	0.48
LVEDVI (ml/m^2)	89 ± 28	89 ± 26	0.47
LVESV (ml)	91 ± 57	88 ± 57	0.81
LVESVI (ml/m^2)	47 ± 28	46 ± 29	0.95
LVSV (ml)	78 ± 21	83 ± 20	0.65
LVSVI (ml/m^2)	45 ± 11	47 ± 11	0.16
LVEF (%)	53 ± 12	54 ± 11	0.44
LVM (g)	110 ± 26	112 ± 42	0.41
LVMI (g/m^2)	62 ± 14	64 ± 22	0.49
ECV (%)	29 ± 4	29 ± 3	0.72
Hematocrit (%)	38 ± 4	38 ± 5	0.93
Septal wall thickness (mm)	9 ± 2	9 ± 3	0.45
Myocardial T1 (ms)	1046 ± 41	1040 ± 37	0.29
Mean blood R1 (ms^{-1})	0.00062 ± 0.00003	0.00062 ± 0.00003	0.58
Mean blood R1* (ms^{-1})	0.00059 ± 0.00004	0.00054 ± 0.00005	0.95

Characteristics are given as means ± standard deviations, or percentages as appropriate. p-values refer to comparison of mean values of derivation and validation cohort. [a]Data missing for LV volumes, EF and mass ($n = 2$), and ECV ($n = 4$) in the derivation cohort. Data missing for ECV ($n = 2$) in the validation cohort

Table 3 Baseline characteristics of the males in the derivation and validation cohorts

Characteristic, males ($n = 200$)	Derivation cohort ($n = 100$)	Validation cohort ($n = 100$)	p-value
Age (years)	49 ± 18	47 ± 18	0.40
Female sex, n (%)	0 (0%)	0 (0%)	1.0
Height (cm)	181 ± 14	180 ± 8	0.81
Weight (kg)	86 ± 14	85 ± 16	0.84
BSA (m^2)	2.0 ± 0.3	2.1 ± 0.2	0.77
LVEDV (ml)	204 ± 64	207 ± 68	0.67
LVEDVI (ml/m^2)	99 ± 29	100 ± 36	0.96
LVESV (ml)	103 ± 62	101 ± 64	0.71
LVESVI (ml/m^2)	50 ± 29	49 ± 34	0.56
LVSV (ml)	99 ± 27	106 ± 24	0.047*
LVSVI (ml/m^2)	49 ± 16	52 ± 11	0.02*
LVEF (%)	51 ± 12	54 ± 11	0.06
LVM (g)	166 ± 45	162 ± 51	1.0
LVMI (g/m^2)	80 ± 20	80 ± 21	0.78
ECV (%)	27 ± 3	27 ± 4	0.60
Hematocrit (%)	42 ± 4	43 ± 4	0.41
Septal wall thickness (mm)	11 ± 2	11 ± 2	0.58
Myocardial T1 (ms)	1015 ± 39	1005 ± 46	0.10
Mean blood R1 (ms^{-1})	0.00066 ± 0.00004	0.00066 ± 0.00003	0.57
Mean blood R1* (ms^{-1})	0.00063 ± 0.00004	0.00063 ± 0.00004	0.98

Characteristics are given as mean ± standard deviations, or percentages as appropriate. p-values refer to comparison of derivation and validation cohort. *marks significant results

and females was eliminated by blood correction in the healthy volunteers (1012 ± 33.7 ms vs 1023 ± 39.0 ms, $p = 0.20$).

Differences in native myocardial T1

To ascertain if the partial-volume effect or hematocrit range contributed to the differences in native myocardial T1, the patients with the highest and lowest quartiles of wall thickness and hematocrit were examined in the derivation and validation cohorts, respectively. Patients with the thickest (>11.4 mm) and thinnest (<8.4 mm) myocardium had no difference in native myocardial T1 in the derivation cohort (1036 ± 44 ms vs 1028 ± 39 ms, $p = 0.30$). In the validation cohort, there was no difference in native myocardial T1 between patients with the thickest (>11.1 mm) and thinnest (<8.5 mm) myocardium (1026 ± 46 ms vs 1023 ± 38 ms, $p = 0.76$).

Table 4 Correlations and multivariate linear regression coefficients

Characteristic	Univariate r	Multivariate beta	Multivariate beta, final model	Global R^2
Derivation cohort (n = 200)				0.26 ($p < 0.001$)
Hematocrit (%)	−0.37 ($p < 0.001$)	0.00 ($p = 0.98$)		
Mean blood R1 (ms^{-1})	−0.45 ($p < 0.001$)	−0.28 ($p = 0.003$)	−0.28 ($p = 0.001$)	
Mean blood R1* (ms^{-1})	−0.45 ($p < 0.001$)	−0.28 ($p = 0.002$)	−0.28 ($p = 0.001$)	
Septal wall thickness (mm)	0.07 ($p = 0.33$)	-	-	
Validation cohort ($n = 200$)				
Hematocrit (%)	−0.39 ($p < 0.001$)			
Mean blood R1 (ms^{-1})	−0.49 ($p < 0.001$)			
Mean blood R1* (ms^{-1})	−0.44 ($p < 0.001$)			
Septal wall thickness (mm)	0.07 ($p = 0.32$)	-	-	

All blood measurements correlated with myocardial T1, however hematocrit was not significant in multivariate regression analysis, and therefore not included in the final model.

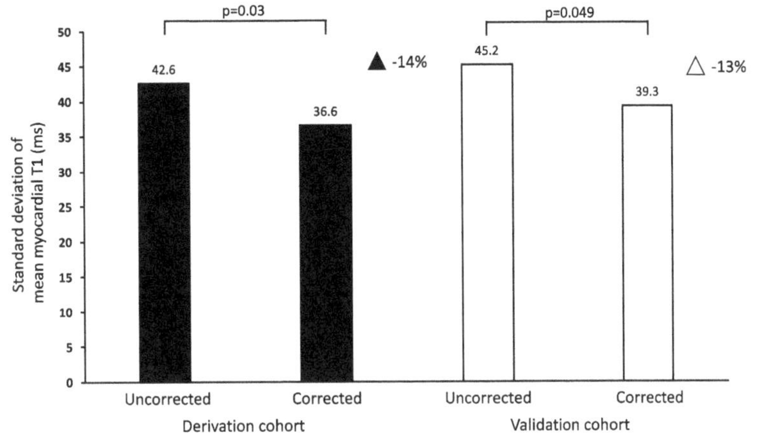

Fig. 3 Standard deviation of corrected and uncorrected myocardial T1. The figure shows the SD of mean myocardial T1 in ms for uncorrected and blood corrected measurements, in the derivation cohort (black) and the validation cohort (white). The triangles denote reduction in variability in percent. *P*-values denote F-test

Patients with the highest (>43%) and lowest (<37%) hematocrit, differed significantly in myocardial T1 in the derivation cohort (1017 ± 44 ms vs 1054 ± 43 ms, $p < 0.001$). There was also a difference in myocardial T1 in the validation cohort, between patients with the highest (>44%) and lowest (<37%) hematocrit (993 ± 41 ms vs 1046 ± 30 ms, $p < 0.001$). These differences disappeared following blood correction, in both the derivation cohort (1033 ± 36 ms vs 1034 ± 36 ms, $p = 0.87$) and in the validation cohort (1012 ± 43 ms vs 1020 ± 31 ms, $p = 0.35$).

The reduction in SD allows for detection of differences with a smaller population in research studies. A reduction of 13% in SD reduces the sample size for identifying a 50 ms difference in myocardial T1 from 26 patients to 20 patients (23% reduction in sample size).

Discussion

We have demonstrated that correcting for blood characteristics decreases the variability of native myocardial T1 in a clinical population, and reduces gender differences in healthy volunteers. Blood correction was achieved by

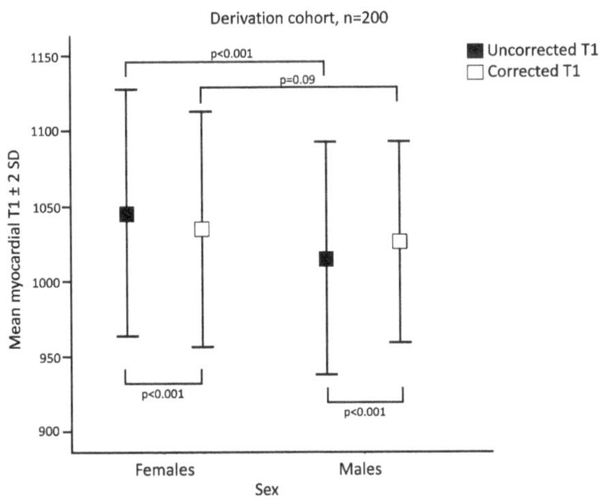

Fig. 4 Mean myocardial T1 values for females compared to males, derivation cohort. The figure displays the mean ± 95% limits of agreement for females and males, prior to correction (black) and after blood correction (white). The mean myocardial T1 values differed between the sexes prior to blood correction, but the differences were eliminated after correction. *P*-values denote paired and unpaired *t*-test as appropriate

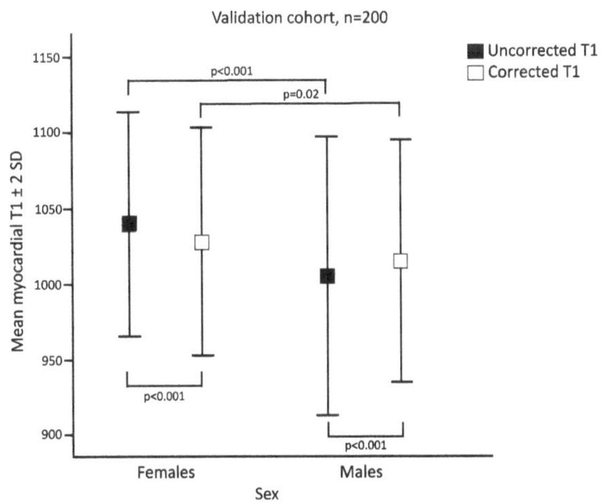

Fig. 5 Mean myocardial T1 values for females compared to males, validation cohort. The figure displays the mean ± 95% limits of agreement for females and males, prior to correction (black) and after blood correction (white). The mean myocardial T1 values differed significantly prior to blood correction, and the differences were reduced, however not eliminated following correction. *P*-values denote paired and unpaired *t*-test as appropriate

using the average of LV and RV blood (mean blood R1 and mean blood R1*), resulting in a 13% reduction in variability for native myocardial T1 measurements in the validation cohort. Correction for hematocrit did not provide an incremental reduction in SD beyond image-based blood characteristics. The use of the LV and RV blood highlights the feasibility of implementing an automatic blood pool mask [27], in order for inline reconstruction of a blood corrected T1 map.

Importance of blood correction

There are several physiological factors that influence the variation of blood T1 values, such as hematocrit [18], sex [10], age [19] and oxygen pressure [18, 20]. Also, technical aspects such as CMR magnetic field strength [12, 28, 29], off-resonance effects [30], and adiabatic inversion pulse imperfections [31] affect T1 values. Currently there is no reference standard for measuring myocardial T1 in vivo [32], and the extent of the effect of blood T1 on myocardial T1 is unknown. Furthermore, myocardial T1 values have been found to differ over the cardiac cycle, and this can be attributed to myocardial contraction compressing the vasculature [33] with reduced native myocardial T1 values during systole due to less blood (with longer T1) present in the myocardium [12]. Systolic readout has been proposed to reduce myocardial T1 variability by reducing partial volume effects since the myocardium is thicker in systole, and could theoretically include less intramyocardial blood [22, 34, 35]. Notably, in our data myocardial T1 values did not vary with end-diastolic myocardial thickness, but did vary with hematocrit. This suggests that measuring the native myocardial T1 values in a conservatively placed ROI in the mid-mural third of the septum in a clinical population reduces contamination from the blood pool. However, the results are surprising, considering that hematocrit did not independently contribute to native myocardial T1 values in the multivariate regression analysis. Hematocrit is not the only factor contributing to blood T1, and therefore the T1 of the blood is a better correction measure to use for native myocardial T1. Previous studies have assumed linear relationships between myocardial T1 values and blood T1 [22, 36]. In this study, we chose to correct for blood R1 and R1*. R1 is linearly related to the concentration of differing T1 species such as a contrast agent or blood, as opposed to T1. However, there could potentially be other relationships between native myocardial T1 values and other correction factors. This highlights the complexity of T1 mapping, but also stresses the importance of post-processing methods to increase precision and enhance clinical diagnostic use. To make the blood correction method clinically applicable we chose to correct for hematocrit, as this is determined prior to imaging in our clinical routine, for the purpose of performing extracellular volume fraction (ECV) mapping. Other parameters that could have been considered are ferritin or hepcidin. However, this was not performed in the current study. Furthermore, the blood in the RV is less oxygenated than in the LV, and therefore more paramagnetic than in the LV [18]. As the LV myocardium is directly perfused by the coronary arteries from the aorta, the use of mean blood T1 and T1* could potentially degrade the blood correction model. However, mean T1 and T1* values were chosen in order to make blood correction feasible by implementing an automatic (LV and RV) blood pool mask [27] for inline reconstruction of a blood corrected T1 map.

Furthermore, Reiter et al. [22] showed that sex differences in normal T1 values can be eliminated by blood correction. We also showed that sex differences were eliminated by blood correction in the derivation cohort, and in healthy volunteers. However, the sex differences in the validation cohort were reduced, but not eliminated following blood correction. This could be due to different distributions of physiological factors in different populations such as age, hematocrit, and oxygen pressure, as the means of these factors did not differ between the males or females in the validation and derivation cohorts in this study. This shows that blood correction provides improved precision in native myocardial T1, but not to the extent that it completely eliminates sex differences in clinical patients, even though the remaining difference had a very small magnitude. Further studies may be of value to better understand these mechanisms.

MOLLI sequences and myocardial T1 variability

Several different methods to quantitatively measure T1 relaxation times are currently in clinical use [37]. The original MOLLI pulse sequence with acquisition over 17 successive heart beats has become a commonly used T1 mapping method [1]. The original MOLLI sequence has high precision, however the accuracy declines with longer T1 values, and is particularly susceptible to higher heart rates [38]. Variations of MOLLI have been purposed to reduce breath-hold duration, and reduce heart rate sensitivity such as the 5(3s)3 [30, 39] scheme. The 5(3s)3 protocol has high precision, but somewhat limited accuracy for shorter T1 values [38]. The Shortened MOLLI (ShMOLLI) scheme consists of sequential inversion-recovery acquisitions of nine successive heart beats [29] and uses a conditional fitting algorithm to account for the short recovery period between inversion pulses. The conditional fitting discards data, sacrificing precision without improving accuracy [38]. T1 mapping can also be performed with saturation recovery single-shot acquisition (SASHA) [40] which mitigates the underestimation of T1 values by MOLLI, however with a reduced precision [38]. SASHA was modified to mitigate heart rate dependency with saturation pulse prepared heart-rate-independent inversion recovery (SAPPHIRE) [41], however, this approach still has a lower precision in measuring myocardial T1 compared to MOLLI [42]. The myocardial T1 values in the patients in our study were 1023 ± 42.6 ms and 1030 ± 45.2 ms, which closely corresponds to the myocardial T1 found in the healthy volunteers in our study (1027 ± 37 ms), both acquired using a MOLLI sequence. However, this is longer and more variable than 962 ± 25 ms in healthy volunteers imaged with ShMOLLI [10]. The mean differences in T1 are related to the inherent differences between the sequences, and the differences in variability are likely related to differences in ROI placement strategy. Furthermore, the blood correction model did not decrease myocardial T1 variability in healthy volunteers, however it did eliminate gender differences. This is probably due to fact that healthy volunteers have a greater homogeneity in myocardial T1 values, but also blood T1 values. It is possible that the resultant blood correction reduction, even in a study powered to reduce variability in healthy volunteers, would be so small that it's not clinically relevant. Therefore, the necessary study design to illustrate the clinical performance of blood correction in native T1 mapping is to study patients with variable T1 in both blood and myocardium.

Furthermore, T1 values differ over CMR magnetic field strength, both for blood and myocardium. Blood correction assuming linear correlation has been performed successfully at 3 T, however the changes in variability following blood correction were not evaluated [36]. Therefore, blood correction is feasible for 3 T as well, however the optimal correction model would have to be evaluated in dedicated clinical cohorts and healthy volunteers.

Clinical implications

The proposed validated blood correction method might have clinical significance for diseases that are characterized by a change in native myocardial T1 values, such as amyloidosis, iron-overload cardiomyopathy, Anderson-Fabry disease and other non-ischemic heart diseases. With increased diagnostic precision, these diseases could potentially be identified earlier when only subtle differences in the myocardial T1 may be present. The range of myocardial T1 values was decreased by 25% in the derivation cohort. This suggests that blood correction helps in determining the true biological variability in myocardial T1 values, making it easier to differentiate pathological myocardial T1 values from normal myocardial T1 values. Native T1 mapping has shown diagnostic promise in amyloidosis [5, 43], as native myocardial T1 increases with amyloid deposition and inflammation [44]. Amyloidosis can be apparent in late gadolinium enhancement (LGE) images, but the patterns are often diffuse and globally distributed [45]. This can pose a challenge when selecting the inversion time for LGE imaging, since normal myocardium may be absent. However, native T1 mapping is not dependent upon normal myocardium for determining normality, and can therefore provide a useful imaging method in amyloidosis. Furthermore, native myocardial T1 mapping has been shown to be an independent predictor of survival in amyloidosis [46]. By correcting for myocardial blood content, the differences between normal and diseased myocardium might increase and allow for earlier clinical detection of disease.

Anderson-Fabry is a disease with accumulation of glycosphingolipids within lysosomes, causing progressive fibrosis in certain tissues [47]. Native T1 mapping has shown promising results for identifying these patients since native myocardial T1 decreases, and might be used as a surrogate measure for the disease [7]. With less variability in native myocardial T1 values following blood correction, diagnostic precision increases. Therefore, the diagnostic accuracy provided by native T1 mapping of cardiac involvement by Anderson-Fabry disease may improve.

Furthermore, differences in myocardial T1 values at RV insertion points between patients with and without pulmonary hypertension (PH) were highlighted by blood correction [36], suggesting that blood correction can increase diagnostic precision for diseases with more subtle changes in native myocardial T1.

Limitations

This study included patients with known or suspected heart disease to develop and validate a blood correction method. Patients were used in order to yield the clinical ranges of myocardial and blood T1 values necessary for determining meaningful correlations. As patients were used, this also sometimes resulted in changes in the MOLLI acquisition parameters with varying FoV size and phase encoding lines, which can influence the accuracy of the T1 measurement. However, the strategy used underscores that the resulting blood correction model is valid for clinical use, since adjusting image acquisition parameters is a part of the clinical routine. Furthermore, only septal myocardial T1 values were acquired, and not all segments according to American Heart Association (AHA) segmentation scheme, which has been used in other studies [36, 48]. Notably, it is not known how the blood correction model in this study affects the rest of the myocardium. However, Reiter et al. [22] studied all segments of the left ventricle and identified negligible differences in myocardial T1 throughout the left ventricle. This suggests that the same blood correction could be applied for the entire left ventricular myocardium.

Conclusions

Blood correction improves the precision of native myocardial T1 measurement by 13% and reduces gender differences. Image-based correction of native myocardial T1 values for R1 and R1* of blood is valid for clinical use and may improve disease detection in the clinical evaluation of native myocardial T1, and reduce sample size needs for clinical research.

Abbreviations

AHA: American Heart Association; BSA: Body surface area; bSSFP: Balance steady state free precession; CMR: Cardiovascular magnetic resonance; ECV: Extracellular volume fraction; EDV: End diastolic volume; EF: Ejection fraction; ESV: End systolic volume; FoV: Field of view; LGE: Late gadolinium enhancement; LV: Left ventricle; LVM: Left ventricular mass; MBV: Myocardial blood volume; MOLLI: Modified Look-Locker inversion recovery; PAT: Parallel acquisition technique; ROI: Region of interest; RV: Right ventricle; SD: Standard deviation; SV: Stroke volume; TE: Echo time; TR: Repetition time

Acknowledgements

We would like the acknowledge Jenny Rasck, technologist, and Karin Loiske, technologist, PhD, Karolinska University Hospital Solna, for their help with patient image acquisition.

Funding

The research was funded in part by the Swedish Research Council, Swedish Heart and Lung Foundation, the Stockholm County Council and Karolinska Institutet. Karolinska University Hospital has a research and development agreement regarding CMR with Siemens.

Authors' contributions

JN participated in the design of the study, performed all image, data and statistical analysis, contributed to the interpretation of data and drafted the manuscript. ML participated in the interpretation of data and revised the manuscript. GA and PS were in charge of image acquisition and revised the manuscript. SR performed all image and data acquisition of the healthy volunteers. JM, PK, AS participated in the study design, the interpretation of data and revised the manuscript. MU conceived the study, participated in its design and interpretation of data, and helped to draft the manuscript. All authors read and approved the final manuscript.

Competing interests

The authors declare that they have no competing interests.

Author details

[1]Department of Clinical Physiology, Karolinska Institutet and Karolinska University Hospital, Stockholm, Sweden. [2]Department of Medicine, Unit of Cardiology, Karolinska Institutet and Karolinska University Hospital, Stockholm, Sweden. [3]Institute of Cardiovascular Science, University College London, London, UK. [4]National Heart, Lung, and Blood Institute, National Institutes of Health, Bethesda, MD, USA.

References

1. Messroghli DR, Radjenovic A, Kozerke S, Higgins DM, Sivananthan MU, Ridgway JP. Modified Look-Locker inversion recovery (MOLLI) for high-resolution T1 mapping of the heart. Magn Reson Med. 2004;52(1):141–6.
2. Dall'Armellina E, Piechnik SK, Ferreira VM, Si QL, Robson MD, Francis JM, et al. Cardiovascular magnetic resonance by non contrast T1-mapping allows assessment of severity of injury in acute myocardial infarction. J Cardiovasc Magn Reson. 2012;14:15.
3. Ferreira VM, Piechnik SK, Dall'Armellina E, Karamitsos TD, Francis JM, Ntusi N, et al. T(1) mapping for the diagnosis of acute myocarditis using CMR: comparison to T2-weighted and late gadolinium enhanced imaging. JACC Cardiovasc Imaging. 2013;6(10):1048–58.
4. Ferreira VM, Piechnik SK, Dall'Armellina E, Karamitsos TD, Francis JM, Ntusi N, et al. Native T1-mapping detects the location, extent and patterns of acute myocarditis without the need for gadolinium contrast agents. J Cardiovasc Magn Reson. 2014;16:36.
5. Karamitsos TD, Piechnik SK, Banypersad SM, Fontana M, Ntusi NB, Ferreira VM, et al. Noncontrast T1 mapping for the diagnosis of cardiac amyloidosis. JACC Cardiovasc Imaging. 2013;6(4):488–97.
6. Ferreira VM, Piechnik SK, Dall'Armellina E, Karamitsos TD, Francis JM, Choudhury RP, et al. Non-contrast T1-mapping detects acute myocardial edema with high diagnostic accuracy: a comparison to T2-weighted cardiovascular magnetic resonance. J Cardiovasc Magn Reson. 2012;14:42.
7. Sado DM, White SK, Piechnik SK, Banypersad SM, Treibel T, Captur G, et al. Identification and assessment of Anderson-Fabry disease by cardiovascular magnetic resonance noncontrast myocardial T1 mapping. Circ Cardiovasc Imaging. 2013;6(3):392–8.
8. Amano Y, Takayama M, Kumita S. Contrast-enhanced myocardial T1-weighted scout (Look-Locker) imaging for the detection of myocardial damages in hypertrophic cardiomyopathy. J Magn Reson Imaging. 2009; 30(4):778–84.
9. Mahmod M, Piechnik SK, Levelt E, Ferreira VM, Francis JM, Lewis A, et al. Adenosine stress native T1 mapping in severe aortic stenosis: evidence for a role of the intravascular compartment on myocardial T1 values. J Cardiovasc Magn Reson. 2014;16:92.
10. Piechnik SK, Ferreira VM, Lewandowski AJ, Ntusi NA, Banerjee R, Holloway C, et al. Normal variation of magnetic resonance T1 relaxation times in the human population at 1.5 T using ShMOLLI. J Cardiovasc Magn Reson. 2013;15:13.
11. Messroghli DR, Walters K, Plein S, Sparrow P, Friedrich MG, Ridgway JP, et al. Myocardial T1 mapping: application to patients with acute and chronic myocardial infarction. Magn Reson Med. 2007;58(1):34–40.
12. Kawel N, Nacif M, Zavodni A, Jones J, Liu S, Sibley CT, et al. T1 mapping of the myocardium: intra-individual assessment of the effect of field strength, cardiac cycle and variation by myocardial region. J Cardiovasc Magn Reson. 2012;14:27.
13. Morgenstern C, Holjes U, Arnold G, Lochner W. The influence of coronary pressure and coronary flow on intracoronary blood volume and geometry of the left ventricle. Pflugers Arch. 1973;340(2):101–11.
14. McCommis KS, Goldstein TA, Zhang H, Misselwitz B, Gropler RJ, Zheng J. Quantification of myocardial blood volume during dipyridamole and doubtamine stress: a perfusion CMR study. J Cardiovasc Magn Reson. 2007;9(5):785–92.
15. Tohka J. Partial volume effect modeling for segmentation and tissue classification of brain magnetic resonance images: A review. World J Radiol. 2014;6(11):855–64.
16. Lu H, Clingman C, Golay X, van Zijl PC. Determining the longitudinal relaxation time (T1) of blood at 3.0 Tesla. Magn Reson Med. 2004;52(3): 679–82.
17. Fullerton GD, Potter JL, Dornbluth NC. NMR relaxation of protons in tissues and other macromolecular water solutions. Magn Reson Imaging. 1982;1(4):209–26.
18. Silvennoinen MJ, Kettunen MI, Kauppinen RA. Effects of hematocrit and oxygen saturation level on blood spin-lattice relaxation. Magn Reson Med. 2003;49(3):568–71.
19. Varela M, Hajnal JV, Petersen ET, Golay X, Merchant N, Larkman DJ. A method for rapid in vivo measurement of blood T1. NMR Biomed. 2011; 24(1):80–8.
20. Tadamura E, Hatabu H, Li W, Prasad PV, Edelman RR. Effect of oxygen inhalation on relaxation times in various tissues. J Magn Reson Imaging. 1997;7(1):220–5.
21. Wansapura J, Gottliebson W, Crotty E, Fleck R. Cyclic variation of T1 in the myocardium at 3 T. Magn Reson Imaging. 2006;24(7):889–93.
22. Reiter U, Reiter G, Dorr K, Greiser A, Maderthaner R, Fuchsjager M. Normal Diastolic and Systolic Myocardial T1 Values at 1.5-T MR Imaging: Correlations and Blood Normalization. Radiology. 2013;131225.
23. Hill VL, Simpson VZ, Higgins JM, Hu Z, Stevens RA, Metcalf JA, et al. Evaluation of the Performance of the Sysmex XT-2000i Hematology Analyzer With Whole Bloods Stored at Room Temperature. Lab Med. 2009;40(12):709–18.
24. Xue H, Greiser A, Zuehlsdorff S, Jolly MP, Guehring J, Arai AE, et al. Phase-sensitive inversion recovery for myocardial T1 mapping with motion correction and parametric fitting. Magn Reson Med. 2013;69(5):1408–20.
25. Xue H, Shah S, Greiser A, Guetter C, Littmann A, Jolly MP, et al. Motion correction for myocardial T1 mapping using image registration with synthetic image estimation. Magn Reson Med. 2012;67(6):1644–55.
26. Du Bois D, Du Bois EF. A formula to estimate the approximate surface area if height and weight be known. 1916. Nutrition. 1989;5(5):303–11. discussion 12–3.

27. Kellman P, Wilson JR, Xue H, Ugander M, Arai AE. Extracellular volume fraction mapping in the myocardium, part 1: evaluation of an automated method. J Cardiovasc Magn Reson. 2012;14:63.
28. Lee JJ, Liu S, Nacif MS, Ugander M, Han J, Kawel N, et al. Myocardial T1 and extracellular volume fraction mapping at 3 tesla. J Cardiovasc Magn Reson. 2011;13:75.
29. Piechnik SK, Ferreira VM, Dall'Armellina E, Cochlin LE, Greiser A, Neubauer S, et al. Shortened Modified Look-Locker Inversion recovery (ShMOLLI) for clinical myocardial T1-mapping at 1.5 and 3 T within a 9 heartbeat breathhold. J Cardiovasc Magn Reson. 2010;12:69.
30. Kellman P, Herzka DA, Arai AE, Hansen MS. Influence of Off-resonance in myocardial T1-mapping using SSFP based MOLLI method. J Cardiovasc Magn Reson. 2013;15:63.
31. Kellman P, Herzka DA, Hansen MS. Adiabatic inversion pulses for myocardial T1 mapping. Magn Reson Med. 2014;71(4):1428–34.
32. Moon JC, Messroghli DR, Kellman P, Piechnik SK, Robson MD, Ugander M, et al. Myocardial T1 mapping and extracellular volume quantification: a Society for Cardiovascular Magnetic Resonance (SCMR) and CMR Working Group of the European Society of Cardiology consensus statement. J Cardiovasc Magn Reson. 2013;15(1):92.
33. Gregg DE, Sabiston Jr DC. Effect of cardiac contraction on coronary blood flow. Circulation. 1957;15(1):14–20.
34. Ferreira VM, Wijesurendra RS, Liu A, Greiser A, Casadei B, Robson MD, et al. Systolic ShMOLLI myocardial T1-mapping for improved robustness to partial-volume effects and applications in tachyarrhythmias. J Cardiovasc Magn Reson. 2015;17:77.
35. Tessa C, Diciotti S, Landini N, Lilli A, Del Meglio J, Salvatori L, et al. Myocardial T1 and T2 mapping in diastolic and systolic phase. Int J Cardiovasc Imaging. 2015;31(5):1001–10.
36. Reiter U, Reiter G, Kovacs G, Adelsmayr G, Greiser A, Olschewski H, et al. Native myocardial T1 mapping in pulmonary hypertension: correlations with cardiac function and hemodynamics. Eur Radiol. 2017;27(1):157–66.
37. Haaf P, Garg P, Messroghli DR, Broadbent DA, Greenwood JP, Plein S. Cardiac T1 Mapping and Extracellular Volume (ECV) in clinical practice: a comprehensive review. J Cardiovasc Magn Reson. 2016;18(1):89.
38. Kellman P, Hansen MS. T1-mapping in the heart: accuracy and precision. J Cardiovasc Magn Reson. 2014;16:2.
39. Kellman P, Arai AE, Xue H. T1 and extracellular volume mapping in the heart: estimation of error maps and the influence of noise on precision. J Cardiovasc Magn Reson. 2013;15:56.
40. Chow K, Flewitt JA, Green JD, Pagano JJ, Friedrich MG, Thompson RB. Saturation recovery single-shot acquisition (SASHA) for myocardial T(1) mapping. Magn Reson Med. 2014;71(6):2082–95.
41. Weingartner S, Akcakaya M, Basha T, Kissinger KV, Goddu B, Berg S, et al. Combined saturation/inversion recovery sequences for improved evaluation of scar and diffuse fibrosis in patients with arrhythmia or heart rate variability. Magn Reson Med. 2014;71(3):1024–34.
42. Roujol S, Weingartner S, Foppa M, Chow K, Kawaji K, Ngo LH, et al. Accuracy, precision, and reproducibility of four T1 mapping sequences: a head-to-head comparison of MOLLI, ShMOLLI, SASHA, and SAPPHIRE. Radiology. 2014;272(3):683–9.
43. Fontana M, Banypersad SM, Treibel TA, Maestrini V, Sado DM, White SK, et al. Native T1 mapping in transthyretin amyloidosis. JACC Cardiovasc Imaging. 2014;7(2):157–65.
44. Robbers LF, Baars EN, Brouwer WP, Beek AM, Hofman MB, Niessen HW, et al. T1 mapping shows increased extracellular matrix size in the myocardium due to amyloid depositions. Circ Cardiovasc Imaging. 2012;5(3):423–6.
45. White JA, Kim HW, Shah D, Fine N, Kim KY, Wendell DC, et al. CMR imaging with rapid visual T1 assessment predicts mortality in patients suspected of cardiac amyloidosis. JACC Cardiovasc Imaging. 2014;7(2):143–56.
46. Banypersad SM, Fontana M, Maestrini V, Sado DM, Captur G, Petrie A, et al. T1 mapping and survival in systemic light-chain amyloidosis. Eur Heart J. 2015;36(4):244–51.
47. O'Mahony C, Elliott P. Anderson-Fabry disease and the heart. Prog Cardiovasc Dis. 2010;52(4):326–35.
48. Liu A, Wijesurendra RS, Francis JM, Robson MD, Neubauer S, Piechnik SK, et al. Adenosine Stress and Rest T1 Mapping Can Differentiate Between Ischemic, Infarcted, Remote, and Normal Myocardium Without the Need for Gadolinium Contrast Agents. JACC Cardiovasc Imaging. 2016;9(1):27–36.

8

Myocardial perfusion cardiovascular magnetic resonance: optimized dual sequence and reconstruction for quantification

Peter Kellman[1*], Michael S. Hansen[1], Sonia Nielles-Vallespin[1], Jannike Nickander[2], Raquel Themudo[2], Martin Ugander[2] and Hui Xue[1]

Abstract

Background: Quantification of myocardial blood flow requires knowledge of the amount of contrast agent in the myocardial tissue and the arterial input function (AIF) driving the delivery of this contrast agent. Accurate quantification is challenged by the lack of linearity between the measured signal and contrast agent concentration. This work characterizes sources of non-linearity and presents a systematic approach to accurate measurements of contrast agent concentration in both blood and myocardium.

Methods: A dual sequence approach with separate pulse sequences for AIF and myocardial tissue allowed separate optimization of parameters for blood and myocardium. A systems approach to the overall design was taken to achieve linearity between signal and contrast agent concentration. Conversion of signal intensity values to contrast agent concentration was achieved through a combination of surface coil sensitivity correction, Bloch simulation based look-up table correction, and in the case of the AIF measurement, correction of T2* losses. Validation of signal correction was performed in phantoms, and values for peak AIF concentration and myocardial flow are provided for 29 normal subjects for rest and adenosine stress.

Results: For phantoms, the measured fits were within 5% for both AIF and myocardium. In healthy volunteers the peak [Gd] was 3.5 ± 1.2 for stress and 4.4 ± 1.2 mmol/L for rest. The T2* in the left ventricle blood pool at peak AIF was approximately 10 ms. The peak-to-valley ratio was 5.6 for the raw signal intensities without correction, and was 8.3 for the look-up-table (LUT) corrected AIF which represents approximately 48% correction. Without T2* correction the myocardial blood flow estimates are overestimated by approximately 10%. The signal-to-noise ratio of the myocardial signal at peak enhancement (1.5 T) was 17.7 ± 6.6 at stress and the peak [Gd] was 0.49 ± 0.15 mmol/L. The estimated perfusion flow was 3.9 ± 0.38 and 1.03 ± 0.19 ml/min/g using the BTEX model and 3.4 ± 0.39 and 0.95 ± 0.16 using a Fermi model, for stress and rest, respectively.

Conclusions: A dual sequence for myocardial perfusion cardiovascular magnetic resonance and AIF measurement has been optimized for quantification of myocardial blood flow. A validation in phantoms was performed to confirm that the signal conversion to gadolinium concentration was linear. The proposed sequence was integrated with a fully automatic in-line solution for pixel-wise mapping of myocardial blood flow and evaluated in adenosine stress and rest studies on $N = 29$ normal healthy subjects. Reliable perfusion mapping was demonstrated and produced estimates with low variability.

Keywords: Myocardial perfusion, Flow, Perfusion quantification, Arterial input function, Gadolinium

* Correspondence: kellman@nih.gov
[1]National Heart, Lung, and Blood Institute, National Institutes of Health, DHHS, 10 Center Drive MSC-1061, Bethesda, MD 20892, USA
Full list of author information is available at the end of the article

Background

Myocardial perfusion can be evaluated with dynamic cardiovascular magnetic resonance (CMR) during the passage of a bolus of contrast agent. Most commonly, perfusion CMR is evaluated qualitatively, but objective quantitative evaluation would be more desirable. The potential benefits of quantification are: objective assessment, simpler and faster analysis, and the ability to detect disease with a global reduction in flow such as multi-vessel obstructive disease or microvascular disease. Quantification of myocardial blood flow using CMR was first proposed over 20 years ago [1, 2], yet qualitative interpretation of images remains the primary means available to clinicians. The desired output of a quantitative perfusion study is a map of myocardial blood flow in units of ml/g/min.

Quantification requires knowledge of the amount of contrast agent in the myocardial tissue and the arterial input function (AIF) driving the delivery of this contrast agent. Accurate quantification is challenged by the lack of linearity between the measured signal and contrast agent concentration. Ideally these measurements would consist of input and response curves in units of contrast agent concentration. Current, commercially available, myocardial perfusion sequences have not been optimized to yield accurate concentration curves and the observed signal intensity curves are not linearly related to the concentrations of contrast agent, i.e., there is a non-linear relationship between signal intensity and contrast agent concentration, which leads to quantification biases.

The main sources of non-linearity and bias are: spatial signal variations caused by the sensitivity profiles of the surface coils, imperfect saturation of magnetization during contrast bolus passage, T2* decay (and signal loss) caused by high contrast agent concentrations in the blood pool, and the non-linear signal response inherent due to saturation recovery that depends on the parameters of the imaging protocol. It has been proposed that some of the non-linearity of the AIF response curve can be mitigated by imaging the AIF during a separate injection of a bolus with lower concentration (the dual bolus approach)[3], but this approach has some practical drawbacks as it requires multiple injections and acquisitions. Moreover, there are other potential bias sources with his approach, since changes in breathing, etc. between the two measurements may introduce new sources of variation. Consequently, it is desirable to acquire the AIF curve simultaneously with the tissue response curve.

A dual sequence [4] approach, which separately optimizes the imaging protocols for blood and myocardium has been proposed. This approach may be more easily incorporated into a clinical workflow. The proposed dual sequence was optimized for perfusion quantification and was evaluated using a recently developed fully automatic in-line solution for pixel-wise mapping of myocardial blood flow [5]. This work characterizes the sources of non-linearity and presents a systematic approach to accurate measurements of contrast agent concentration in both blood and tissue of interest.

Methods

Sequence

A saturation recovery (SR) sequence was used for myocardial perfusion imaging during the passage of a bolus of gadolinium based contrast agent as depicted in Fig. 1 which is illustrated for a subject with single vessel disease. Baseline images were acquired prior to bolus administration and continued through the first pass. Typically, images were acquired for 60-90 heartbeats depending on the cardiac output. Proton density (PD) weighted images were acquired at the start.

A multi-slice 2D SR dual imaging sequence is diagrammed in Fig. 2. Low resolution blood pool images used for estimating the AIF were acquired every heartbeat immediately following the R-wave trigger. Higher resolution images were acquired following the AIF and may be sampled every RR or every second RR if greater spatial coverage is desired. The sequence uses a pulse sequel for saturation [6] for each image. The image readout is single shot using parallel imaging acceleration to reduce the imaging duration. The AIF uses a FLASH readout, whereas the higher resolution myocardial images may be either b-SSFP or FLASH, selected by the user. The measurement begins with the acquisition of PD weighted images used for surface coil intensity correction and normalization of signal values. The PD images are acquired using a low flip angle FLASH readout without SR preparation to minimize artifacts of b-SSFP at low flip angle [7]. An optional chemical shift fat suppression may be used to mitigate artifacts due to the presence of fat around the heart. Fat suppression is used in this study.

Saturation efficiency is very important in quantification since the conversion of signal intensities to gadolinium concentration depends on a known signal recovery and independence of the signal from slice to slice that is achieved by resetting the magnetization to zero for each image. With high saturation efficiency it is also possible to prescribe a mixture of long and short axis views without cross-talk between slices due to the readout. The SR preparation using the 6-pulse design [6] was chosen since it had excellent saturation efficiency over a wide range of off-resonance and effective transmitter flip angle (FA) which may vary across the heart. A BIR-4 design [6] achieved excellent saturation performance with a shorter duration but was found empirically to have specific absorption rate (SAR) limitation at higher

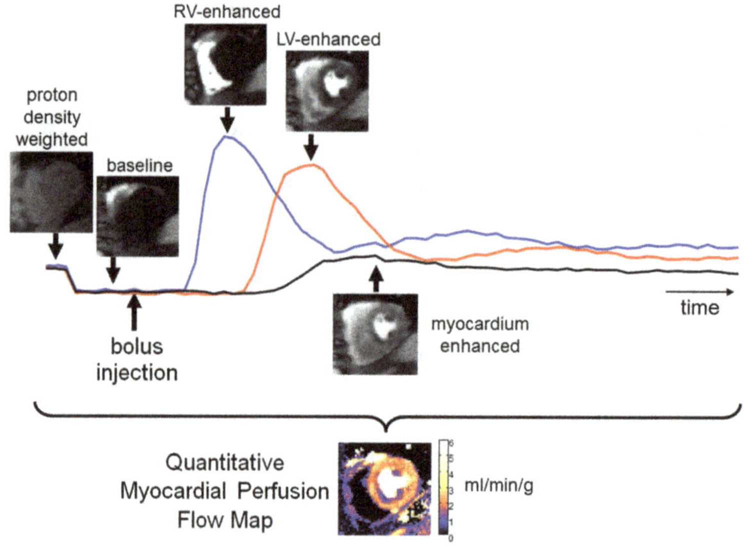

Fig. 1 Illustration of first-pass contrast enhanced myocardial perfusion imaging showing different phases of image contrast during passage of the bolus for a subject with single vessel disease. Proton density weighted images are acquired at the start of acquisition prior to administering the contrast agent bolus. The complete time series of images are automatically processed to estimate pixel-wise myocardial blood flow maps which show regions of low flow in different color than normal flow, thereby reducing the time required to analyze the raw images. The time intensity signals represent the intensities of RV blood pool (*blue*), LV blood pool (*red*), and myocardium (*black*) regions. Note that flow map values are only valid for myocardium tissue and not blood pool regions or in non-tissue

heart rates particularly at higher field strength such as 3 Tesla. The 6-pulse design consisted of non-selective RF pulses with tailored flip angles separated by gradient spoilers. The voltage of the RF pulses was maximized in order to reduce the pulse duration, and the duration was modulated to achieve the specified FAs. The pulse amplitude corresponded to approx. 27 μT at 1.5 T and was reduced to approx. 11 μT at 3 T to reduce the SAR. To ensure that the sequence would not terminate at run time due to average SAR monitor responding to actual changes in the heart rate, a post-scan acquisition delay of up to 100 s was allowed to increase the averaging interval. The performance of the SR preparation in both blood and myocardium was characterized by simulation for different gadolinium contrast concentrations. At 1.5 T, the SR preparation was 26 ms including 1 ms pre- and 4 ms post-spoiler gradients.

Signal intensities were converted to gadolinium concentration, [Gd], in order to linearize the relationship of signal and [Gd] and to be able to have a common

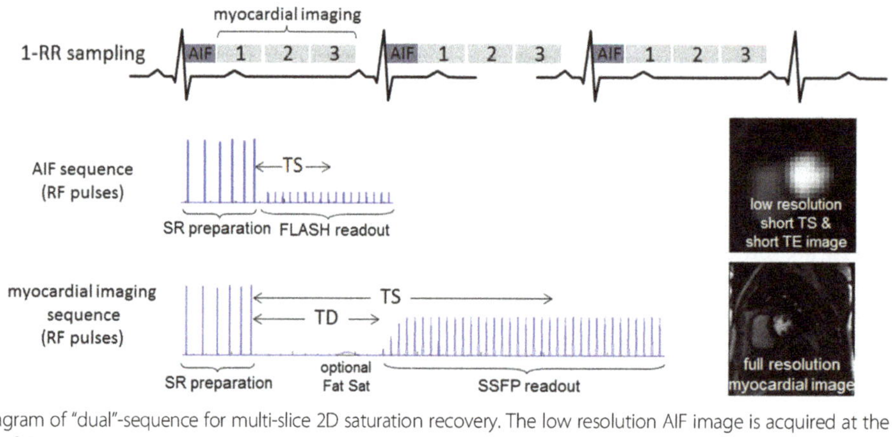

Fig. 2 Overview diagram of "dual"-sequence for multi-slice 2D saturation recovery. The low resolution AIF image is acquired at the R-wave triggered followed by multiple full resolution myocardial perfusion images. Each image has a saturation recovery RF preparation consisting of a sequence of RF pulses and gradient spoilers followed by single shot image readout. The myocardial perfusion images have an optional chemical shift fat saturation. The AIF uses a FLASH readout, whereas the full resolution myocardial images may be either b-SSFP or FLASH. The AIF is acquired for a single slice every RR interval, whereas the myocardial perfusion images may be sampled every RR or every other RR interval to increase the overall number of slices. TD and TS are the trigger delay and saturation time, respectively

scaling between the AIF and myocardial signals which are acquired using different protocols. Cernicanu, et al. [8] proposed a method for conversion of normalized signal intensities using an analytic expression for readout using a gradient recalled echo (GRE) protocol. This formulation was extended to the dual sequence using a numerical Bloch calculation [9] which permitted application to b-SSFP readout of myocardium and FLASH readout of the AIF.

Proton density weighted images were acquired at the start of the scan for both AIF and myocardial image slices using a FLASH sequence without the SR preparation. The timing of the PD images matched the SR prepared images such that the images were acquired at the same cardiac phase. The images were used to correct the surface coil variation and were used as the signal normalization for look-up table (LUT) linearization. LUT calculations assumed that the native tissue T1 for the PD is prior to contrast ($T1_0$), therefore it was important that the PD signal intensity was sufficiently independent of the actual T1 since acquisition of rest perfusion scans typically follow the stress scans after only several minutes at which time the actual T1 is not fully recovered, i.e., the actual gadolinium concentration [Gd] > 0. The dependence of PD signal amplitude versus [Gd] for myocardium and blood tissue was calculated through simulation. This led to a selection of readout FA = 5°. Note that coil sensitivity maps, used both in parallel imaging reconstruction and adaptive coil combination, consisted of the average of all time frames including PD weighted images, therefore the number of PD frames acquired was set equal to the parallel imaging acceleration factor of the myocardial imaging (in this case, $R = 3$). The first PD image was used for normalization to avoid signal loss caused by previous heartbeat images.

Arterial input function

The AIF was acquired immediately after the R-wave trigger and was selected as the most basal of the slices prescribed in the first slice group. The AIF used the 6-pulse sequel for saturation preparation as described above followed by a dual echo low FA FLASH readout. The protocol parameters are listed in Table 1. A short readout (64 point) with wide bandwidth (3900 Hz/pixel) and short duration RF pulses (250 μs, time-bandwidth product = 2.0) were used to achieve low T2* losses (TE_1 = 0.76 ms). T2* dephasing loss has been a known concern in estimating AIF and conversion to [Gd] and approaches to this problem have focused either on minimizing the loss by choosing adequately short echo time (TE) [10] or on correcting for T2* loss based on modeling the relationship between T1 and T2* [11, 12]. In this work, the dual sequence approach was modified to incorporate a 2 echo acquisition for measurement of T2* during the bolus passage. A dual echo acquisition with monopolar readout was used to acquire a second echo (TE_2 = 1.76 μs) which was used for direct estimation of T2* during the first pass. The ratio of the 2 echo signals S1/S2 = S0 exp((T2-T1)/T2*) was used to calculate the signal amplitude S0 without T2* loss. This was performed for a blood pool region signal after left ventricle (LV) blood pool segmentation.

Table 1 Protocol parameters for AIF imaging sequence at 1.5 T

	FLASH
TE	0.76 & 1.76 ms
TR	2.45 ms
FA	5°
Matrix	64×34
FOV (typical)	360x270x10 mm^3
PE order	Linear
Parallel imaging	TPAT2
TI	23.8 ms
SR prep	6-pulse (26 ms incl. spoilers)
Imaging duration	42 ms
Total duration	68.2 ms

Blood pool segmentation was performed on the motion corrected low resolution AIF image series to extract arterial input function intensities signals for both echoes. First, the AIF PD image is used to detect the noise background. Since the noise standard deviation (SD) is unity after the SNR unit reconstruction [13], a simple threshold of 3 SD's was used. For all foreground pixels as determined by the noise mask, the time intensity curves are analyzed using a scale-space based detector [14]. Pixels with top 10% upslope and AUC values are picked as the candidates for LV blood pool mask. A connected component analysis is then used to separate RV and LV pixels based on the time to peak enhancement. The final LV blood pool mask is calculated using a further erosion step which seeks to drop border pixels which are a mixture of blood and myocardial tissue.

In order to shorten the imaging duration, 2-fold acceleration was achieved using parallel imaging with temporal generalized autocalibrating partially parallel acquisitions (TGRAPPA) [15]. In order to minimize the non-linear response due to saturation at high gadolinium concentration a short saturation delay (TS) is desired, where TS is defined as the time from saturation to the k-space center. There is a tradeoff between the image signal-to-noise ratio (SNR), which is reduced at low TS, and linearity, which is improved at low TS. Early designs used a centric readout ordering to minimize TS [16, 17]. In centric ordering the saturation delay is nearly the trigger delay (TD), which may be as short as the gradient spoiler following the RF saturation (4 ms). The difficulty with centric order is 2-fold: 1) the SNR of the baseline images is too low, and 2) the k-space weighting during the saturation recovery leads to a strong high pass spatial filter that enhances the edge of the blood pool. The high pass spatial filter is problematic for accurate calculation of gadolinium concentration since the effective TS is a function of spatial frequency and will vary depending on how the blood region is segmented. For this reason, a linear acquisition ordering was chosen. Although not perfectly linear at high [Gd], it was sufficiently linear to enable LUT correction.

Using a low resolution image and parallel imaging factor 2, the k-space center was typically at $N = 9$ pulses. The sensitivity of the blood signal to in-flowing spins was estimated by comparing the signal after 9-pulses compared to the signal assuming all spins were new.

Conversion of the signal to gadolinium concentration, [Gd], was performed by LUT based on Bloch signal calculations. In this way, the LUT corrected signal was directly proportional to [Gd] and importantly was in the same units as the LUT corrected myocardial signal which was acquired with a different imaging protocol. The LUT was applied to the normalized signal SR/PD where SR and PD were the saturation recovery and proton density weighted images, respectively. It was important that the normalized signal SR/PD was not strongly dependent on the actual transmitted FA. The sensitivity of the LUT to transmit FA was calculated through simulation.

The readout of the PD image for the AIF may influence the initial magnetization of the 1st myocardial image which is at the same slice location since there is no SR preparation for the PD image. For this reason, a low PD FA is used (5°) which minimizes this effect. After 17 RF pulses (time bandwidth 2.0), the magnetization is reduced approximately 2%, as calculated by Bloch simulation.

Myocardial Imaging

The 2D multi-slice myocardial imaging sequence used the same 6-pulse sequel saturation preparation, followed by a trigger delay (TD) and single shot readout. The single shot readout was either FLASH or b-SSFP. Protocol parameters at 1.5 T are listed in Table 2 and may vary slightly at 3 T. The readout used parallel imaging with 3-fold acceleration using TGRAPPA, and there were 3 PD frames without SR using a FLASH readout at the start of the sequence. An optional chemical shift fat saturation may be used without any penalty in the timing since the TD accommodated the fat saturation RF pulse. Although the gadolinium concentration in the myocardium is typically < 1 mmol/L, the signal response is still somewhat non-linear and therefore, the normalized signal SR/PD was corrected by a LUT which converts the myocardial signal to gadolinium concentration units,

Table 2 Protocol parameters for myocardial perfusion CMR sequence at 1.5 T

	FLASH	SSFP
PD frames	3	
PD FA	5° (FLASH)	
TE	1.0 ms	1.04 ms
TR	2.1 ms	2.5 ms
Bandwidth	1085 Hz/pixel	
FA	14°	50°
Matrix	192×111 (1.9×2.4 mm^2)	
Partial Fourier	3/4	
Asymmetric echo	weak	
FOV (typical)	360x270x8 mm^3	
PE order	Linear	
Parallel imaging	TPAT3	
TS/TD	100/62 ms	95/40 ms
SR prep	6-pulse (26 ms including spoilers)	
Fat saturation	optional	
Imaging duration	59 ms	70 ms
Total duration	143 ms/slice	142 ms/slice
3 slices + AIF	497 ms (>120 bpm)	495 ms (>120 bpm)

[Gd]. The sensitivity of the LUT correction to the actual transmitted FA was calculated by simulation. The b-SSFP FA was limited to 50° in order to reduce sensitivity of LUT correction to variations in actual transmitted FA and well as to reduce the average SAR.

The duration of actual signal shot image was 70 ms for SSFP protocol using factor 3 acceleration and Partial Fourier factor of ¾ with the latter part of k-space omitted. There is a trade-off between contrast-to-noise ratio (CNR), spatial coverage (number of slices per RR), and linearity as illustrated in Fig. 3. The protocol was designed to work at a heart rate of 120 bpm which is commonly seen for patients under adenosine stress. It was possible to acquire the AIF plus 3 slices at 120 bpm with the proposed protocol using TS = 95 ms, or AIF plus 2 slices using TI = 160 with increased CNR. It is also possible to prescribe 2x the number of slices by acquiring slices at 2RR intervals. Although there is a gain CNR with longer TS, there is also a loss in performance when using 2RR sampling since there will be fewer samples of the myocardial signal during the first pass measurement.

Image reconstruction & flow estimation

Image reconstruction and processing steps are diagrammed in Fig. 4. Parallel imaging was used to accelerate the acquisition of both AIF and myocardial images. This helped to minimize cardiac motion contribution to dark

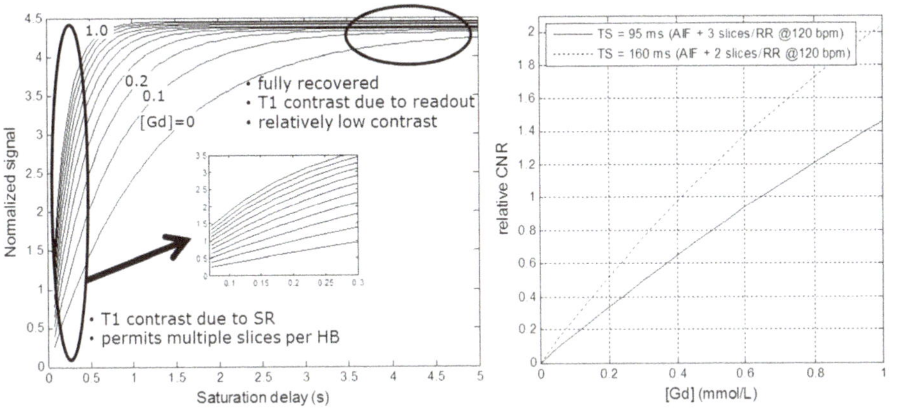

Fig. 3 Normalized saturation recovery myocardial signal (SR/PD) for b-SSFP protocol (Table 2) versus saturation delay (TS) for various values of tissue gadolinium concentration, [Gd] (left). With short TS protocols it is possible to acquire multiple slices per heart beat with T1 contrast. The contrast to noise ratio increases with TS, with increasing signal non-linearity and eventually at very long TS there is low contrast as the signal recovers. The CNR vs [Gd] is plotted for 2 values of TS (right) corresponding to T2 = 95 and 160 ms, corresponding to 3 and 2 slices/RR at a heart rate of 120 bpm. The increased TS can achieve approx. 40% higher CNR at the cost of less spatial coverage

rim artifacts (DRA) [18, 19] that appear as false perfusion defects, and to achieve adequate spatial coverage. Parallel imaging used TGRAPPA reconstruction with coil maps estimated by integrating the complete dataset [15]. All acquisitions were with normal free breathing and parallel imaging auto-calibration was performed on the complete dataset resulted in images free of aliasing artifacts. Individual coil images are adaptively combined to minimize noise bias prior to magnitude detection.

Raw filtering was used to reduce edge ringing [20] (Gibb's ringing) and to mitigate contamination of the measurements due to fat. In the low resolution AIF, a true Hanning window (i.e., without modification as in Tukey windows) was used to mitigate the influence of fat on the blood pool. For the low resolution AIF images the chest wall fat may be only 10–20 pixels from the LV blood pool. The Hanning window point spread function is <0.02% at a distance greater than 10 pixels whereas an un-windowed reconstruction would be <3.5% at this distance. The loss in resolution at full width half maximum is approx. 60%. In the higher resolution myocardial images, a truncated Gaussian filter was used, truncated to a width of 1.5 standard deviations. The first sidelobe was reduced to 36% compared to unweighted with a mainlobe broadening of 16% at full width half maximum.

Reconstruction and processing were implemented within the Gadgetron software framework [21] and were in-line and fully automatic. All images were respiratory motion corrected using a non-rigid image registration [22]. All images were reconstructed in SNR units [13] to facilitate image scaling, SNR measurements, and calculation of fixed threshold noise masks.

Myocardial blood flow was calculated multiple tissue models: 1) a Fermi model [2], and 2) a blood tissue exchange (BTEX) model originally developed by Bassingthwaighte [23] which is a distributed model described by the partial differential equations (PDE):

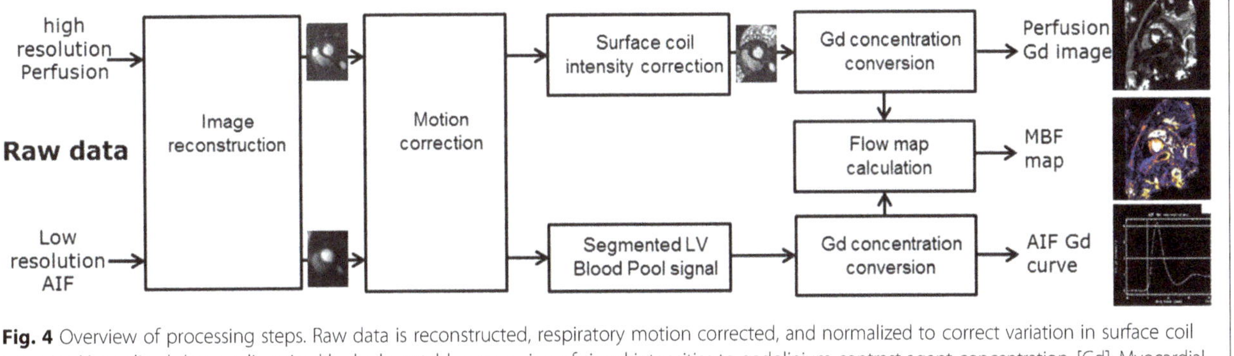

Fig. 4 Overview of processing steps. Raw data is reconstructed, respiratory motion corrected, and normalized to correct variation in surface coil intensity. Normalized data are linearized by look-up-table conversion of signal intensities to gadolinium contrast agent concentration, [Gd]. Myocardial blood flow is estimated from the AIF and myocardial pixel time series [Gd] values

$$\frac{\partial C_p}{\partial t} = \frac{-FL}{V_p} \cdot \frac{\partial C_p}{\partial x} + \frac{PS}{V_p} \cdot (C_{isf} - C_p) + D_p \cdot \frac{\partial^2 C_p}{\partial x^2} \quad (1)$$

$$\frac{\partial C_{isf}}{\partial t} = -\frac{PS}{V_{isf}} \cdot (C_{isf} - C_p) + D_{isf} \cdot \frac{\partial^2 C_{isf}}{\partial x^2} \quad (2)$$

where subscripts p and isf correspond to plasma and interstitial fluid, respectively, C the contrast agent concentration, F is the blood flow, PS is the permeability surface area product for the capillaries, V_p and V_{isf} are the intracapillary plasma and interstitial fluid volume, respectively, D is the axial diffusion coefficient, L is the capillary length, and x is the distance along the capillary. These equations follow Bassingthwaighte [23] Eqs. (1) and (3) with the term for regional consumption ignored, assuming a single term for capillary leakage dominated by the gaps in the capillary wall, and that the gadolinium based contrast agent is extracellular. The BTEX implementation solved for 4 unknown parameters: myocardial blood flow, interstitial volume, plasma volume, and the permeability surface area product that governs the extraction efficiency, with fixed values for other parameters. The PDE was applied to the AIF to calculate the myocardial response for each set of model parameters, and the parameters with the minimum mean squared error were used as the estimate. The Fermi model was fit to the first pass only and the BTEX model was fit to the entire measurement. The influence of T2* correction of the AIF on myocardial blood flow was analyzed.

Phantom validations

The sequence was simulated by Bloch equations to calculate the transverse magnetization as a function of all the protocol and tissue parameters in order to construct the LUT corrections for both the AIF and myocardial imaging protocols. Input to the LUT was the normalized signal SR/PD, where PD used the FLASH protocol and SR used either a b-SSFP or FLASH protocol. LUT were validated by phantom measurement by comparing the estimates of [Gd] after LUT correction with the known [Gd] using least squares fitting. A set of gadolinium doped saline phantoms were constructed at concentrations up to 10 mmol/L using both Gadoterate meglumine (Dotarem, Guerbet LLC) and Gadobutrol (Gadavist, Bayer Healthcare). LUT estimates of [Gd] vs known [Gd] were calculated with and without T2* correction. The phantom T1 values were measured using an inversion recovery GRE sequence at multiple inversion times (TI) with TR = 10s such that the longitudinal magnetization was fully relaxed after each RF excitation, and T1 was estimated by 3-parameter fitting to the mono-exponential inversion recovery S = A-Bexp(-TI/T1). The phantom T2 values were measured using a spin echo sequence (TR = 10s) with varying echo times (TE) and using T2 estimates from a 2-parameter fit to the mono-exponential decay curve, S = Aexp(-TE/T2). The coefficients for relaxivity rates (r1 and r2) were calculated from the T1 and T2 measurements vs known [Gd] using linear fitting, i.e., $R1 = R1_0 + r1[Gd]$ with R1 = 1/T1.

In-vivo data measurements

The proposed sequence and in-line flow mapping was performed at stress and rest on 29 healthy normal volunteers (11 men and 18 women, mean age 25.4 ± 5.7 years) at the Karolinska University Hospital, Stockholm, Sweden. Studies were approved by the local Ethics Committee. Anonymized data was analyzed at NIH with approval by the NIH Office of Human Subjects Research OHSR (Exemption #13156). All imaging was performed at 1.5 T (Magnetom AERA, Siemens, software version VE11A). Gadolinium (Gd) contrast agent (Gadobutrol) was administered as a bolus with 0.5 dose (0.05 mmol/kg) at 4 mL/s with 20 mL saline flush. One cannula was used for administration of adenosine and another cannula for the administration of contrast agent. Adenosine was administered by continuous infusion for approximately 8 min at a dose of 140 μg/kg/min to allow for additional research scans at stress just prior to contrast administration. The SSFP protocol was used in this study with fat saturation enabled.

In-vivo studies were performed to test the sequence and LUT conversion of signal intensities. Peak [Gd] was measured for the AIF blood pool signal and myocardium, as well as peak SNR in the myocardium from SNR scaled signal intensities. Blood pool T2* values at peak [Gd] were measured as well as the influence of T2* correction on estimates of myocardial blood flow. Duration of the bolus first pass was measured automatically from the AIF signal from the foot of the curve on the upslope of the AIF to the foot of the downslope. The improvement in linearity of the AIF after conversion to gadolinium concentration was measured by the ratio of the AIF peak to valley following the peak, for the raw signal intensities and for the LUT corrected [Gd].

Results

Simulations and Look-up table calculations

Performance of the 6-pulse saturation recovery preparation is shown in Fig. 5. Over the target design range of ±150 Hz and 17.5–29.6 μT (65–110% of effective FA) (dotted white box), the residual magnetization was < 0.5% in the myocardium for [Gd] up to 1 mmol/L, and for blood was < 0.5% up to 2.5 mmol/L, < 1% up to 5 mmol/L, and < 2.5% up to 10 mmol/L.

LUT's relating the normalized signal (SR/PD) and [Gd] were calculated for ±20% variation in transmitted B1 from nominal (Fig. 6). The error in [Gd] due to the LUT using the assumed specified FA rather than actual was

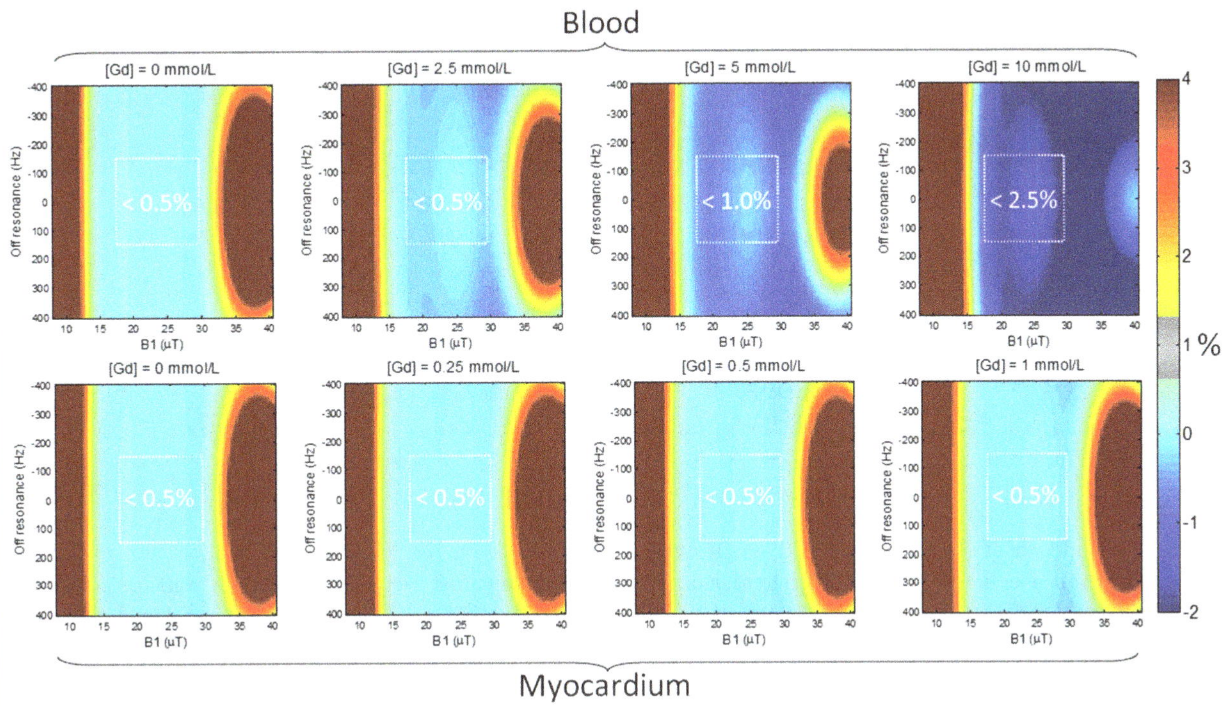

Fig. 5 Performance of saturation recovery preparation for blood and myocardium vs off-resonance and transmitter B1 for varying [Gd]. Over the target design range of ±150 Hz and 17.5–29.6 μT (65–110% of effective FA) (dotted white box), the residual magnetization was < 0.5% in the myocardium for [Gd] up to 1 mmol/L, and for blood was < 0.5% up to 2.5 mmol/L, < 1% up to 5 mmol/L, and < 2.5% up to 10 mmol/L

<10% over this range up to 1 mmol/L and <3% in the blood up to 10 mmol/L.

The T1 weighting of the PD images had < 1% variation in signal intensity over 0-2 mmol/L in the myocardium, and <1% over 0-1 mmol/L in the blood. The [Gd] in blood was < 1 mmol/L for a rest study following stress by several minutes, therefore using a fixed value of native $T1_0$ had <1% effect on the LUT. The effect of in-flow on the AIF LUT was calculated to be <4% assuming all spins were refreshed every RF pulse.

Phantom measurements

Measurement of r1 and r2 relaxivities was made for both Gadobutrol (Gadovist®) and Gadoterate meglumine (Dotarem®) doped saline phantoms. For Gadobutrol, the measured values for r1 and r2 were 5.5 L/mmol/s and 6.8 L/mmol/s, respectively and for Gadoterate meglumine the measured values were 4.6 L/mmol/s and 5.7 L/mmol/s, respectively. The measured [Gd] versus actual [Gd] is shown with and without T2* correction (Fig. 7). The linear fit for Gadobutrol was $[Gd]_{estimate} = 0.99\ [Gd] + 0.0002$ with

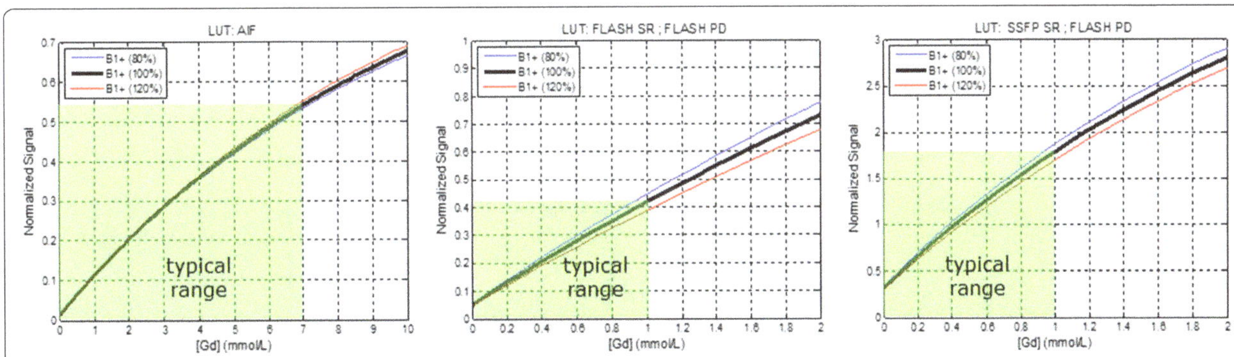

Fig. 6 Look-up-tables (LUT) relating the normalized signal (SR/PD) and gadolinium concentration, [Gd], for arterial input function (left), myocardium using SR-FLASH (center), and myocardium using SR-SSFP (right) for protocols in Tables 1 and 2. Typical ranges of [Gd] are highlighted by green shading. Sensitivity to actual transmitted flip angle is indicated by plotting variation of ±20% in B1+ which was <10% at 1 mmol/L in the myocardium, and <3% in the blood up to 10 mmol/L

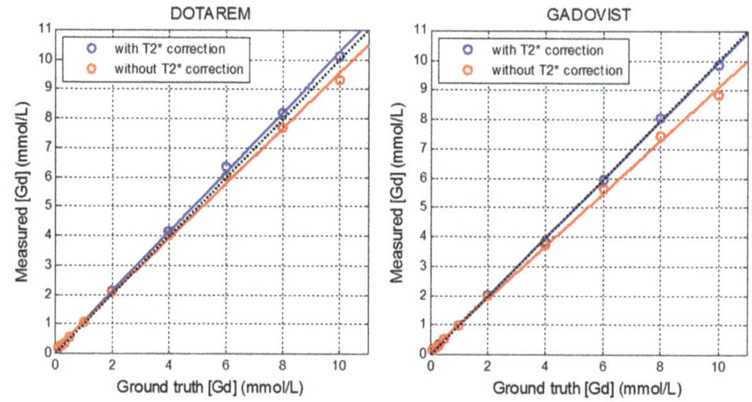

Fig. 7 Measured [Gd] vs true [Gd] for phantoms estimated with and without T2* correction for the AIF protocol with the line of identity shown as dotted black line

T2* correction and was $[Gd]_{estimate} = 0.90\ [Gd] + 0.08$, without T2* correction. The linear fit for Gadoterate meglumine was $[Gd]_{estimate} = 1.02\ [Gd] + 0.07$ with T2* correction and was $[Gd]_{estimate} = 0.94\ [Gd] + 0.12$, without T2* correction. Measurements of [Gd] for the myocardial signal protocol are shown in Fig. 8 for TS = 95 ms. For TS = 95 ms the fits were 1.004[Gd] + 0.005 and 1.04[Gd] + 0.01 for SSFP protocol with Gadobutrol and Gadoterate meglumine, respectively, and were 0.96[Gd] + 0.01 and 0.96[Gd] + 0.02 for the FLASH protocol with Gadobutrol and Gadoterate meglumine, respectively. The measurements were made for TS = 65 to 125 ms in steps of 10 ms. For SSFP, the slopes of the fits were within 4% of unity slope for all TS values and both agents and for FLASH were within 5%.

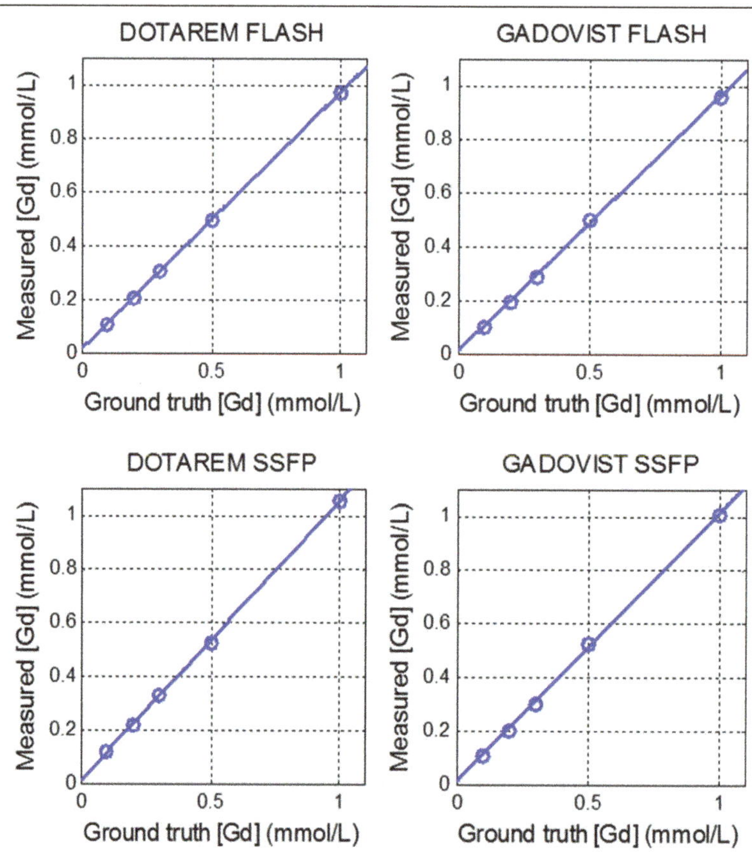

Fig. 8 Measured [Gd] versus true [Gd] for phantoms for the FLASH and SSFP myocardial imaging protocols with TS = 95 ms

Invivo AIF data

Adenosine stress studies were conducted on 29 normal healthy volunteers. The peak [Gd] was 3.5 ± 1.2 mmol/L (m ± SD) for stress and 4.4 ± 1.2 mmol/L for rest as measured in the AIF. The T2* in the LV blood pool at peak AIF [Gd] was 10.0 ± 2.4 ms at stress and 9.9 ± 1.7 ms at rest. The duration of the 1st pass was 10.3 ± 2.1 s at stress and 14.7 ± 3.2 s at rest. Example AIF images for echo 1 and echo 2 are shown in Fig. 9 for stress, and normalized AIF signal curves are shown in Fig. 10. In this example, the T2* corrected signal was approximately 8% higher than the echo 1 peak signal, which led to approximately 10% greater [Gd] after LUT correction. For 29 subjects, the peak to valley ratio was 5.6 for the raw signal intensities without correction, and was 8.3 for the LUT corrected AIF in gadolinium concentration units. The valley is indicated by the arrow in Fig. 10 stress signal intensity plot. This represents approximately 48% improvement in linearity.

Invivo myocardium data

The SNR of the myocardial time intensity was measured on a pixel-wise basis using SNR scaled reconstruction and measured at peak myocardial enhancement. Peak myocardial SNR was 21.8 ± 7.6 at stress and the peak [Gd] was 0.49 ± 0.15 mmol/L. Example of myocardial stress perfusion images are shown before and after normalization (Fig. 11) and myocardial blood flow maps are shown in Fig. 12. Images are well saturated as observed at baseline. Influence of T2* correction on flow comparing myocardial blood flow estimates with and without T2* correction is shown in Fig. 13. Without T2* correction the myocardial perfusion estimates of blood flow are overestimated by 10%. Estimates of perfusion stress flow using the BTEX model was 3.93 ± 0.38 and rest flow was 1.03 ± 0.19 ml/min/g (N = 29). Estimates for extraction fraction were 0.5 ± 0.04 and 0.85 ± 0.03, at stress and rest, respectively. Estimates of the permeability surface area product (PS) were 1.55 ± 0.2 and 1.33 ± 0.21 (ml/min/g), at stress and rest, respectively. Estimates for the interstitial volume fraction (%) were 27.4 ± 5.9 and 24.8 ± 5.9, at stress and rest, respectively. Estimates for the blood volume fraction (ml/g) were 13.0 ± 0.85 and 9.2 ± 0.76, at stress and rest, respectively. Estimates of perfusion flow using the Fermi model fit over the 1st pass were 3.4 ± 0.39 and 0.95 ± 0.16 ml/min/g, at stress and rest, respectively.

Raw images for a typical case corresponding to the example in Figs. 10 and 12 are provided as supplemental data as movies to include raw AIF images at stress and rest for both echo times before [see Additional file 1] and after respiratory MOCO [see Additional file 2], and the multislice stress and rest myocardium images including raw images [see Additional file 3], MOCO images [see Additional file 4], and MOCO images including surface coil correction [see Additional file 5].

Discussion

The dual sequence approach was chosen for automated, in-line perfusion mapping since it is readily integrated into a clinical workflow. Unlike the dual bolus method, simultaneous measurement of the AIF and myocardial signals avoids physiological variation between bolus injections such as those due to differences in respiration. Another benefit of the dual sequence is that it decouples the measurement of the AIF from the myocardial imaging protocol so that they may be independently optimized. The inherent non-linear response of SR on

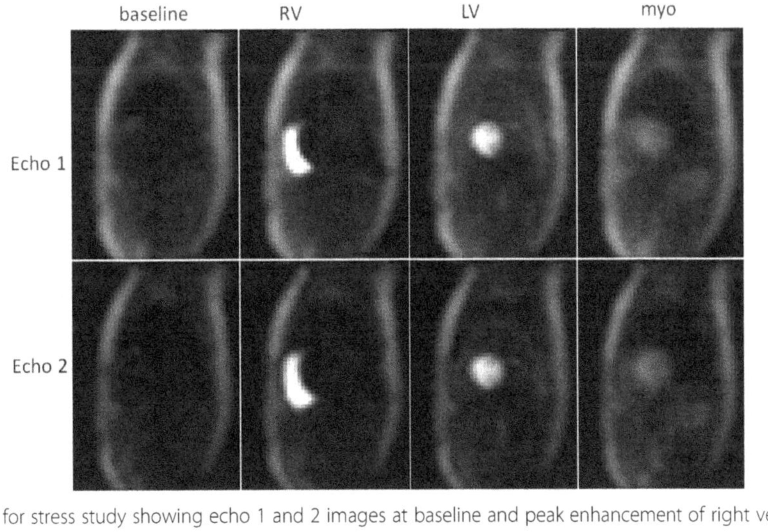

Fig. 9 Example AIF images for stress study showing echo 1 and 2 images at baseline and peak enhancement of right ventricle (RV), left ventricle (LV) and myocardium (myo)

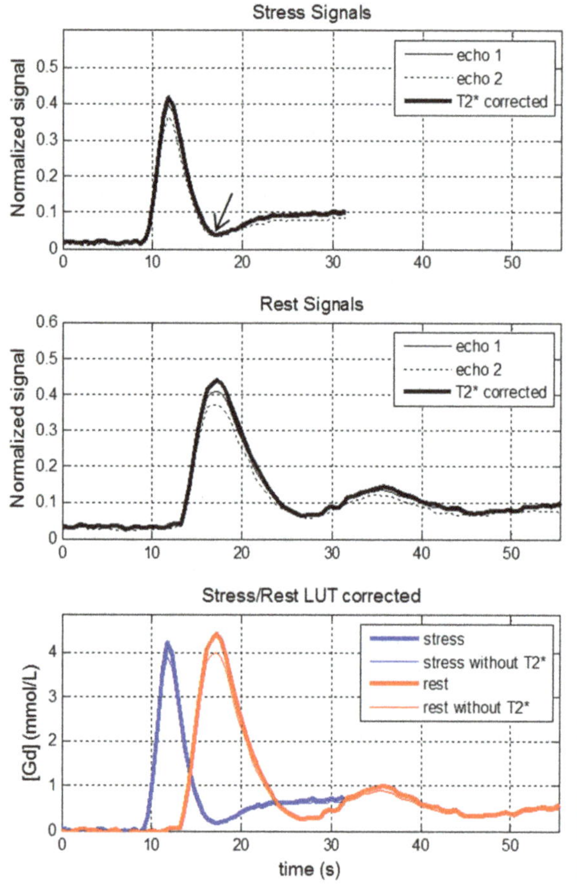

Fig. 10 Example of AIF signals for a stress/rest study showing normalized signals (SR/PD) for echo 1 and echo 2 and T2* corrected for stress (top) and rest (middle). The estimated [Gd] (bottom) is shown with and without T2* correction

the AIF was minimized by design of the protocol and post-processing. Earlier dual sequence AIF protocols used centric ordered acquisition to minimize the TS for improved linearity, but this leads to a high pass spatial filtering of the blood pool signal which becomes dependent on gadolinium concentration [10] and creates a dependence on the AIF and how the blood pool is segmented, i.e., the edges of the blood pool will have a longer effective saturation delay. Use of a linear ordering leads to a more homogeneous blood pool image. The saturation delay was minimized by use of parallel imaging acceleration to reduce the number of phase encodes lines actually acquired. The AIF signal with linear phase encoder order was slightly more non-linear than centric but could be corrected by a look-up-table approach based on Bloch signal calculations of the normalized signal (SR/PD). In this way, the blood pool signal could be automatically segmented and the AIF could be reliably estimated. Parallel imaging was used to accelerate the acquisition of myocardial perfusion images in order to reduce the single shot duration and thereby mitigate dark rim artifacts to some extent. Gibb's ringing was suppressed by raw filtering [24].

T2* correction

It is difficult to make direct comparison between the T2* values reported here and many of the previously reported measurements since many of the previous publications used different Gd contrast agents (e.g., Magnevist), administered different concentrations of [Gd] (0.05-0.1 mmol/kg), and used different infusion rates (3-7 mL/s). Additionally, several publications measured the signal loss with specific sequence parameters and not actual measurement of T2* with multiple echo times. Thus effects of in-flow due to FA, phase encode acquisition order, slice thickness, will vary between

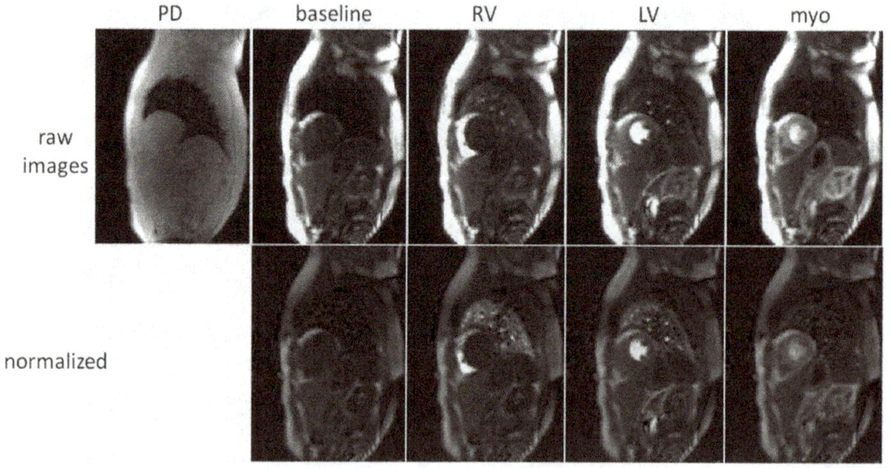

Fig. 11 Example of myocardial stress perfusion images for a stress study before (top) and after (bottom) intensity normalization using the PD image

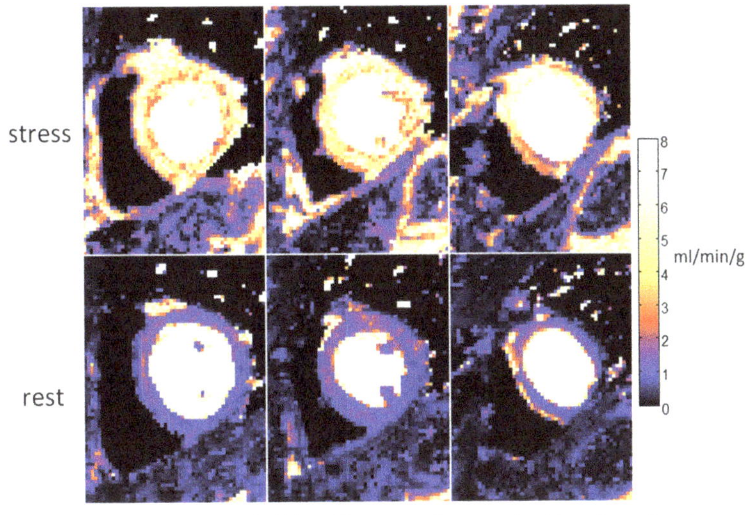

Fig. 12 Example of stress (top) and rest (bottom) myocardial blood flow maps for normal subject. Stress flow is appox. 4.1 mmol/min/g and rest flow is approx. 1.2 mmol/min/g

sequences. Finally, not all work was done at 1.5 T. These factors make the direct comparison difficult. The paper by de Bazelaire [15] predicts a value of T2* of 7.5 ms at a peak concentration of [Gd] = 4 mmol at 3 T, and does not give values for 1.5 T which are expected to be longer. By comparison the T2* reported here at 1.5 T for estimated concentration of approx. 4 mmol was approx. 10 ms. Prior work with Magnevist at 1.5 T, 0.1 mmol/kg dose, 5 mmol/s infusion [25] reported T2* values of approx. 9 ms at peak [Gd] concentration. It is also important to adequately shim the volume to minimize intravoxel de-phasing such that the measured value represents the intrinsic T2*.

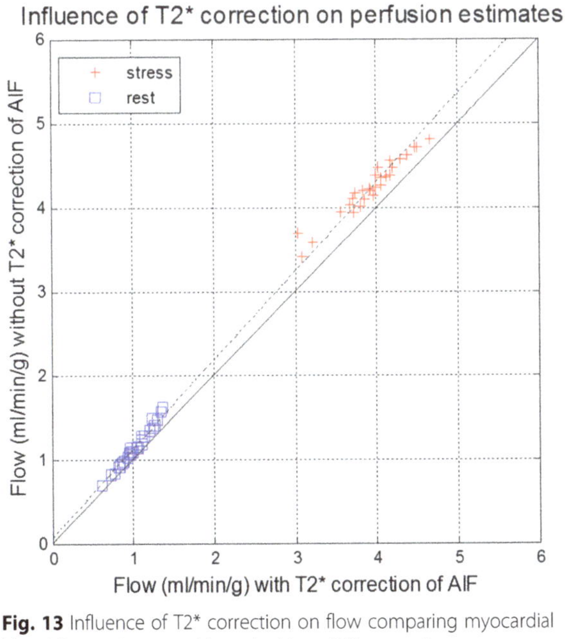

Fig. 13 Influence of T2* correction on flow comparing myocardial blood flow estimates with and without T2* correction

The correction of T2* in the AIF avoid underestimating the peak [Gd]. Underestimation the input function [Gd] will result in an overestimation of the flow. This is true in general for all perfusion models (BTEX, Fermi, exponential) that are implemented based on the absolute [Gd] signals.

Conversion to [Gd]

The conversion to gadolinium concentration units facilitated the use of the dual sequence which used a FLASH readout for the AIF and could support either FLASH or SSFP for myocardial perfusion imaging. The relaxivities (r1 and r2) were measured in Gd doped saline phantoms. Although the estimated concentration is dependent on the accuracy of these values, which may be slightly different in blood plasma, the quantified myocardial blood flow has been found through simulation to be quite insensitive since they affect the scale of both blood and myocardium. In-vivo values of blood T2* were significantly lower than for saline phantoms at a given [Gd] as previously reported [26]. The average blood T2* at 1.5 T was approximately 10 ms at 4 mmol/L peak [Gd], whereas the T2* was approximately 25 ms in saline at the same concentration. The T2* decreases with field strength [26] and values as low as 4 ms are likely to be encountered at 3 T using a dose of 0.05 mmol/kg leading to higher signal losses and greater importance for T2* correction. The conversion to [Gd] in the presence of error in FA due to unknown B1 was analyzed through simulation to cause small errors in [Gd] which in turn will result in an error in estimated flow of < 15% for ±20% variation in B1.

Tissue models

The in-line automated perfusion mapping software has the capability of calculating perfusion estimates based on several different widely used models with differing complexity including the Fermi model [2] and distributed BTEX model [23]. The distributed BTEX model explicitly estimates the permeability surface area (PS) product which is used to calculate an extraction fraction to account for the flow dependent leakage of Gd from the vascular space into the interstitium. The BTEX model has been used in ^{13}N-Ammonia PET and validated against microspheres [27]. There is growing interest in distributed tissue models for perfusion [28–30]. A more comprehensive comparison of models will be the subject of a detailed study. Despite significant differences in models, the mean values for perfusion estimates compare reasonably well with other reported values in normal subjects. In a study by Broadbent, et al. [28], perfusion was estimated using both Fermi and a distributed parameter (DP) model. Values for stress and rest perfusion estimates and myocardial flow reserve in that study were 3.8/1.5/2.7 for Fermi and 3.5/1.5/2.5 for DP, as compared to 3.4/0.95/3.6 for Fermi and 3.9/1.03/3.8 for BTEX in the present study. In a study of 10 normal subjects, Hsu, et al. [31] reported values of 3.39/1.02/3.3 using a Fermi tissue model.

Saturation preparation

The 6-pulse saturation preparation achieved > 99% saturation over a wide range of off-resonance, effective transmitter FA, and gadolinium concentration. Excellent saturation mitigates slice to slice cross-talk and allows the user to prescribe a mixture of short and long axis slices. There is possibility of slight cross talk between intersecting slices for the initial non-saturated PD frames, but this is quite small due to the low FA of PD weighted acquisition protocol. The 6-pulse is designed conservatively, and has recently been reduced to a 5-pulse design to reduce the overall duration and SAR. The newly design preparation has recently been evaluated and perform with >99% saturation over a design range of 50–110% nominal B1+. This newly designed SR preparation is 14.7 ms including crushers which translated to a total AIF duration of 57 ms. Using this 5-pulse design allows for slight increase of the saturation delay from 95 to 105 ms, thereby increasing the SNR while maintaining 3-slices up to 120 bpm.

Conclusion

A dual sequence for myocardial perfusion CMR and arterial input function measurement has been optimized for quantification of myocardial blood flow. A validation in phantoms was performed to confirm that the signal conversion to gadolinium concentration was linear. The proposed sequence was integrated with a fully automatic in-line solution for pixel-wise mapping of myocardial blood flow and evaluated in adenosine stress and rest studies on $N = 29$ normal healthy subjects. Reliable perfusion mapping was demonstrated and produced estimates with low variability.

Additional files

Additional file 1: Example raw AIF images for both echos at stress (top) and rest (bottom).

Additional file 2: Example MOCO AIF images for both echos at stress (top) and rest (bottom).

Additional file 3: Example raw myocardium images at stress (top) and rest (bottom).

Additional file 4: Example MOCO myocardium images at stress (top) and rest (bottom).

Additional file 5: Example normalized MOCO myocardium images at stress (top) and rest (bottom).

Abbreviations

[Gd]: Gadolinium concentration; AIF: Arterial input function; CMR: Cardiovascular magnetic resonance; CNR: Contrast-to-noise ratio; DRA: Dark rim artifact; FA: Flip angle; FLASH: Fast low angle shot; LGE: Late gadolinium enhancement; LUT: Look-up table; MOCO: Motion correction; PD: Proton density; RF: Radio frequency; SAR: Specific absorption ratio; SR: Saturation recovery; SSFP: Steady state free precession; TD: Trigger delay; TS: Saturation delay

Acknowledgements

We acknowledge Kelvin Chow for his design of the saturation recovery preparation.

Funding

Supported by the National Heart, Lung and Blood Institute, National Institutes of Health by the Division of Intramural Research.

Authors' contributions

PK and HX conceived of the study, developed the sequence and Bloch simulations, performed processing and analysis, and drafted the manuscript. SNV contributed to sequence development, and MSH contributed to the image reconstruction framework and data analysis. JN, RT, and MU acquired normal volunteer data. All authors participated in revising the manuscript and read and approved the final manuscript.

Competing interests

The authors declare that they have no competing interests

Author details

[1]National Heart, Lung, and Blood Institute, National Institutes of Health, DHHS, 10 Center Drive MSC-1061, Bethesda, MD 20892, USA. [2]Department of Clinical Physiology, Karolinska Institutet and Karolinska University Hospital, Stockholm, Sweden.

References

1. Wilke N, Simm C, Zhang J, Ellermann J, Ya X, Merkle H, et al. Contrast-enhanced first pass myocardial perfusion imaging: correlation between myocardial blood flow in dogs at rest and during hyperemia. Magn Reson Med. 1993;29:485–97.
2. Jerosch-Herold M, Wilke N, Stillman AE, Wilson RF. Magnetic resonance quantification of the myocardial perfusion reserve with a Fermi function model for constrained deconvolution. Med Phys. 1998;25:73.
3. Christian TF, Aletras AH, Arai AE. Estimation of absolute myocardial blood flow during first-pass MR perfusion imaging using a dual-bolus injection technique: comparison to single-bolus injection method. J Magn Reson Imaging. 2008;27:1271–7.
4. Gatehouse PD, Elkington AG, Ablitt NA, Yang G-Z, Pennell DJ, Firmin DN. Accurate assessment of the arterial input function during high-dose myocardial perfusion cardiovascular magnetic resonance. J Magn Reson Imaging. 2004;20:39–45.
5. Xue H, Hansen MS, Nielles-vallespin S, Arai AE, Kellman P. Inline quantitative myocardial perfusion flow mapping. JCMR/ISMRM Work. 2016;18:4–6.
6. Chow K, Kellman P, Spottiswoode BS, Nielles-Vallespin S, Arai AE, Salerno M, et al. Saturation pulse design for quantitative myocardial T1 mapping. J Cardiovasc Magn Reson. 2015;17:84.
7. Nielles-Vallespin S, Kellman P, Hsu L-Y, Arai AE. FLASH proton density imaging for improved surface coil intensity correction in quantitative and semi-quantitative SSFP perfusion cardiovascular magnetic resonance. J Cardiovasc Magn Reson. 2015;17:16.
8. Cernicanu A, Axel L. Theory-based signal calibration with single-point T1 measurements for first-pass quantitative perfusion MRI studies. Acad Radiol. 2006;13:686–93.
9. Sekihara K. Steady-state magnetizations in angles and short repetition intervals. IEEE Trans Med Imaging. 1987;MI-6:157–64.
10. Gatehouse P, Lyne J, Smith G, Pennell D, Firmin D. T2* effects in the dual-sequence method for high-dose first-pass myocardial perfusion. J Magn Reson Imaging. 2006;24:1168–71.
11. Sánchez-González J, Fernandez-Jiménez R, Nothnagel ND, López-Martín G, Fuster V, Ibañez B. Optimization of dual-saturation single bolus acquisition for quantitative cardiac perfusion and myocardial blood flow maps. J Cardiovasc Magn Reson. 2015;17:21.
12. de Bazelaire C, Rofsky NM, Duhamel G, Zhang J, Michaelson MD, George D, et al. Combined T2* and T1 measurements for improved perfusion and permeability studies in high field using dynamic contrast enhancement. Eur Radiol. 2006;16:2083–91.
13. Kellman P, McVeigh ER. Image reconstruction in SNR units: a general method for SNR measurement. Magn Reson Med. 2005;54:1439–47.
14. Xue H, Zuehlsdorff S, Kellman P, Arai A, Nielles-Vallespin S, Chefdhotel C, et al. Unsupervised inline analysis of cardiac perfusion MRI. Lect. Notes Comput. Sci. (including Subser. Lect. Notes Artif. Intell. Lect. Notes Bioinformatics). 2009;5762 LNCS:741–9.
15. Breuer FA, Kellman P, Griswold MA, Jakob PM. Dynamic autocalibrated parallel imaging using temporal GRAPPA (TGRAPPA). Magn Reson Med. 2005;53:981–5.
16. Kim D. Influence of the k-space trajectory on the dynamic T1-weighted signal in quantitative first-pass cardiac perfusion MRI at 3 T. Magn Reson Med. 2008;59:202–8.
17. Elkington AG, He T, Gatehouse PD, Prasad SK, Firmin DN, Pennell DJ. Optimization of the arterial input function for myocardial perfusion cardiovascular magnetic resonance. J Magn Reson Imaging. 2005;21:354–9.
18. Zhao L, Salerno M, Kramer CM, Meyer CH. The contribution of cardiac motion to dark rim artifacts in myocardial perfusion scans. Proc ISMRM. 2010;18:3626.
19. Storey P, Chen Q, Li W, Edelman RR, Prasad PV. Band artifacts due to bulk motion. Magn Reson Med. 2002;48:1028–36.
20. Di Bella EVR, Parker DL, Sinusas AJ. On the dark rim artifact in dynamic contrast-enhanced MRI myocardial perfusion studies. Magn Reson Med. 2005;54:1295–9.
21. Hansen MS, Sørensen TS. Gadgetron: an open source framework for medical image reconstruction. Magn Reson Med. 2013;69:1768–76.
22. Chefd'Hotel C, Hermosillo G, Faugeras O. Flows of diffeomorphisms for multimodal image registration. IEEE Int Symp Biomed Imaging. 2002;753–756.
23. Bassingthwaighte JB, Wang CY, Chan IS. Blood-tissue exchange via transport and transformation by capillary endothelial cells. Circ Res. 1989;65:997–1020.
24. Zhou Z, Bi X, Wei J, Yang H-J, Dharmakumar R, Arsanjani R, et al. First-pass myocardial perfusion MRI with reduced subendocardial dark-rim artifact using optimized Cartesian sampling. J Magn Reson Imaging. 2017;45(2):542–55. doi:10.1002/jmri.25400.
25. Kellman P, Aletras AH, Hsu L-Y, McVeigh ER, Arai AE. T2* measurement during first-pass contrast-enhanced cardiac perfusion imaging. Magn Reson Med. 2006;56:1132–4.
26. Kalavagunta C, Michaeli S, Metzger GJ. In vitro Gd-DTPA relaxometry studies in oxygenated venous human blood and aqueous solution at 3 and 7 T. Contrast Media Mol Imaging. 2014;9:169–76.
27. Alessio A, Bassingthwaighte JB, Glenny R, Caldwell J. Validation of an axially distributed model for quantification of myocardial blood flow using 13 N-ammonia PET. J Nucl Cardiol. 2013;20:64–75.
28. Broadbent DA, Biglands JD, Larghat A, Sourbron SP, Radjenovic A, Greenwood JP, et al. Myocardial blood flow at rest and stress measured with dynamic contrast-enhanced MRI: comparison of a distributed parameter model with a Fermi function model. Magn Reson Med. 2013;70:1591–7.
29. Chung S, Shah B, Storey P, Iqbal S, Slater J, Axel L. Quantitative Perfusion Analysis of First-Pass Contrast Enhancement Kinetics: Application to MRI of Myocardial Perfusion in Coronary Artery Disease. PLoS One [Internet]. 2016;11: e0162067. Available from: http://dx.plos.org/10.1371/journal.pone.0162067
30. Kunze KP, Rischpler C, Hayes C, Ibrahim T, Laugwitz K-L, Haase A, et al. Measurement of extracellular volume and transit time heterogeneity using contrast-enhanced myocardial perfusion MRI in patients after acute myocardial infarction. Magn Reson Med. 2016. doi:10.1002/mrm.26320. [Epub ahead of print]
31. Hsu L-Y, Rhoads KL, Holly JE, Kellman P, Aletras AH, Arai AE. Quantitative myocardial perfusion analysis with a dual-bolus contrast-enhanced first-pass MRI technique in humans. J Magn Reson Imaging. 2006;23:315–22.

Longitudinal assessment of right ventricular structure and function by cardiovascular magnetic resonance in breast cancer patients treated with trastuzumab

Ashita Barthur[1], Christine Brezden-Masley[2,3], Kim A. Connelly[3,4,5], Vinita Dhir[2], Kelvin K. W. Chan[6], Rashida Haq[2], Anish Kirpalani[1,3], Joseph J. Barfett[1,3], Laura Jimenez-Juan[7], Gauri R. Karur[1], Djeven P. Deva[1,3*] and Andrew T. Yan[3,4,5*]

Abstract

Background: There are limited data on the effects of trastuzumab on the right ventricle (RV). Therefore, we sought to evaluate the temporal changes in right ventricular (RV) structure and function as measured by cardiovascular magnetic resonance (CMR), and their relationship with left ventricular (LV) structure and function in breast cancer patients treated with trastuzumab.

Methods: Prospective, longitudinal, observational study involving 41 women with HER2+ breast cancer who underwent serial CMR at baseline, 6, 12, and 18 months after initiation of trastuzumab. A single blinded observer measured RV parameters on de-identified CMRs in a random order. Linear mixed models were used to investigate temporal changes in RV parameters.

Results: Of the 41 women (age 52 ± 11 years), only one patient experienced trastuzumab-induced cardiotoxicity. Compared to baseline, there were small but significant increases in the RV end-diastolic volume at 6 months ($p = 0.002$) and RV end-systolic volume at 6 and 12 months ($p < 0.001$ for both), but not at 18 months ($p = 0.82$ and 0.13 respectively). RV ejection fraction (RVEF), when compared to baseline (58.3%, 95% CI 57.1–59.5%), showed corresponding decreases at 6 months (53.9%, 95% CI 52.5–55.4%, $p < 0.001$) and 12 months (55%, 95% CI 53.8–56.2%, $p < 0.001$) that recovered at 18 months (56.6%, 95% CI 55.1–58.0%, $p = 0.08$). Although the temporal pattern of changes in LVEF and RVEF were similar, there was no significant correlation between RVEF and LVEF at baseline ($r = 0.29$, $p = 0.07$) or between their changes at 6 months ($r = 0.24$, $p = 0.17$).

Conclusion: In patients receiving trastuzumab without overt cardiotoxicity, there is a subtle but significant deleterious effect on RV structure and function that recover at 18 months, which can be detected by CMR. Furthermore, monitoring of LVEF alone may not be sufficient in detecting early RV injury. These novel findings provide further support for CMR in monitoring early cardiotoxicity.

Keywords: Right ventricle, Cardiovascular magnetic resonance, Cardiotoxicity, Trastuzumab

* Correspondence: devad@smh.ca; yana@smh.ca
[1]Department of Medical Imaging, St. Michael's Hospital, University of Toronto, Toronto, ON, Canada
[3]Keenan Research Centre, Li Ka Shing Knowledge Institute, St. Michael's Hospital, University of Toronto, Toronto, ON, Canada
Full list of author information is available at the end of the article

Background

Breast cancer is the most common cancer and second most common cause of cancer death among women in North America [1, 2]. At least 20% of invasive breast cancers demonstrate human epidermal growth factor receptor type 2 (HER2) over-expression which adversely affects prognosis [3]. Recent guidelines recommend evaluation of HER2 status in all invasive breast cancers at diagnosis or recurrence for consideration of trastuzumab therapy [4]. Cardiac dysfunction, defined as a symptomatic decline in left ventricular ejection function (LVEF) of >5% from baseline or an asymptomatic reduction of >10% from baseline to <55%, has been recognized as a potential dose-limiting toxicity of trastuzumab therapy [5]. Cardiac dysfunction occurs in up to 34% patients on trastuzumab and anthracyclines leading to adverse cardiac events [6], and is mediated by HER2 receptor inhibition in cardiomyocytes [7, 8]. RV dysfunction is known to be a poor prognosticator in a variety of other cardiovascular diseases [9–16]. However, there are limited data regarding trastuzumab induced toxicity affecting the right ventricle (RV) [17, 18]. The initial studies on cardiotoxic effects in breast cancer patients utilized radionuclide ventriculography [19, 20] and echocardiography [21–24], which have limited accuracy in evaluating RV owing to its shape and position, in addition to inherent drawbacks of each modality [25].

Methods

Aim

To evaluate the temporal changes in RV structure and function as measured by cardiovascular magnetic resonance (CMR) over 18 months, and to examine the relationship between the LV and RV structure and function in breast cancer patients treated with trastuzumab.

Study protocol

This prospective cohort study comprised of 41 consecutive eligible women from the medical oncology departments of 2 tertiary care hospitals, who were newly diagnosed with HER2 positive breast cancer between Jan 2010 and Dec 2013. The study was approved by the Research and Ethics Boards of both hospitals. Written informed consent was obtained from each participant. We included women older than 18 years; with histologically confirmed invasive breast cancer and HER 2 over-expression; planned to be treated with trastuzumab; with a baseline LVEF ≥50% by radionuclide ventriculography. Those with previous treatment with trastuzumab, other anti-HER2 agent, pre-existing symptomatic heart failure (NYHA Class III or IV), recent acute coronary syndrome or coronary revascularization within the last 6 months, permanent atrial fibrillation, contraindications to MRI and pregnant and/or nursing patients were excluded.

All participants were scheduled for CMR at baseline (prior to the initiation of trastuzumab therapy) and at 6, 12 and 18 months following initiation of therapy. Blood samples were obtained for measurements of serum NT-BNP and high-sensitivity troponin I (hs-TnI) as biomarkers of cardiotoxicity.

Trastuzumab and chemotherapy regimen

Chemotherapy consisted of anthracycline or non-anthracycline regimen at the discretion of the treating oncologist. Participants received 18 cycles (12 months) of trastuzumab therapy.

Cardiotoxicity

All patients underwent serial radionuclide ventriculography for monitoring of LVEF, as part of standard of care. In the event of cardiotoxicity based on LVEF measurement by radionuclide ventriculography, trastuzumab treatment was withheld for 3 weeks [26]. After 3 weeks, if the repeat radionuclide ventriculography scan showed improvement in LVEF, then trastuzumab was re-initiated. Both the medical oncologist and patient were blinded to the results of the CMR.

CMR

CMR was performed at baseline, 6, 12 and 18 months. All CMR was performed with a 1.5 T scanner (Intera, Philips Medical Systems, Best, the Netherlands, or GE Signa Excite Cv, Milwaukee, WI) using a phased-array cardiac coil and retrospective electrocardiographic gating. Standard protocols using validated, commercially available sequences were used. Images were obtained with breath-hold at end-expiration. Segmented, balanced steady-state free-precession sequence was used for cine acquisition with the following typical parameters: TR 4 ms, TE 2 ms, slice thickness 8 mm, field of view 320–330 x 320–330 mm, matrix size 256x196, temporal resolution of <40 ms (depending on the heart rate) and flip angle 50 degrees. Following administration of intravenous gadolinium contrast, phase sensitive inversion recovery sequences were obtained. CMR scans were analyzed with CVi 42 software (Circle Cardiovascular, Calgary, Alberta, Canada).

A single blinded experienced reader measured all RV parameters on de-identified CMR scans in a random order. LV measurements and late gadolinium enhancement (LGE) assessment were made independently by another blinded experienced reader.

Both the LV and RV were analyzed only by volumetric measurements on the short-axis cine steady state free precision images. The LV and RV were contoured according to the current practice at our institution using semi-automated tracing of the endocardial borders at end diastole and end systole, which corresponded to the cardiac phases with the largest and smallest ventricular volumes, respectively. Papillary muscles and trabeculations were considered part of the blood pool and not as a part of the RV mass. RV end-diastolic and end-systolic volumes (RVEDV and RVESV) were determined by summing the volume across slices without geometric assumptions, and EF is calculated as (EDV-ESV)/EDV x100% [27]. The normal reference range for RVEF in women was defined as 51–71% [28].

Statistical analysis

The sample size calculation was based on the detection of clinically meaningful changes in LV volume and LVEF, between baseline and 12 months, using the simple paired *t*-test approach. 38 subjects would provide at least 95% power to detect a 10-ml mean change in LV volumes, or a 3% mean change in LVEF. This sample size of 38 patients also achieves 95% power to detect an intraclass correlation of 0.80 between LVEF measurements by CMR and radionuclide ventriculography (when the null hypothesis is 0.50) at a significance level of 0.05. However, because the impact of trastuzumab on RV volume and RVEF changes were not known and our study is the first study to longitudinally assess the changes in RV parameters in breast cancer patients treated with trastuzumab over 18 months, the sample size was not based on expected changes in RV volume or RVEF. Mean and standard deviation (or median and interquartile range) are reported for continuous variables. Mixed linear models were performed to test for longitudinal changes in RV and LV parameters over time. This method has the advantage of allowing all available data over time to be analyzed, unlike repeated measures ANOVA which allows only complete case analysis. We selected the unstructured covariance based on the Akaike's information criterion. Sidak adjustment was utilized for pairwise comparisons of the three time points (6, 12, 18 months) with the baseline measurement. We also tested for potential interaction between anthracycline use and time in the mixed linear model. We calculated the Pearson correlation coefficients between RV and LV parameters. To examine the non-linear relationship between biomarker and RVEF, we used the non-parametric Kendall tau-b (τ) correlation test. To explore whether cardiovascular risk factors might impact on RV volume and RVEF, we compared the changes in RVEDV, RVESV and RVEF at 6 months in the group with versus the group without any cardiovascular risk factors (hypertension, diabetes, dyslipidemia or smoking). To assess intra-observer reproducibility, we calculated the intraclass correlation coefficients for RVEDV and RVESV. A two-sided *p*-value <0.05 was defined as significant. Statistical analysis was performed using SPSS version 22 (IBM Corp., Armonk, NY).

Results

In total, 41 women who received trastuzumab underwent CMR at baseline; 33 of them completed the 18 months follow up, and the remaining 8 patients did not undergo all the CMRs either due to tissue expanders, change in treatment or personal reasons. Table 1 shows the baseline characteristics of the study population. Amongst these, 23 patients received anthracycline based chemotherapy. There were no patients with heart failure at baseline.

Only 1 patient experienced cardiotoxicity for which trastuzumab was subsequently withheld for one cycle. No patient developed new clinical heart failure or died due to heart failure during the study follow up.

RVEDV, RVESV, and RVEF changed significantly over the course of the study (Figs. 1, 2 and 3). Although the mean RVEF remained normal (≥51%) throughout the study, 8/35 patients (23%) showed a decline in RVEF to less than the lower limits of normal (<51%) at 6 months; only 2 of these patients had a decrease from baseline of more than 10%. At 12 months, 4/34 (12%) patients had an RVEF below the lower limit of normal, with only one patient demonstrating a persistent drop in RVEF of more than 10% when compared to baseline.

By pairwise comparisons with the baseline, there was a significant increase in RVEDV only at 6 months (129.9 ml, 95% CI 122–137.7 ml, $p = 0.002$) but not at 12 months (127 ml, 95% CI 118.3–135.7 ml, $p = 0.09$) and 18 months (123.3 ml, 95% CI 115–131.7 ml, $p = 0.82$) (Fig. 1), whereas the increase in RVESV were significant at both 6 months (59.9 ml, 95% CI 55.3–64.4 ml, $p < 0.001$) and 12 months (56.7 ml, 95% CI 52.6–60.8 ml, $p < 0.001$) but not at 18 months (53.4 ml, 95% CI 49.5–57.3 ml, $p = 0.14$) (Fig. 2). Analogous to the changes in RVESV, we noted a significant decline in the mean RVEF at 6 months (53.9%, 95% CI 52.5–55.4%, $p < 0.001$) and 12 months (55%, 95% CI 53.8–56.2%, $p < 0.001$), which became non-significant at 18 months (56.6%, 95% CI 55.1–58.0%, $p = 0.08$) (Fig. 3). When indexed RV volumes were analysed, the overall temporal changes and pattern remained the same (data not shown).

The mean LVEF at baseline was normal (60.4 ± 4.2%). Although the mean LVEF remained normal throughout the study, there was a significant decrease in LVEF at 6 and 12 months (58.3 ± 5.1%, 57.9 ± 4.8%, respectively, both $p < 0.05$) compared to baseline. The changes in LVEF and RVEF paralleled each other during treatment; both were significantly lower at 6 and 12 months and both recovered by 18 months (Fig. 4). Overall, RVEF and LVEF showed weak and non-significant correlation at baseline ($r = 0.29$, $p = 0.07$). Likewise, the changes in

Table 1 Baseline characteristics of the study population

	n (%), Total n = 41
Demographics	
Age	52 ± 11
BMI, kg/m2	26.8 ± 6.3
Cardiovascular risk factors	
Hypertension	10 (24.4%)
Diabetes	4 (9.8%)
Hypercholesterolemia	3 (7.3%)
Coronary artery disease	1 (2.4%)
Smoking	10 (24.4%)
Medications:	
Beta-blocker	3 (9%)
ACE inhibitor	3 (9%)
NYHA class III/IV	0
Cancer-related variables	
Breast cancer site	
Left	27 (65.9%)
Stage of disease	
Early	27 (68%)
Locally invasive	13 (32%)
Type of surgery	
Breast-conserving surgery	22 (53.7%)
Mastectomy	19 (46.3%)
Chemotherapeutic regimen	
Anthracycline based	23 (56.1%)
Left sided radiation	12 (29.3)
Biomarkers:	
High sensitivity-troponin I, ng/mL (n = 37)[a]	<0.006 (<0.006–0.012)
NT-BNP, ng/mL (n = 39)[a]	57 (33–128)
LV parameters	
LVEDV, ml	129.7 ± 24.9
LVESV, ml	51.5 ± 12
LVEF, %	60.4 ± 4.2
RV parameters	
RVEDV, ml	121 ± 24
RVESV, ml	51 ± 11
RVEF, %	58.3 ± 3.8

Data presented as frequency (percentages) or mean ± standard deviation unless otherwise specified
[a]median (interquartile range)

LVEF and RVEF over 6 months showed only a weak and non-significant correlation ($r = 0.24$, $p = 0.17$, Fig. 5).

There was no significant interaction between anthracycline and time for RVEF ($p = 0.12$), RVEDV ($p = 0.52$), and RVESV ($p = 0.25$). This suggests that the temporal changes in RVEF, RVEDV, and RVESV were similar between the anthracycline and non-anthracycline groups.

The median (interquartile range) for NT-BNP was 57(33–128) at baseline, 39(30.3–86.5) at 6 months, 47.5(29.3–74.8) at 12 months and 61(36.8–111.8) at 18 months. There was no significant correlation between changes in NT-BNP and RVEF at 6 months ($\tau = 0.11$, $p = 0.42$). There was no significant change in the hs-TnI [median(interquartile range)] from baseline <0.006 ng/ml (<0.006–0.012) to 6 months <0.006 ng/ml(<0.006– < 0.006) or 12 months <0.006 ng/ml(<0.006– < 0.006).

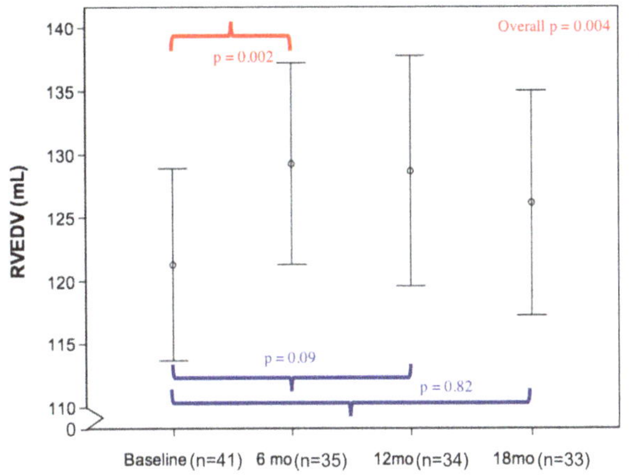

Fig. 1 Longitudinal measurements of RVEDV over 18 months. There were significant changes in RVEDV over time ($p = 0.004$). By Sidak-adjusted pairwise comparisons with the baseline, the mean RVEDV showed a small but significant increase at 6 months ($p = 0.002$), that was no longer significant at 18 months ($p = 0.82$). Data shown as mean and 95% confidence intervals (*vertical bars*)

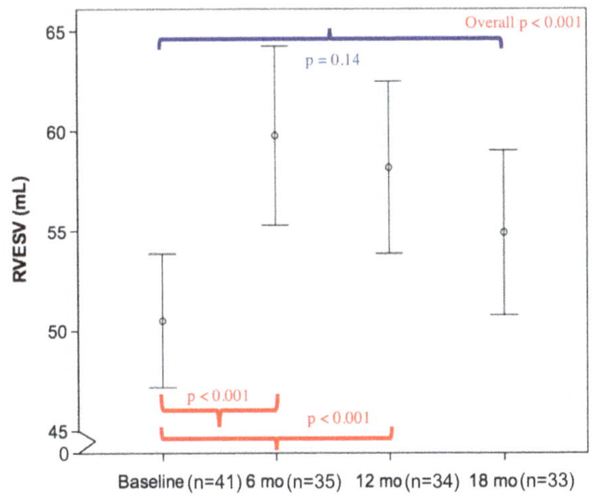

Fig. 2 Longitudinal measurements of RVESV over 18 months. There were significant changes in RVESV over time ($p < 0.001$). By Sidak-adjusted pairwise comparisons with the baseline, the mean RVESV showed a small but significant increase at 6 and 12 months (both $p < 0.001$), that was no longer significant at 18 months ($p = 0.14$). Data shown as mean and 95% confidence intervals (*vertical bars*)

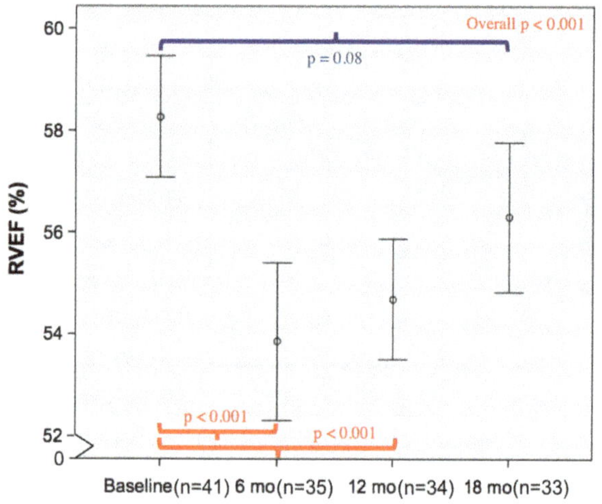

Fig. 3 Longitudinal measurements of RVEF over 18 months. There were significant changes in RVEF over time ($p < 0.001$). By Sidak-adjusted pairwise comparisons with the baseline, the mean RVEF showed a small but significant decrease at 6 and 12 months ($p < 0.001$ for both), that was no longer significant at 18 months ($p = 0.08$). Data shown as mean and 95% confidence intervals (*vertical bars*)

There was no significant difference in changes in RVEF, RVEDV or RVESV at 6 months between the group with any cardiovascular risk factor ($n = 15$) and with no risk factors ($n = 20$).

Only 2 patients demonstrated LGE. One patient had an ischemic pattern of LGE (attributable to a previous myocardial infarction) which was seen at baseline and did not change or develop new focus of LGE during the study. The other patient showed a non-specific inferior RV hinge point LGE at 12 months that was not subsequently evident at 18 months.

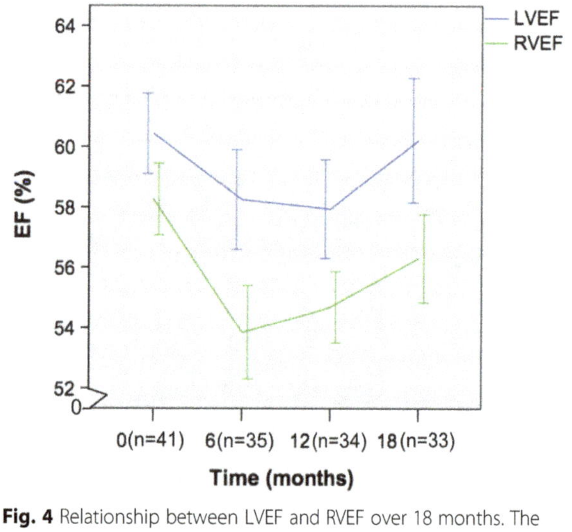

Fig. 4 Relationship between LVEF and RVEF over 18 months. The changes in LVEF and RVEF paralleled each other over time. Both the LVEF and RVEF showed significant changes at 6 and 12 months that recover at 18 months

There was excellent intra-observer reproducibility; the intra-class correlation coefficients for absolute agreement were 0.97 for RVEDV and 0.98 for RVESV (both $p < 0.001$).

Discussion

In this prospective longitudinal study of 41 consecutive patients treated with trastuzumab over 18 months with rigorous blinding strategies, we found small, but significant increases in RV volumes, with a corresponding subtle reduction in RVEF during trastuzumab therapy. These changes were no longer significant after completion of trastuzumab therapy (18 months). The pattern of temporal changes in LVEF and RVEF paralleled each other but showed only weak and non-significant correlation. By demonstrating that CMR can detect even subclinical RV changes in breast cancer patients treated with trastuzumab, our study provides further support for the use of CMR in research and clinical practice.

The cardiotoxic effect of trastuzumab in breast cancer patients has been explained on the basis of HER2 receptors in cardiomyocytes. Trastuzumab blocks these HER2 receptors in the cardiomyocytes rendering both RV and LV vulnerable to type II or reversible cardiotoxicity [7, 8]. Theoretically, the thinner structure of the RV with lesser myofibrils may make it more vulnerable to cardiotoxicity induced by trastuzumab [18, 24]. A decrease in RV function and RV hypertrophy have been associated with an increased risk of morbidity and mortality in other diseases such as heart failure, post myocardial infarction, congenital heart disease and dilated cardiomyopathy [12–16]. Furthermore, changes in RV function over time have been shown to confer incremental prognostic value in dilated cardiomyopathy [16].

RV dysfunction has been demonstrated as RV wall motion abnormalities [20] or functional abnormalities [18, 24] in patients receiving anthracyclines and trastuzumab. Initial studies evaluating trastuzumab induced RV dysfunction utilized 2D-echocardiography, which has limited accuracy in assessing RV size and function owing to its shape and position, and other inherent drawbacks including operator dependency and need for a good acoustic window for accurate measurements [29]. Furthermore, the results based on these echocardiography studies have been inconsistent [30]. Lange et al. used 2D-echocardiography at baseline, 3 and 6 months after trastuzumab which showed no difference in global RV function [21], while Kilicaslan et al. demonstrated a reduction in RV function at 6 months, similar to our results [22]. Another 2D-echocardiography based study by Calleja et al. retrospectively analyzed 30 breast cancer patients with cardiotoxicity who received

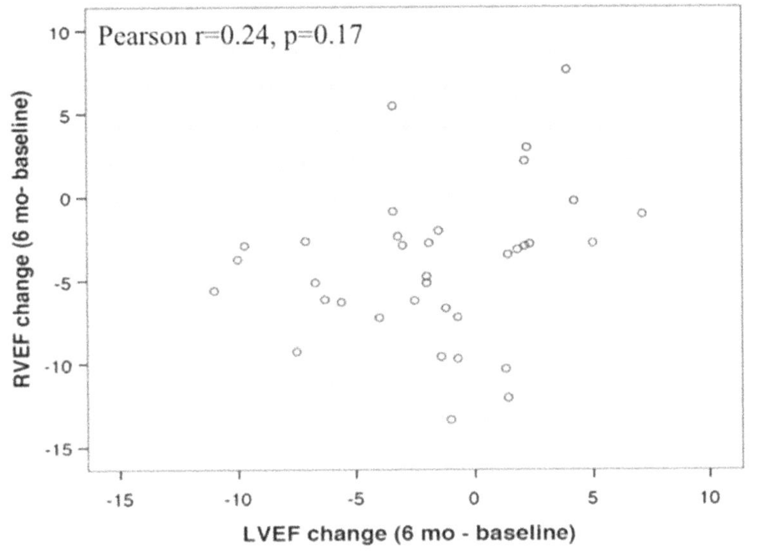

Fig. 5 Relationship between changes in RVEF and LVEF over 6 months

trastuzumab [23]. RV dysfunction based on RV fractional area change, RV global longitudinal strain and RV free wall peak systolic longitudinal strain was seen in 40% of their patients, whereas it was seen in 23% of our study participants. Most of these previous studies utilized conventional, M mode, and Doppler echocardiography derived measurements such as tricuspid annular plane systolic excursion, RV fractional area change, RV myocardial performance index to evaluate RV function. 2D-echocardiography based RV strain, although angle independent and gives information regarding global and regional strain, provides only longitudinal strain information on the apical 4 chamber view. Another important inherent limitation is loss of speckles due to motion outside the imaging plane and excessive motion of the RV lateral wall. Also, the use of different techniques, intervendor variability and lack of reference values make CMR derived RV parameters likely more robust [31]. Although 3D-echocardiography based RV strain has been used to assess RV regional wall motion abnormality in patients with tetralogy of Fallot, there was no validation of this technique with references such as 2D-echocardiography based strain or CMR [32]. Other studies have shown newer techniques like 3D-echocardiography based strain parameters to have relatively low reproducibility in comparison with 2D-echocardiography and CMR [31]. CMR has the advantage of excellent endocardial definition, accurate volumetric measurements with no geometric assumptions, and is therefore the reference standard for RV volumes and RVEF.

To the best of our knowledge, there have been only two published studies utilizing CMR to evaluate the effects of trastuzumab therapy on the RV [17, 18]. However, it is difficult to draw conclusions from these previous studies as trastuzumab was only utilized in a third (15/46) of patients in one study [18], while only 9 of 16 patients in the other study were evaluated by CMR [17]. Furthermore, neither study had follow-up beyond 1 year. The RVEDV, RVESV and RVEF remained unchanged over the time period in the small study of 9 patients [17]. In contrast, Grover et al. demonstrated a significant decline in RV function at 4 months that persisted at 12 months; thereafter RV function was not re-assessed [18]. Our results supported their findings of decline in RV function during treatment. Importantly, we have also demonstrated a recovery of RVEF at 18 months (6 months post completion of trastuzumab therapy) which has not been reported previously. Furthermore, to the best of our knowledge, no study has reported the relationship between the temporal changes in the RVEF and LVEF among patients receiving trastuzumab. Our study revealed only a weak and non-significant correlation between change in LVEF and RVEF over time. This suggests that early RV changes cannot be reliably detected by monitoring LV *alone*.

Previous studies have assessed longitudinal changes in NT-BNP but not relationship between NT-BNP and RVEF. Similar to results by Grover et al. and Nakano et al., we did not find a significant change in NT-BNP before and after initiation of trastuzumab therapy. In addition, we observed no significant correlation between NT-BNP and RVEF and RV volumes. This novel finding implies that NT-BNP may not be a useful biomarker for subclinical changes in RV function. This may be explained by the only subtle changes in RV structure and function in our participants, who were not selected based on presence of overt cardiotoxicity. It is also plausible that most of the BNP originates from the LV rather than the RV. These findings further support the use of CMR as a unique non-invasive imaging modality to detect the early or subclinical RV changes, for which biomarkers may not be a reliable surrogate.

Several study limitations should be noted. Our study cohort was relatively small, but it is the largest longitudinal study published to date of trastuzumab-treated patients using CMR, and adds to the existing literature which has been scarce. A few patients did not complete all 4 scheduled CMR scans over 18 months, but the linear mixed model allowed all available CMR data to be analyzed. We did not evaluate short term (1–4 months) and long term effects (>18 months) on the RV. Nevertheless, the aim of our study was to accurately assess the temporal changes in RV over 18 months, and compare it to the LV, which is unique to our study. We utilized RVEF and not RV strain to evaluate RV function due to its thin free wall. Our study did not have adequate power to examine the significance of cardiovascular risk factors and to assess clinical outcomes, but RVEF is expected to carry prognostic value as in other disease states [12–16]. While we speculate that the small subclinical RV changes that we observed in our cohort *without* overt cardiotoxicity are likely not clinically significant, future studies are needed to precisely determine the prognostic and therapeutic implications of the *spectrum and progression* of RV changes. Importantly, this study demonstrates the potential of CMR to detect the *early* and subtle changes in RV function, even *before* the development of overt cardiotoxicity.

As a multicenter study with utilization of two vendors for the performance of CMR and broader representation of patients, our study has greater generalizability in routine clinical practice in the real world. Furthermore, in contrast to previous studies, this prospective cohort study employed a rigorous blinding strategy, in which a single observer was blinded to all the clinical data, time of occurrence, and the LV parameters, thereby reducing bias. The demonstration of the detrimental effect of trastuzumab on the RV during the course of treatment, with recovery 6 months post completion of treatment, is novel and biologically plausible. The observation of weak and non-significant correlation between the pattern of temporal changes in LVEF and RVEF has also not been reported in the existing literature. Importantly, it illustrates that monitoring of LVEF alone may not reveal subtle changes in RV structure and function during trastuzumab therapy. Our findings support the recent American Society of Echocardiography guidelines [33] which recommend routine follow up of RV and LV during cancer therapy. An accurate and reproducible imaging technique such as CMR may be particularly valuable in this setting.

Our study raises several important questions for future research. Although it remains to be determined whether RV dysfunction provides incremental prognostic information specifically in this patient population, the current definition of cardiotoxicity (arbitrarily based on a decline in LVEF only) may not always adequately reflect cardiac injury. While isolated RVEF decline may not warrant treatment discontinuation, its prevalence and clinical significance need to be elucidated. Currently, AHA/ACC practice guidelines for heart failure recommend angiotensin converting enzyme inhibitors or angiotensin receptor blockers and beta-blockers for asymptomatic LV dysfunction (stage B heart failure). It would be important to determine whether these neurohormonal modulators would also be cardioprotective for the RV. With emerging sequences such as T1 and T2 mapping and extracellular volume assessment, there is potential for CMR to provide comprehensive assessment of cardiotoxicity. Further studies should determine whether these "imaging biomarkers" may furnish greater or incremental utility beyond the serum biomarkers (TnI and NT-BNP) in monitoring cardiotoxicity.

Conclusion

There were small but significant increases in RV volumes, with a corresponding subtle reduction in RVEF during trastuzumab therapy. The pattern of temporal changes in LVEF and RVEF paralleled each other but revealed only weak and non-significant correlation. In addition to accurate assessment of LV function and scar, CMR is a unique, safe, and promising modality to reliably monitor deterioration in RV function. Further studies are required to determine its prognostic and therapeutic implications.

Abbreviations

CI: Confidence interval; CMR: Cardiovascular magnetic resonance; EDV: End-diastolic volume; EF: Ejection fraction; ESV: End-systolic volume; HER2: Human epidermal growth factor receptor 2; hs-TnI: High-sensitivity troponin I; LGE: Late gadolinium enhancement; LV: Left ventricle; NT-BNP: N-terminal prohormone of brain natriuretic peptide; NYHA: New York Heart Association (NYHA); RV: Right ventricle

Acknowledgements

We thank all the study coordinators and patients who participated in this study, and Rosane Nisenbaum who assisted in data management.

Funding

This study was supported by an operating grant from the Canadian Institutes of Health Research and an industry partnered grant from Roche Canada. The study sponsors had no role in the study design, data collection or analysis, interpretation of the findings, writing the manuscript or the decision to submit the manuscript for publication.

Authors' contributions

AB Study conception and design, data analysis and interpretation, drafting and revision of the manuscript. CBM Study conception and design, data analysis and interpretation, revision of the manuscript. KAC Data analysis and interpretation, manuscript revision. VD analysis and interpretation, manuscript revision. KKWC Data analysis and interpretation, manuscript revision. RH analysis and interpretation, manuscript revision. AK analysis and interpretation, manuscript revision. JJB Data analysis and interpretation, manuscript revision. LJJ analysis and interpretation, manuscript revision. GRK analysis and interpretation, manuscript revision. DPD Study conception and design, data analysis and interpretation, revision of the manuscript. ATY Study conception and design, data analysis and interpretation, manuscript revision. All authors read and approved the final manuscript.

Competing interests

AB, none; CBM, none; KAC, none; VD, none; KKWC, none; RH, none; AK, none; JJB, none; LJJ, none; GK, none; DPD, none; ATY, none.

Author details

[1]Department of Medical Imaging, St. Michael's Hospital, University of Toronto, Toronto, ON, Canada. [2]Division of Hematology/Oncology, St. Michael's Hospital, University of Toronto, Toronto, ON, Canada. [3]Keenan Research Centre, Li Ka Shing Knowledge Institute, St. Michael's Hospital, University of Toronto, Toronto, ON, Canada. [4]Terrence Donnelly Heart Centre, St. Michael's Hospital, University of Toronto, Toronto, ON, Canada. [5]Division of Cardiology, St. Michael's Hospital, University of Toronto, Toronto, ON, Canada. [6]Sunnybrook Health Sciences Centre, University of Toronto, Cancer Care Ontario, Canadian Center for Applied Research in Cancer Control, Toronto, ON, Canada. [7]Department of Medical Imaging, Sunnybrook Health Sciences Centre, University of Toronto, Toronto, ON, Canada.

References

1. American Cancer Society. Cancer Facts & Figures 2015. Cancer Facts Fig 2015. 2015;1–9.
2. Canadian Cancer Society. Canadian Cancer Statistics Special topic : Predictions of the future burden of cancer in Canada. Public Heal Agency Canada. 2015;1–151.
3. Krishnamurti U, Silverman JF. HER2 in breast cancer: a review and update. Adv Anat Pathol. 2014;21:100–7.
4. Ramakrishna N, Temin S, Chandarlapaty S, Crews JR, Davidson NE, Esteva FJ, Giordano SH, Gonzalez-Angulo AM, Kirshner JJ, Krop I, Levinson J, Modi S, Patt DA, Perez EA, Perlmutter J, Winer EP, Lin NU. Recommendations on disease management for patients with advanced human epidermal growth factor receptor 2-positive breast cancer and brain metastases: American society of clinical oncology clinical practice guideline. J Clin Oncol. 2014;32: 2100–8.
5. Seidman A, Hudis C, Pierri MK, Shak S, Paton V, Ashby M, Murphy M, Stewart SJ, Keefe D. Cardiac dysfunction in the trastuzumab clinical trials experience. J Clin Oncol. 2002;20:1215–21.
6. Cardinale D, Colombo A, Torrisi R, Sandri MT, Civelli M, Salvatici M, Lamantia G, Colombo N, Cortinovis S, Dessanai MA, Nolè F, Veglia F, Cipolla CM. Trastuzumab-induced cardiotoxicity: clinical and prognostic implications of troponin I evaluation. J Clin Oncol. 2010;28:3910–6.
7. Ewer MS, Lippman SM. Type II chemotherapy-related cardiac dysfunction: time to recognize a new entity. J Clin Oncol. 2005;23:2900–2.
8. Tan-Chiu E, Yothers G, Romond E, Geyer CE, Ewer M, Keefe D, Shannon RP, Swain SM, Brown A, Fehrenbacher L, Vogel VG, Seay TE, Rastogi P, Mamounas EP, Wolmark N, Bryant J. Assessment of cardiac dysfunction in a randomized trial comparing doxorubicin and cyclophosphamide followed by paclitaxel, with or without trastuzumab as adjuvant therapy in node-positive, human epidermal growth factor receptor 2-overexpressing breast can. J Clin Oncol. 2005;23:7811–9.
9. Chrysohoou C, Antoniou C-K, Kotrogiannis I, Metallinos G, Aggelis A, Andreou I, Brili S, Pitsavos C, Stefanadis C. Role of right ventricular systolic function on long-term outcome in patients with newly diagnosed systolic heart failure. Circ J. 2011;75(September):2176–81.
10. Guendouz S, Rappeneau S, Nahum J, Dubois-Rande J-L, Gueret P, Monin J-L, Lim P, Adnot S, Hittinger L, Damy T. Prognostic significance and normal values of 2D strain to assess right ventricular systolic function in chronic heart failure. Circ J. 2012;76:127–36.
11. Haddad F, Doyle R, Murphy DJ, Hunt SA. Right ventricular function in cardiovascular disease, part II: pathophysiology, clinical importance, and management of right ventricular failure. Circulation. 2008;117:1717–31.
12. Ghio S, Gavazzi A, Campana C, Inserra C, Klersy C, Sebastiani R, Arbustini E, Recusani F. TL: independent and additive prognostic value of right ventricular systolic function and pulmonary artery pressure in patients with chronic heart failure. J Am Coll Cardiol. 2001;37:183–8.
13. Kawut SM, Barr RG, Lima JAC, Praestgaard A, Johnson WC, Chahal H, Ogunyankin KO, Bristow MR, Kizer JR, Tandri H, Bluemke DA. Right ventricular structure is associated with the risk of heart failure and cardiovascular death: the multi-ethnic study of atherosclerosis (MESA)-right ventricle study. Circulation. 2012;126:1681–8.
14. Sabe MA, Sabe SA, Kusunose K, Flamm SD, Griffin BP, Kwon DH. Predictors and prognostic significance of right ventricular ejection fraction in patients with ischemic CardiomyopathyClinical perspective. Circulation. 2016;134:656–65.
15. Gulati A, Ismail TF, Jabbour A, Alpendurada F, Guha K, Ismail NA, Raza S, Khwaja J, Brown TDH, Morarji K, Liodakis E, Roughton M, Wage R, Pakrashi TC, Sharma R, Carpenter JP, Cook SA, Cowie MR, Assomull RG, Pennell DJ, Prasad SK. The prevalence and prognostic significance of right ventricular systolic dysfunction in nonischemic dilated cardiomyopathy. Circulation. 2013;128:1623–33.
16. Merlo M, Gobbo M, Stolfo D, Losurdo P, Ramani F, Barbati G, Pivetta A, Di Lenarda A, Anzini M, Gigli M, Pinamonti B. GS: The Prognostic Impact of the Evolution of Right Ventricular Function in Idiopathic Dilated Cardiomyopathy. JACC Cardiovasc Imaging. 2016;9:1034–42.
17. Nakano S, Takahashi M, Kimura F, Senoo D, Saeki T, Ueda S, Tanno J, Senbonmatsu T, Kasai T, Nishimura S. Cardiac magnetic resonance imaging-based myocardial strain study for evaluation of cardiotoxicity in breast cancer patients treated with trastuzumab: a pilot study to evaluate the feasibility of the method. Cardiol J. 2016;23:270–80.
18. Grover S, Leong DP, Chakrabarty A, Joerg L, Kotasek D, Cheong K, Joshi R, Joseph MX, Depasquale C, Koczwara B, Selvanayagam JB. Left and right ventricular effects of anthracycline and trastuzumab chemotherapy: a prospective study using novel cardiac imaging and biochemical markers. Int J Cardiol. 2013;168:5465–7.
19. Cottin Y, Touzery C, Coudert B, Richebourg S, Cohen M, Toubeau M, Louis P, Wolf JE, Brunotte F. Diastolic or systolic left and right ventricular impairment at moderate doses of anthracycline? A 1-year follow-up study of women. Eur J Nucl Med. 1996;23:511–6.
20. Barendswaard EC, Prpic H, Van der Wall EE, Camps JA, Keizer HJ, Pauwels EK. Right ventricle wall motion abnormalities in patients treated with chemotherapy. Clin Nucl Med. 1991;16:513–6.
21. Lange SA, Ebner B, Wess A, Kögel M, Gajda M, Hitschold T, Jung J. Echocardiography signs of early cardiac impairment in patients with breast cancer and trastuzumab therapy. Clin Res Cardiol. 2012;101:415–26.
22. Kılıçaslan B, Özdoğan Ö, Demir Pişkin G, Kahya Eren N, Dursun H. Echocardiographic signs of right ventricle changes after trastuzumab treatment in breast cancer patients with erb-2 overexpression. Anatol J Cardiol. 2015;15:143–8.
23. Calleja A, Poulin F, Khorolsky K, Bedard PL, Shariat M, Amir E, Rakowski H, McDonald M, Delgado D, Thavendiranathan P. Right ventricular dysfunction in patients with breast cancer experiencing cardiotoxicity during trastuzumab therapy. J Oncol. 2015;65:A940.
24. Tanindi A, Demirci U, Tacoy G, Buyukberber S, Alsancak Y, Coskun U, Yalcin R, Benekli M. Assessment of right ventricular functions during cancer chemotherapy. Eur J Echocardiogr. 2011;12:834–40.
25. Goetschalckx K, Rademakers F, Bogaert J. Right ventricular function by MRI. Curr Opin Cardiol. 2010;25:451–5.
26. Mackey JR, Clemons M, Côté MA, Delgado D, Dent S, Paterson A, Provencher L, Sawyer MB, Verma S. Cardiac management during adjuvant trastuzumab therapy: recommendations of the Canadian Trastuzumab Working Group. Curr Oncol. 2008;15:24–35.
27. Schulz-Menger J, Bluemke DA, Bremerich J, Flamm SD, Fogel MA, Friedrich MG, Kim RJ, Von Knobelsdorff-Brenkenhoff F, Kramer CM, Pennell DJ, Plein S, Nagel E. Standardized image interpretation and post processing in cardiovascular magnetic resonance: society for cardiovascular magnetic resonance (SCMR) board of trustees task force on standardized post

processing. J Cardiovasc Magn Reson. 2013;15:1.
28. Kawel-Boehm N, Maceira A, Valsangiacomo-Buechel ER, Vogel-Claussen J, Turkbey EB, Williams R, Plein S, Tee M, Eng J, Bluemke DA. Normal values for cardiovascular magnetic resonance in adults and children. J Cardiovasc Magn Reson. 2015;17:29.
29. Marcus FI, McKenna WJ, Sherrill D, Basso C, Bauce B, Bluemke DA, Calkins H, Corrado D, Cox MGPJ, Daubert JP, Fontaine G, Gear K, Hauer R, Nava A, Picard MH, Protonotarios N, Saffitz JE, Yoerger Sanborn DM, Steinberg JS, Tandri H, Thiene G, Towbin JA, Tsatsopoulou A, Wichter T, Zareba W. Diagnosis of arrhythmogenic right ventricular cardiomyopathy/dysplasia: proposed modification of the task force criteria. Circulation. 2010;121:1533–41.
30. Tadic M, Cuspidi C, Ivanovic B. How does trastuzumab treatment affect the right ventricle in females with breast cancer? Anatol J Cardiol. 2015;15:149–50.
31. Tadic M. Multimodality evaluation of the right ventricle: an updated review. Clin Cardiol. 2015;38:770–6.
32. Atsumi A, Ishizu T, Kameda Y, Yamamoto M, Harimura Y, Machino-Ohtsuka T, Kawamura R, Enomoto M, Seo Y, Aonuma K. Application of 3-dimensional speckle tracking imaging to the assessment of right ventricular regional deformation. Circ J. 2013;77(July):1760–8.
33. Plana JC, Galderisi M, Barac A, Ewer MS, Ky B, Scherrer-Crosbie M, Ganame J, Sebag IA, Agler DA, Badano LP, Banchs J, Cardinale D, Carver J, Cerqueira M, Decara JM, Edvardsen T, Flamm SD, Force T, Griffin BP, Jerusalem G, Liu JE, Magalhães A, Marwick T, Sanchez LY, Sicari R, Villarraga HR, Lancellotti P. Expert consensus for multimodality imaging evaluation of adult patients during and after cancer therapy: a report from the American society of echocardiography and the European association of cardiovascular imaging. J Am Soc Echocardiogr. 2014;27:911–39.

10

Impaired right ventricular contractile function in childhood obesity and its association with right and left ventricular changes: a cine DENSE cardiac magnetic resonance study

Linyuan Jing[1,2], Arichanah Pulenthiran[1,2], Christopher D. Nevius[1,2], Abba Mejia-Spiegeler[1,2], Jonathan D. Suever[1,2], Gregory J. Wehner[3], H. Lester Kirchner[2], Christopher M. Haggerty[1,2] and Brandon K. Fornwalt[1,2,4*]

Abstract

Background: Pediatric obesity is a growing public health problem, which is associated with increased risk of cardiovascular disease and premature death. Left ventricular (LV) remodeling (increased myocardial mass and thickness) and contractile dysfunction (impaired longitudinal strain) have been documented in obese children, but little attention has been paid to the right ventricle (RV). We hypothesized that obese/overweight children would have evidence of RV remodeling and contractile dysfunction.

Methods: One hundred and three children, ages 8–18 years, were prospectively recruited and underwent cardiovascular magnetic resonance (CMR), including both standard cine imaging and displacement encoding with stimulated echoes (DENSE) imaging, which allowed for quantification of RV geometry and function/mechanics. RV free wall longitudinal strain was quantified from the end-systolic four-chamber DENSE image. Linear regression was used to quantify correlations of RV strain with LV strain and measurements of body composition (adjusted for sex and height). Analysis of variance was used to study the relationship between RV strain and LV remodeling types (concentric remodeling, eccentric/concentric hypertrophy).

Results: The RV was sufficiently visualized with DENSE in 70 (68%) subjects, comprising 36 healthy weight (13.6 ± 2.7 years) and 34 (12.1 ± 2.9 years) obese/overweight children. Obese/overweight children had a 22% larger RV mass index (8.2 ± 0.9 vs 6.7 ± 1.1 g/m$^{2.7}$, $p < 0.001$) compared to healthy controls. RV free wall longitudinal strain was impaired in obese/overweight children (−16 ± 4% vs −19 ± 5%, $p = 0.02$). Ten (14%) out of 70 children had LV concentric hypertrophy, and these children had the most impaired RV longitudinal strain compared to those with normal LV geometry (−13 ± 4% vs −19 ± 5%, $p = 0.002$). RV longitudinal strain was correlated with LV longitudinal strain ($r = 0.34$, $p = 0.004$), systolic blood pressure ($r = 0.33$, $p = 0.006$), as well as BMI z-score ($r = 0.28$, $p = 0.02$), waist ($r = 0.31$, $p = 0.01$), hip ($r = 0.40$, $p = 0.004$) and abdominal ($r = 0.38$, $p = 0.002$) circumference, height and sex adjusted.

(Continued on next page)

* Correspondence: bkf@gatech.edu
[1]Department of Imaging Science and Innovation, Geisinger Health System, 100 North Academy Avenue, Danville 17822-4400, PA, USA
[2]Biomedical and Translational Informatics Institute, Geisinger Health System, Danville, PA, USA
Full list of author information is available at the end of the article

(Continued from previous page)

Conclusions: Obese/overweight children have evidence of RV remodeling (increased RV mass) and RV contractile dysfunction (impaired free wall longitudinal strain). Moreover, RV longitudinal strain correlates with LV longitudinal strain, and children with LV concentric hypertrophy show the most impaired RV function. These results suggest there may be a common mechanism underlying both remodeling and dysfunction of the left and right ventricles in obese/overweight children.

Keywords: DENSE, Right ventricle, Strain, Pediatric obesity

Background

Childhood obesity is a rapidly growing public health problem. Recent studies in the United States show that 17% of children and adolescents (2–19 years) are obese, while 5.8% are severely obese [1]. A longitudinal study which followed over two million adolescents into adulthood showed that pediatric obesity is linked to increased risk of mortality in adulthood [2]. Although the exact mechanisms are not well understood, evidence suggests that this premature mortality is likely attributed to early onset of cardiovascular diseases [3].

Prior research has focused primarily on changes in the structure and function of the left ventricle (LV) in obese/overweight children using echocardiography or cardiovascular magnetic resonance (CMR). Major findings include: LV remodeling, evidenced by increased LV myocardial mass and wall thickness [4–6]; contractile dysfunction, measured by impaired LV longitudinal and circumferential strain [6–8]; and diastolic dysfunction, indicated by reduced early (E) and late (A) relaxation velocity as well as decreased E/A ratio [4, 5]. Moreover, approximately 25% of obese children have LV concentric hypertrophy [9], the type of remodeling that is most closely related to early mortality in adults [10]. A recent CMR study showed that obese children with LV concentric hypertrophy demonstrate the most impaired LV longitudinal and circumferential strains, despite normal ejection fraction [6].

Despite mounting evidence of LV remodeling and dysfunction, little is known about the right heart in obese children. There is growing appreciation that right ventricular (RV) dysfunction is related to adverse outcomes [11–13]. RV remodeling (larger RV mass and volumes) and impaired systolic and diastolic function have been documented in overweight and obese adults [14–17]. Moreover, there is evidence of potential links between LV and RV function in obese adults [14]. Thus, obese children with LV concentric hypertrophy and impaired LV strain/function may also suffer from RV remodeling and impaired RV function. Information on RV geometry and function could facilitate the identification of obese children who are at high risk of adverse outcomes, as well as provide new insights into the etiology underlying cardiac dysfunction in the setting of pediatric obesity.

Only a few studies have investigated obesity-related changes in RV geometry and function in children, but the findings are conflicting [4, 5, 18–21]: both no change and a decrease in RV systolic function were reported. These conflicting reports may result from the fact that all previous studies have utilized echocardiography (tissue Doppler imaging) to quantify RV function. This methodology suffers from poor image quality and high angle dependency of the imaging plane, especially in the RV [22]. These limitations preclude direct and comprehensive characterization of RV structure and function with echocardiography. Magnetic resonance imaging has excellent image quality and is the gold standard for reproducibly imaging the RV [23]. Moreover, cine displacement encoding with stimulated echoes (DENSE), an advanced CMR technique, encodes displacement of myocardial tissue into CMR phase images, providing adequate resolution to quantify displacement and strain of the RV [24]. To our knowledge, no study has investigated changes in RV structure and function in obese children using CMR. We hypothesized that obese children would have enlarged RV mass as well as impaired contractile function (strain), and that these changes would be associated with LV remodeling and function.

Methods

Study population

Children ages 8–18 years were prospectively recruited from University of Kentucky (the High BMI Diagnostic Clinic, and the Center for Clinical and Translational Science volunteer database) and Geisinger Medical Center. Children were categorized based on their body mass index (BMI) percentiles defined by the United States Centers for Disease Control and Prevention (CDC) growth charts [25]: obese (BMI ≥95th percentile), overweight (BMI 85th–95th percentile) and healthy weight (BMI 5th–85th percentile). Exclusion criteria included diabetes, diagnosed hypertension, history of heart disease, contraindications for CMR, or a waist circumference >125 cm due to the circumference limitation of the bore of the CMR scanner. Children with conditions that could potentially alter right heart function (e.g. obstructive sleep apnea, pulmonary hypertension or lung disease) were excluded. A subgroup (two-thirds) of the subjects were included in a previous study focused on LV remodeling and function (strain) [6].

Clinical assessment

At the time of the CMR scan, height and weight, each averaged from two readings, were measured, and BMI (weight/height^2 in kg/m^2) percentiles were determined. Measurements of the waist, abdominal, and hip circumferences were taken twice with a tailor's scale, and the average values were reported. After being seated for at least 10 min, an appropriately sized cuff was used to measure resting blood pressure by auscultation three times, 5 min apart. The average of the last two readings was reported. All children had a normal 12-lead electrocardiogram (ECG).

CMR imaging

All subjects underwent CMR on a 3 T system (Tim Trio, Siemens Healthcare, Erlangen, Germany) using 6-element chest and 24-element spine coils. All CMRs were conducted solely for research purposes and not for clinical indications. Standard ECG-gated balanced steady-state free-precession (SSFP) images in two- and four-chamber views were acquired during 10–15 s breath-holds. Depending on the size of the heart, a stack of 7–11 short-axis SSFP images spanning both ventricles were acquired for assessment of cardiac geometry. Acquisition parameters were: repetition time (TR) = 3.16–3.37 ms, echo time (TE) = 1.3–1.5 ms, field of view (FOV) = [292–400] × [340–400] mm^2, image matrix = [208–256] × 256, flip angle = 50°, temporal resolution = 16.4–49.9 ms, slice thickness = 8 mm, slice gap = 0–3.7 mm.

Spiral cine DENSE imaging was performed in the two-chamber and four-chamber long-axis views to quantify LV and RV longitudinal strain. A respiratory navigator with an acceptance window of ±3 mm was used to maintain consistent breath-hold position. The acquisition parameters for DENSE images were: 6 or 18 spiral interleaves, in-plane simple displacement encoding (k_e = 0.1 cycles/mm), TE/TR = 1.08/17 ms, flip angle = variable 20°, voxel size = 2.8 × 2.8 × 8 or 1.6 × 1.6 × 8 mm^3, FOV = 360 × 360 or 340 × 340 mm^2, image matrix = 128 × 128 or 214 × 214, temporal resolution = 34 ms (view sharing was used to achieve 17 ms between reconstructed temporal frames). CSPAMM was used for echo suppression.

Image analysis

Endocardial and epicardial boundaries of the RV were manually delineated on end-diastolic and end-systolic frames on all short-axis SSFP slices covering the whole ventricle. Simpson's rule was used to calculate RV end-diastolic (EDV) and end-systolic (ESV) volumes. RV stroke volume (SV = EDV - ESV) and ejection fraction (SV/EDVx100%) were also derived. RV myocardial mass was calculated from the epicardial and endocardial contours on the end-diastolic frame, assuming a myocardial density of 1.05 g/mL, and indexed to height (meters$^{2.7}$).

RV free wall longitudinal strain was quantified from the four-chamber DENSE acquisition (Fig. 1). End-systolic phase images encoding the horizontal (Fig. 1a) and vertical (Fig. 1b) displacements were acquired using 2D spiral cine DENSE. The RV free wall and the interventricular septum were segmented using *DENSEanalysis* [26]. DENSE post-processing was customized [27] to remove temporal smoothing and instantaneously quantify strain using only the end-systolic frame, as determined visually based on the minimum chamber area. Specifically, the displacements for each pixel in the systolic image (black dots in Fig. 1c) relative to end-diastole (grey dots in Fig. 1c) were extracted directly from the

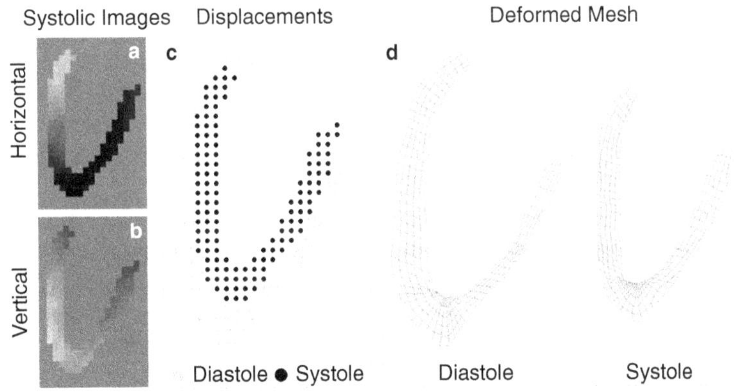

Fig. 1 Right ventricular (*RV*) strain analysis. End-systolic phase images encoding the *horizontal* (**a**) and vertical (**b**) displacements were acquired using 2D spiral cine DENSE. The displacements for each pixel in the end-systolic image (*black dots* in **c**) relative to end-diastole (*grey dots* in **c**) were extracted directly from the phase images. A mesh of the RV myocardium was deformed from diastole to systole using these displacements (**d**), and strains were computed for each mesh element

phase images. Using these displacements, a mesh of the RV myocardium was deformed from diastole to systole (Fig. 1d) and strains were computed for each mesh element. Only RV free wall elements were retained for the analysis. Notably, the analysis of a single time phase in this way was the original approach used for DENSE imaging, prior to the development of the cine version of DENSE [28].

Standard DENSE post-processing was performed to compute LV longitudinal strain in order to study its relationship with RV strain. Analysis included manual segmentation of the LV myocardium, phase unwrapping, tissue tracking throughout the cardiac cycle to derive displacements of the myocardial tissue, and strain calculation as previously described [29, 30]. LV peak longitudinal strain was averaged from the two- and four-chamber views.

To investigate the relationship between RV function/strain and LV remodeling, epicardial and endocardial boundaries of the LV were manually drawn on end-diastolic and end-systolic frames of the SSFP slices. These contours were then used to reconstruct 3D endocardial and epicardial surfaces using a custom algorithm written in MATLAB (The Mathworks, Natick, MA) as previously described [6]. LV volumes, LV myocardial mass (assuming a myocardial density of 1.05 g/mL), and ejection fraction were then calculated from the 3D models. LV myocardial mass was indexed to height (LVMI, grams/meters$^{2.7}$) [31]. Cardiac remodeling types (normal geometry, concentric remodeling, eccentric hypertrophy, concentric hypertrophy) were determined based on previously defined cutoff values for mass/volume ratio (0.69) and LVMI (27.52 g/m$^{2.7}$) in a healthy cohort [6].

Reproducibility

To quantify inter-observer reproducibility of RV longitudinal strain in all subjects, the end-systolic frame of the DENSE images was independently determined, segmented and analyzed by two different investigators. Bland-Altman limits of agreement and bias were computed [32].

Statistics

Continuous variables from obese/overweight and healthy groups were compared with a 2-sample student's t-test and presented as mean ± standard deviation (SD). Fisher's exact test was used to compare the sex distribution between groups. Analysis of covariance (ANCOVA) was used to estimate the differences in cardiac remodeling and function between groups, while accounting for age.

Analysis of Variance (ANOVA) was used to test for a difference in RV strains among different LV remodeling types. Due to the small observed sample sizes, the concentric remodeling and eccentric hypertrophy groups were combined. The concentric hypertrophy group and the combined concentric remodeling/eccentric hypertrophy group were both compared to the normal geometry group using Dunnett's multiple comparison procedure. Pearson's correlation coefficients were used to investigate relationships between LV and RV structural and functional measurements.

A modified coefficient of variation (CoV), which compares the variability of a given variable × relative to its mean, was used to quantify inter-observer reproducibility for RV longitudinal strain [33]. A CoV within 20% was considered reproducible. Given measurements from two observers (Ob1 and Ob2), the CoV was calculated as follows:

$$CoV = \frac{\sum_{i=1}^{N}\left[St.Dev.(X_{Ob1},\, X_{Ob2})_i\right]}{\left|\sum_{i=1}^{N}\left[((X_{Ob1} + X_{Ob2})/2)_i\right]\right|}$$

Multivariable linear regression was used to investigate the relationship between body composition (BMI z-score, waist, hip, abdominal circumference, and waist/hip ratio) and RV remodeling and function. Height and sex were controlled in the model to account for somatic growth and sex differences. Statistical significance was defined as $p \leq 0.05$. All statistical analyses were performed in R [34] (Version 3.3.1 with packages multcomp [35] and car [36]).

Results

Demographics and clinical assessment of the study population

A total of 103 subjects were prospectively recruited and underwent CMR. Of those, two subjects did not complete the CMR study. In 31 (30%) subjects, the RV was either insufficiently visualized or the phase images were not able to be unwrapped properly during post-processing due to poor image quality. The remaining 70 (68%) subjects, including 36 healthy weight and 34 overweight/obese children, were included in subsequent data analysis. Characteristics of these subjects are summarized in Table 1.

Compared to healthy weight children, systolic blood pressure was slightly elevated in the obese/overweight group. In addition, waist, hip, and abdominal circumferences were substantially larger (by 27, 20 and 31%, respectively) in obese/overweight children (all $p < 0.001$). The waist/hip ratio was also higher in obese/overweight children.

We further investigated the characteristics of the 30% of subjects who were excluded from the data analysis. No significant differences were identified in

Table 1 Demographics and Clinical Parameters (mean ± SD) of the Study Population

	Obese/Overweight $n = 34$	Healthy $n = 36$	p
Age (years)	12.1 ± 2.9	13.6 ± 2.7	0.03
Female (%)	56	47	0.49
Weight (kg)	71 ± 23	50 ± 14	<0.001
Height (cm)	155 ± 13	160 ± 17	0.23
Body Mass Index (kg/m²)	29 ± 6	19 ± 2	<0.001
Body Mass Index Percentile	96 ± 4	48 ± 23	<0.001
Body Mass Index z-score	2.0 ± 0.4	−0.1 ± 0.7	<0.001
Heart rate (beats/min)	72 ± 9	70 ± 8	0.09
Systolic blood pressure (mmHg)	116 ± 13	109 ± 8	0.02
Diastolic blood pressure (mmHg)	73 ± 6	71 ± 6	0.32
Mean arterial pressure (mmHg)	87 ± 8	84 ± 6	0.07
Abdominal Circumference (cm)	94 ± 16	72 ± 7	<0.001
Waist Circumference (cm)	85 ± 14	67 ± 6	<0.001
Hip Circumference (cm)	101 ± 16	84 ± 10	<0.001
Waist/Hip Ratio	0.85 ± 0.09	0.80 ± 0.07	0.01

demographic parameters between the excluded subjects and those included for subsequent analysis [see Additional file 1: Table S1]. In addition, the weight group distribution was similar between the two groups: 18 (58%) of the 31 excluded subjects were obese/overweight compared to 34 (49%) out of 70 in the included group, $p = 0.4$.

Right ventricular geometry and function

After adjusting for age, obese/overweight children had a 22% larger RV mass index (8.2 ± 0.9 vs 6.7 ± 1.1 g/m$^{2.7}$, $p < 0.001$), while RV volumes were comparable to healthy controls (Table 2). There was no difference in RV ejection fraction between the two groups. However, RV free wall longitudinal strain was impaired in obese/overweight children compared to healthy weight controls (−16 ± 4% vs −19 ± 5%, $p = 0.02$, Fig. 2).

Association between LV and RV remodeling and function

Consistent with previous studies [4–6], obese/overweight children had a greater LVMI and a higher mass/volume ratio compared to healthy controls (Table 2) after adjusting for age. Furthermore, LVMI correlated with RV mass index (Fig. 3a). Based on cutoff values defined in a previous study [6], ten (14%) subjects had concentric LV hypertrophy, thirteen (19%) subjects had eccentric LV hypertrophy or concentric LV remodeling, and forty-six (66%) had normal LV geometry (Fig. 4). RV free wall longitudinal strain differed among these remodeling groups ($p = 0.01$, Fig. 4), as children with concentric LV hypertrophy had significantly impaired RV strain compared to those with normal LV geometry (−13 ± 4% vs −19 ± 5%, $p = 0.002$). There was no significant difference between the combined concentric remodeling/eccentric hypertrophy group and the normal geometry group (−17 ± 3% vs −19 ± 5%, $p = 0.46$).

In addition, obese/overweight children had impaired LV longitudinal strain (−14 ± 2% vs −15 ± 2%, $p = 0.02$,

Table 2 Cardiac Geometry and Function (mean ± SD)

	Obese/Overweight $n = 34$	Healthy[a] $n = 36$	*p, age adjusted*
LV geometry and function			
LV mass index (g/m$^{2.7}$)	27 ± 4	22 ± 3	**<0.001**
LV end diastolic volume (mL)	135 ± 31	133 ± 41	0.85
LV mass/volume ratio	0.68 ± 0.10	0.60 ± 0.06	**<0.001**
LV ejection fraction (%)	62 ± 5	62 ± 4	0.99
RV geometry and function			
RV end diastolic volume (mL)	149 ± 38	147 ± 46	0.80
RV end systolic volume (mL)	60 ± 17	59 ± 23	0.84
RV stroke volume (mL)	89 ± 23	88 ± 25	0.80
RV mass (g)	27 ± 6	24 ± 7	**0.01**
RV mass index (g/m$^{2.7}$)	8.2 ± 0.9	6.7 ± 1.1	**<0.001**
RV ejection fraction (%)	60 ± 5	61 ± 5	0.68
Strain			
LV longitudinal strain (%)	−14 ± 2	−15 ± 2	**0.02**
RV free wall longitudinal strain (%)	−16 ± 4	−19 ± 5	**0.02**

Abbreviations: *LV* left ventricular, *RV* right ventricular
[a]One of the 36 healthy weight subjects did not complete cine SSFP imaging and was therefore not included in any of the measures of cardiac geometry or ejection fraction

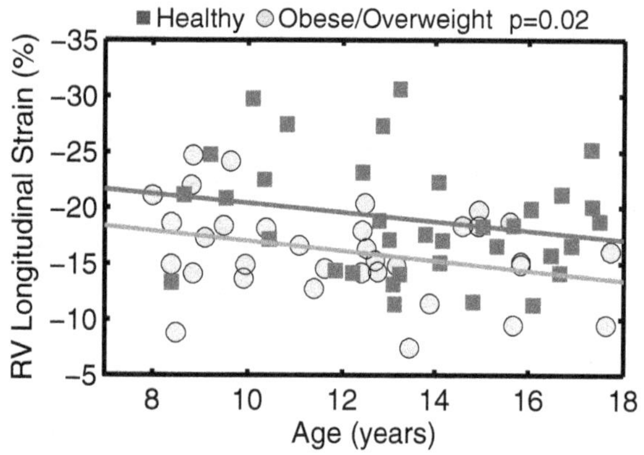

Fig. 2 Obese children across all ages have reduced longitudinal strain in the free wall of the *RV*. There was no difference between the slopes of the two *lines* while the intercepts were significantly different ($p = 0.02$), suggesting a difference in *RV longitudinal strain* independent of age between the *healthy* and *obese/overweight* groups

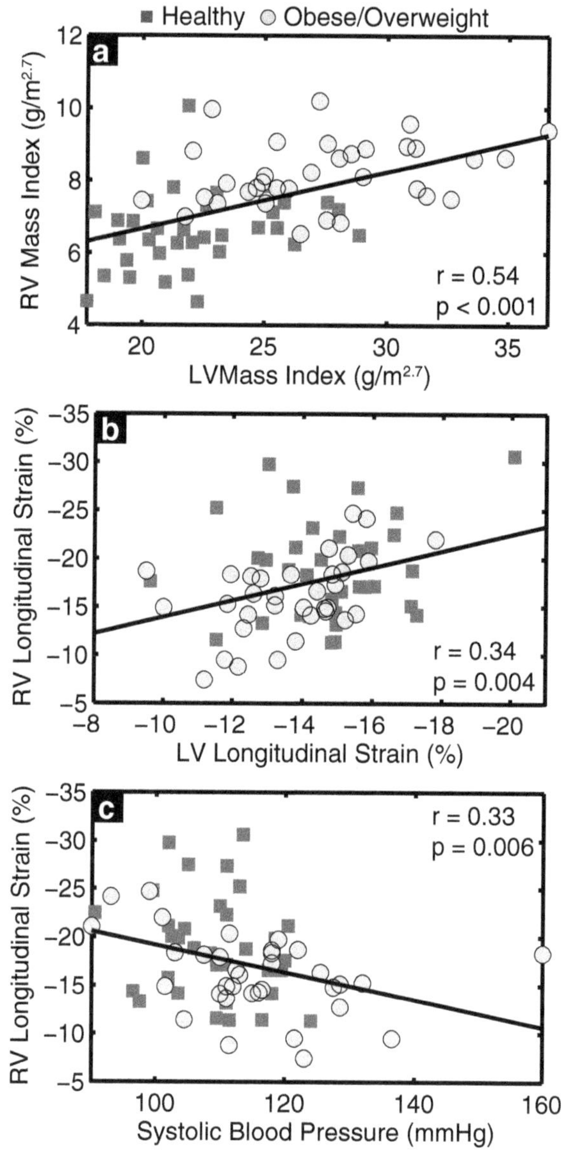

Fig. 3 Right ventricular (*RV*) *mass index* correlated with left ventricular (*LV*) *mass index* (**a**); RV free wall *longitudinal strain* was significantly associated with LV *longitudinal strain* (**b**) and systolic blood pressure (**c**)

Table 2) compared to healthy controls, and the LV longitudinal strain correlated with RV longitudinal strain (Fig. 3b). Finally, systolic blood pressure also correlated with RV longitudinal strain (Fig. 3c).

Correlation between RV function and body composition

Associations of RV function and strain with body composition measurements are summarized in Table 3. Sex and height were included in the multivariate linear regression model to account for somatic growth. Both RV mass index and RV free wall longitudinal strain moderately correlated with most measurements of body composition except waist/hip ratio (Fig. 5), and the correlations were stronger with RV mass index. RV mass index correlated most strongly with BMI z-score ($r = 0.56$, $p < 0.001$), while RV strain was more strongly correlated with abdominal ($r = 0.38$, $p = 0.002$) and hip ($r = 0.40$, $p = 0.004$) circumferences.

Reproducibility

The CoV for inter-observer reproducibility of RV longitudinal strain was 10%. This coefficient corresponds with a bias of 0.57 and 95% limits of agreement of [-5.65, 6.79] % (Fig. 6).

Discussion

We imaged 70 children (36 healthy weight and 34 obese/overweight) with CMR to quantify changes in RV volumes and function in the setting of pediatric obesity. We found that: 1) compared to healthy weight controls, obese/overweight children have increased RV mass index without changes in RV volumes or RV ejection fraction; 2) RV systolic function, measured by free wall longitudinal strain, is impaired by 14% in obese/overweight children 3) There is evidence of a common mechanism underlying RV and LV dysfunction in obese/overweight children, since RV longitudinal strain associates with LV longitudinal strain and RV longitudinal strain is most severely impaired (by 30%) in obese children with LV concentric hypertrophy; 4) RV mass and RV longitudinal strain are related to measures of body composition; 5) inter-observer reproducibility is good for RV longitudinal strain measured with DENSE at end-systole. To our knowledge, this is the first study to comprehensively characterize RV geometry and function in obese children using CMR.

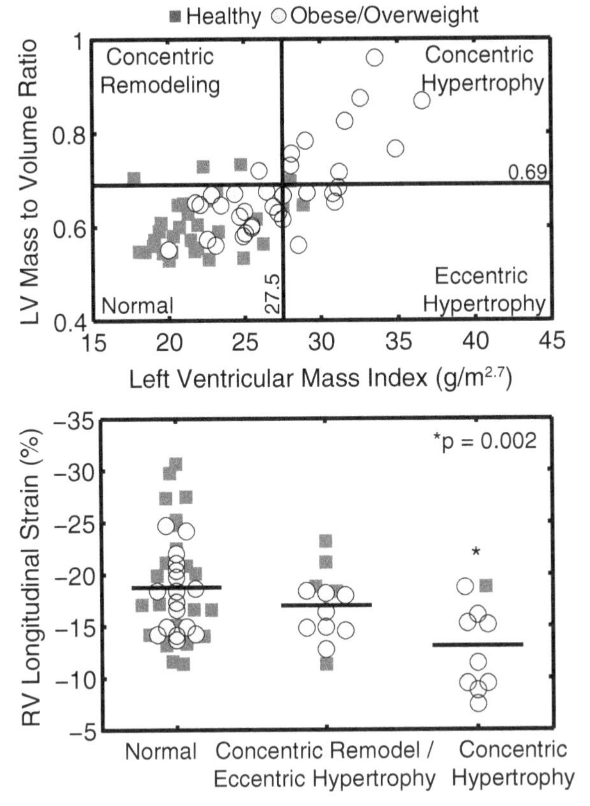

Fig. 4 Children with concentric LV hypertrophy (*top*) had the most impaired *longitudinal strain* in the RV free wall (*bottom*). *The reported *p*-value (0.002) is for the comparison between the *concentric hypertrophy* and *normal geometry* group

RV remodeling and function in pediatric obesity

While RV remodeling (increased mass and volumes) and impaired systolic and diastolic function have been documented in overweight and obese adults, this information is mostly missing and inconclusive in childhood obesity. One study by Labombarda et al. [18] reported enlarged RV end-diastolic dimension in obese children compared to healthy controls, while Mahfouz et al. [19] and Zeybek et al. [20] observed no change in RV dimensions. RV systolic function in obese children was documented by a few studies using tricuspid annular plane systolic excursion (TAPSE) or systolic velocity; however, both no change [4, 18] and decreased function [19, 21] were reported. Only one study [20] quantified RV ejection fraction, a commonly used metric for ventricular function clinically, and found no significant changes in obese children. In the current study, we found increased RV mass index and comparable RV volumes and ejection fraction between obese children and healthy weight controls, suggesting that the RV remodels with preserved ventricular volumes and global systolic function in the early stages of obesity.

Table 3 Correlation between RV Function and Body Composition after Adjusting for Sex and Height

	RV Longitudinal Strain		RV Mass Index	
	r	*p*	*r*	*p*
BMI z-score[a]	0.28	**0.02**	0.56	**<0.001**
Waist circumference	0.31	**0.01**	0.44	**<0.001**
Hip circumference	0.40	**0.004**	0.46	**<0.001**
Abdominal circumference	0.38	**0.002**	0.44	**<0.001**
Waist/Hip Ratio	0.07	0.61	0.26	0.052

Multivariate linear regression was used for each pair of predictor (body composition) and outcome (function) variables with adjustment for sex and height

[a]BMI z-score was only adjusted for sex

Measures of cardiac mechanics, such as strain, are more sensitive metrics of cardiac function than ejection fraction and are more closely related with outcomes such as death [37]. RV free wall strain and strain rate in obese children were documented by several studies using echocardiography, but their findings are again contradictory: Barbosa et al. [4] found increased RV strain and strain rate, while Di Salvo et al. [5] found decreased RV strain and strain rate in obese children. Using the advanced and highly reproducible DENSE CMR technique, our results show a 14% reduction in RV free wall longitudinal strain (Fig. 2, Table 2) in obese/overweight children compared to healthy weight controls. This finding suggests that subclinical RV contractile dysfunction exists in obese/overweight children, despite preserved RV ejection fraction.

It is worth noting that not all obese/overweight children had impaired longitudinal strain. Using previously defined cutoff values of LVMI and LV mass/volume ratio [6], we identified a subgroup of children ($n = 10$, 14%) with LV concentric hypertrophy. These children had the most impaired RV longitudinal strain (by 30%) compared to those with normal LV geometry (Fig. 4), while children with LV concentric remodeling/eccentric hypertrophy had relatively normal RV longitudinal strain. Similar findings about LV longitudinal and circumferential strain have also been reported in obese children [6]. This group of children with LV concentric hypertrophy and reduced LV and RV strain may represent a particularly high-risk phenotype with increased risk of cardiovascular disease and premature death, which deserves further investigation.

Mechanisms for RV remodeling and dysfunction

While this study did not explore the mechanisms underlying the observed ventricular remodeling and dysfunction, which are presently not well understood, the observation of several associations of RV function with LV structure and function are suggestive of common, intrinsic causal factors. For example, insulin resistance is a

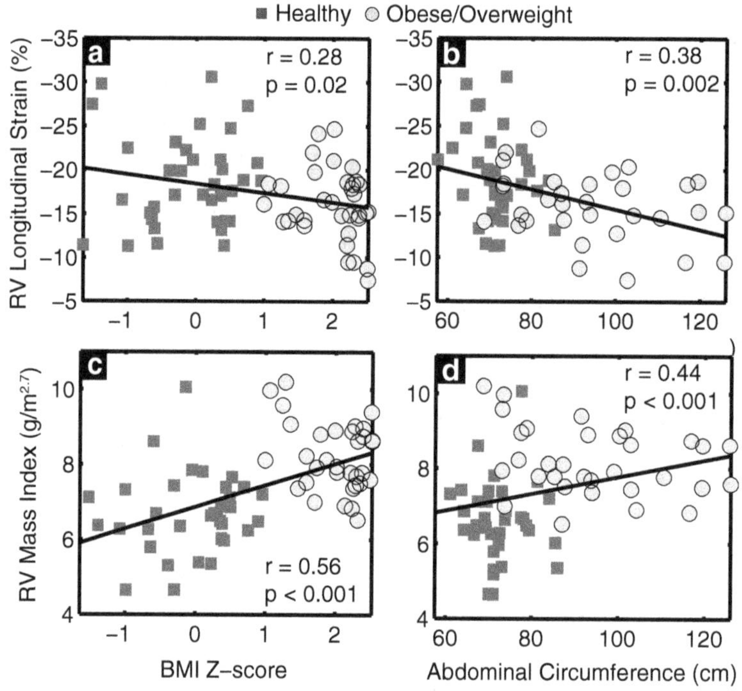

Fig. 5 RV free wall *longitudinal strain* and *RV mass index* moderately correlated with *BMI z-score* (**a** and **c**) and *abdominal circumference* (**b** and **d**)

common comorbidity in childhood obesity and is present in up to 50% of obese children [38]. Hyperinsulinemia in the setting of insulin resistance is a mediator of cardiac growth which could potentially result in hypertrophy and remodeling in both ventricles [39]. Further, hyperinsulinemia could alter contractile function directly [40]. Additionally, we also showed a significant correlation between RV longitudinal strain, RV mass index and measures of body composition independent of somatic growth (Table 3, Fig. 6), suggesting potential impact of excess adipose tissue on RV systolic dysfunction. This contribution of adiposity may be mediated through obesity-related metabolic changes such as insulin resistance and systemic inflammation, which could contribute to RV dysfunction through various growth factors and inflammatory markers [41, 42].

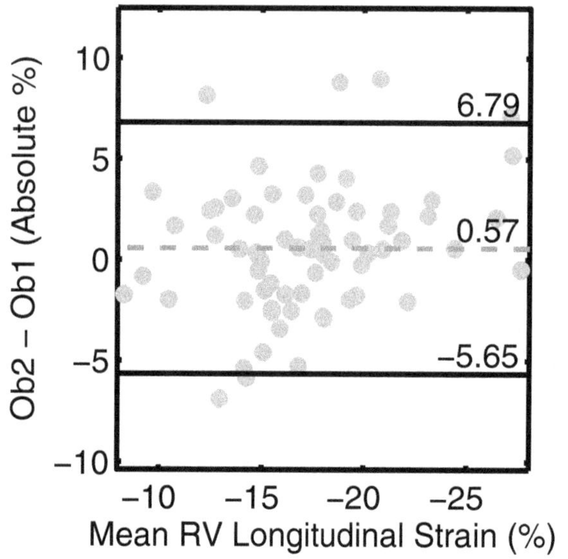

Fig. 6 Bland-Altman *plot* shows good reproducibility for *right* ventricular free wall *longitudinal strain* between two observers. *Ob2*: observer 2; *Ob1*: observer 1

Additional explanations for the observed RV dysfunction include direct mechanical factors. Interactions between the LV and RV [43, 44] are indicated by the facts that obese/overweight children with concentric hypertrophy had the most impaired RV longitudinal strain (Fig. 4), and that LV longitudinal strain and systolic blood pressure were both correlated to RV longitudinal strain (Fig. 3). Pulmonary hypertension and obstructive sleep apnea have a significant effect on RV dysfunction; however, we did not include children who were known to have those conditions. In addition, previous studies have shown no changes in pulmonary artery pressure in obese children [5, 18].

Imaging techniques for the RV

Due to its complex geometry and thin myocardial wall, imaging the RV is inherently difficult. All previous studies of RV function in the setting of obesity have used echocardiographic imaging techniques (Tissue Doppler or 2D speckle tracking), which suffer from poor image quality, limited acoustic windows and angle dependency. Physical interference of excessive adiposity with the imaging signal makes echocardiography even more challenging in obese subjects. CMR overcomes these limitations and is therefore superior to echocardiography for studying both geometry and function (strain) of the RV. As shown in the current study, 68% of subjects had adequate image quality for strain analysis, and the inter-observer reproducibility for RV longitudinal strain by DENSE was good with a coefficient of variation of 10%. To our knowledge, this is the first study to assess and report good reproducibility of RV longitudinal strain in obese children. The superior reproducibility of CMR is therefore favorable for detecting subclinical RV changes in obese children.

Limitations

This study has several limitations. Cross-sectional design of the study precludes determination of onset and development of RV dysfunction in obese children. There was a small difference in age between the healthy weight and obese/overweight groups; however, this difference was accounted for during statistical analysis.

Differences in LV and RV strains between the healthy and obese/overweight groups were relatively small. Despite reasonable inter-observer reproducibility, the limits of agreement were larger than the detected difference between the groups. This could be explained by the fact that we only enrolled uncomplicated obese children in the current study, who are likely to be at the early stage of obesity. Furthermore, due to the limitation of the CMR bore circumference, most severely obese children, who were expected to have the most structural and functional impairment, were excluded from the study.

In addition, 30% of the enrolled subjects were excluded from RV strain analysis due to the poor quality of DENSE images, although demographics of these subjects were similar to those included in the analysis. Potential explanations include inconsistent breathing pattern or subject movement during the scan, which lead to blurry images and mis-registration due to through-plane motion. Future studies with higher resolution and three-dimensional DENSE imaging could improve image quality and therefore, increase the success rate in imaging the RV [24, 45].

Finally, although obesity-related metabolic changes (insulin resistance, systemic inflammation) have been shown to contribute to ventricular remodeling and dysfunction, we did not collect any blood samples to explore the role of insulin resistance and inflammatory biomarkers in RV remodeling and dysfunction observed in the current study. Future studies need to measure insulin resistance and other inflammation markers to elucidate their contribution to RV remodeling and dysfunction in obese children.

Conclusion

Obese/overweight children have increased right ventricular mass and impaired RV contractile function compared to healthy weight children. These changes are associated with left ventricular remodeling, as those children with left ventricular concentric hypertrophy have the most impaired right ventricular longitudinal strain. These results suggest there may be a common mechanism underlying both remodeling and dysfunction of the left and right ventricles in obese/overweight children. Further study is warranted to identify these mechanisms, as well as the prognostic consequences and potential treatment options for these patients with sub-clinical cardiac dysfunction.

Abbreviations

ANCOVA: Analysis of covariance; ANOVA: Analysis of variance; BMI: Body mass index; CMR: Cardiac magnetic resonance; CoV: Coefficient of variation; DENSE: Displacement encoding with stimulated echoes; EDV: End-diastolic volume; ESV: End-systolic volume; LV: Left ventricle; LVMI: Left ventricular mass index; RV: Right ventricle; SD: Standard deviation; SSFP: Steady-state free-precession; SV: Stroke volume

Acknowledgements

Not applicable.

Funding

This project was supported by the NIH via grants P20 GM103527 and UL1 TR000117, and by the American Heart Association Great Rivers Affiliate via grant 14POST20310025. The content is solely the responsibility of the authors and does not necessarily represent the official views of the funding sources.

Authors' contributions

LJ collected and analyzed data, assisted with study design and drafted the manuscript. AP and AM analyzed data and helped with data collection and revision of the manuscript. CN helped with subject recruitment and helped to collect the data and revise the manuscript. JS and GW assisted with data acquisition and analysis, and helped with critical revision of the manuscript. HLK helped with statistical analysis for the study and critical revision of the manuscript. CH contributed to study design, data collection and interpretation, and helped with critical revision of the manuscript. BF conceived the study, participated in study design and implementation, and assisted with critical revision of the manuscript. All authors read and approved the final manuscript.

Competing interests

The authors declare that they have no competing interests.

Author details

[1]Department of Imaging Science and Innovation, Geisinger Health System, 100 North Academy Avenue, Danville 17822-4400, PA, USA. [2]Biomedical and Translational Informatics Institute, Geisinger Health System, Danville, PA, USA. [3]Department of Biomedical Engineering, University of Kentucky, Lexington, KY, USA. [4]Department of Radiology, Geisinger Health System, Danville, PA, USA.

References

1. Ogden CL, Carroll MD, Lawman HG, Fryar CD, Kruszon-Moran D, Kit BK, Flegal KM. Trends in Obesity Prevalence Among Children and Adolescents in the United States, 1988–1994 Through 2013–2014. JAMA. 2016;315:2292.
2. Twig G, Yaniv G, Levine H, Leiba A, Goldberger N, Derazne E, Ben-Ami Shor D, Tzur D, Afek A, Shamiss A, Haklai Z, Kark JD. Body-Mass Index in 2.3 Million Adolescents and Cardiovascular Death in Adulthood. N Engl J Med. 2016;374:2430–40.
3. Cote AT, Harris KC, Panagiotopoulos C, Sandor GGS, Devlin AM. Childhood obesity and cardiovascular dysfunction. J Am Coll Cardiol. 2013;62:1309–19.
4. Barbosa JA, Mota CCC, Simões E Silva AC, Nunes MDCP, Barbosa MM. Assessing pre-clinical ventricular dysfunction in obese children and adolescents: the value of speckle tracking imaging. Eur Heart J Cardiovasc Imaging. 2013;14:882–9.
5. Di Salvo G, Pacileo G, Del Giudice EM, Natale F, Limongelli G, Verrengia M, Rea A, Fratta F, Castaldi B, D'Andrea A, Calabrò P, Miele T, Coppola F, Russo MG, Caso P, Perrone L, Calabrò R. Abnormal myocardial deformation properties in obese, non-hypertensive children: an ambulatory blood pressure monitoring, standard echocardiographic, and strain rate imaging study. Eur Heart J. 2006;27:2689–95.
6. Jing L, Binkley CM, Suever JD, Umasankar N, Haggerty CM, Rich J, Wehner GJ, Hamlet SM, Powell DK, Radulescu A, Kirchner HL, Epstein FH, Fornwalt BK. Cardiac remodeling and dysfunction in childhood obesity: a cardiovascular magnetic resonance study. J Cardiovasc Magn Reson. 2016;18:28.
7. Koopman LP, McCrindle BW, Slorach C, Chahal N, Hui W, Sarkola T, Manlhiot C, Jaeggi ET, Bradley TJ, Mertens L. Interaction between myocardial and vascular changes in obese children: a pilot study. J Am Soc Echocardiogr. 2012;25:401–10. e1.
8. Saltijeral A, Isla LP, Pérez-Rodríguez O, Rueda S, Fernandez-Golfin C, Almeria C, Rodrigo JL, Gorissen W, Rementeria J, Marcos-Alberca P, Macaya C, Zamorano J. Early Myocardial Deformation Changes Associated to Isolated Obesity: A Study Based on 3D-Wall Motion Tracking Analysis. Obesity. 2011;19:2268–73.
9. Dhuper S, Abdullah RA, Weichbrod L, Mahdi E, Cohen HW. Association of obesity and hypertension with left ventricular geometry and function in children and adolescents. Obesity (Silver Spring). 2011;19:128–33.
10. Krumholz HM, Larson M, Levy D. Prognosis of left ventricular geometric patterns in the Framingham Heart Study. J Am Coll Cardiol. 1995;25:879–84.
11. La Gerche A, Claessen G, Dymarkowski S, Voigt JU, De Buck F, Vanhees L, Droogne W, Van Cleemput J, Claus P, Heidbuchel H. Exercise-induced right ventricular dysfunction is associated with ventricular arrhythmias in endurance athletes. Eur Heart J. 2015;36:1998–2010.
12. Kirsch J, Johansen CK, Araoz PA, Brady PA, Williamson EE, Glockner JF. Prevalence of fat deposition within the right ventricular myocardium in asymptomatic young patients without ventricular arrhythmias. J Thorac Imaging. 2010;25:173–8.
13. Vigneault DM, Te Riele ASJM, James CA, Zimmerman SL, Selwaness M, Murray B, Tichnell C, Tee M, Noble JA, Calkins H, Tandri H, Bluemke DA. Right ventricular strain by MR quantitatively identifies regional dysfunction in patients with arrhythmogenic right ventricular cardiomyopathy. J Magn Reson Imaging. 2015;43(5):1132–9.
14. Barbosa MM, Beleigoli AM, De Fatima DM, Freire CV, Ribeiro AL, Nunes MCP. Strain imaging in morbid obesity: insights into subclinical ventricular dysfunction. Clin Cardiol. 2011;34:288–93.
15. Chahal H, McClelland RL, Tandri H, Jain A, Turkbey EB, Hundley WG, Barr RG, Kizer J, Lima JAC, Bluemke DA, Kawut SM. Obesity and right ventricular structure and function. Chest. 2012;141:388–95.
16. Orhan AL, Uslu N, Dayi SU, Nurkalem Z, Uzun F, Erer HB, Hasdemir H, Emre A, Karakus G, Soran O, Gorcsan J, Eren M. Effects of isolated obesity on left and right ventricular function: a tissue Doppler and strain rate imaging study. Echocardiography. 2010;27:236–43.
17. Wong CY, O'Moore-Sullivan T, Leano R, Hukins C, Jenkins C, Marwick TH. Association of subclinical right ventricular dysfunction with obesity. J Am Coll Cardiol. 2006;47:611–6.
18. Labombarda F, Zangl E, Dugue AE, Bougle D, Pellissier A, Ribault V, Maragnes P, Milliez P, Saloux E. Alterations of left ventricular myocardial strain in obese children. Eur Heart J Cardiovasc Imaging. 2013;14:668–76.
19. Mahfouz RA, Dewedar A, Abdelmoneim A, Hossien EM. Aortic and pulmonary artery stiffness and cardiac function in children at risk for obesity. Echocardiography. 2012;29:984–90.
20. Zeybek C, Aktuglu-Zeybek C, Onal H, Altay S, Erdem A, Celebi A. Right ventricular subclinical diastolic dysfunction in obese children: the effect of weight reduction with a low-carbohydrate diet. Pediatr Cardiol. 2009; 30:946–53.
21. Kamal HM, Atwa HA, Saleh OM, Mohamed FA. Echocardiographic evaluation of cardiac structure and function in obese Egyptian adolescents. Cardiol Young. 2012;22:410–6.
22. Grothues F, Smith GC, Moon JCC, Bellenger NG, Collins P, Klein HU, Pennell DJ. Comparison of interstudy reproducibility of cardiovascular magnetic resonance with two-dimensional echocardiography in normal subjects and in patients with heart failure or left ventricular hypertrophy. Am J Cardiol. 2002;90:29–34.
23. Hudsmitht L, Petersent S, Francis J, Robson M, Neubauer S. Normal Human Left and Right Ventricular and Left Atrial Dimensions Using Steady State Free Precession Magnetic Resonance Imaging. J Cardiovasc Magn Reson. 2005;7:775–82.
24. Suever JD, Wehner GJ, Jing L, Powell DK, Hamlet SM, Grabau JD, Mojsejenko D, Andres KN, Haggerty CM, Fornwalt BK. Right Ventricular Strain, Torsion, and Dyssynchrony in Healthy Subjects using 3D Spiral Cine DENSE Magnetic Resonance Imaging. IEEE Trans Med Imaging. 2017;36:1076–85.
25. Kuczmarski RJ, Ogden CL, Guo SS, Grummer-Strawn LM, Flegal KM, Mei Z, Wei R, Curtin LR, Roche AF, Johnson CL. 2000 CDC Growth Charts for the United States: Methods and Development. Vital Heal Stat. 2002;11:1–190.
26. DENSEanalysis [https://www.denseanalysis.com]
27. Framewise DENSEanalysis [https://github.com/fornwaltlab/framewise_strain_plugin]
28. Aletras AH, Balaban RS, Wen H. High-resolution strain analysis of the human heart with fast-DENSE. J Magn Reson. 1999;140:41–57.
29. Kim D, Gilson WD, Kramer CM, Epstein FH. Myocardial tissue tracking with two-dimensional cine displacement-encoded MR imaging: development and initial evaluation. Radiology. 2004;230:862–71.
30. Spottiswoode BS, Zhong X, Hess AT, Kramer CM, Meintjes EM, Mayosi BM, Epstein FH. Tracking myocardial motion from cine DENSE images using spatiotemporal phase unwrapping and temporal fitting. IEEE Trans Med Imaging. 2007;26:15–30.
31. de Simone G, Daniels SR, Devereux RB, Meyer RA RA, Roman MJ, de Divitiis O, Alderman MH. Left ventricular mass and body size in normotensive children and adults: assessment of allometric relations and impact of overweight. J Am Coll Cardiol. 1992;20:1251–60.
32. Bland JM, Altman D. Statistical methods for assessing agreement between two methods of clinical measurement. Lancet. 1986;1:307–10.
33. Haggerty CM, Kramer SP, Binkley CM, Powell DK, Mattingly AC, Charnigo R, Epstein FH, Fornwalt BK. Reproducibility of cine displacement encoding with stimulated echoes (DENSE) cardiovascular magnetic resonance for measuring left ventricular strains, torsion, and synchrony in mice. J Cardiovasc Magn Reson. 2013;15:71.
34. R Core Team: R: A language and environment for statistical computing. 2016.
35. Hothorn T, Bretz F, Westfall P. Simultaneous Inference in General Parametric Models. Biom J. 2008;50:346–63.
36. Fox J, Weisberg S. An {R} Companion to Applied Regression. Second Edi. Thousand Oaks: Sage Publications; 2011.
37. Stanton T, Leano R, Marwick TH. Prediction of all-cause mortality from global longitudinal speckle strain: comparison with ejection fraction and wall motion scoring. Circ Cardiovasc Imaging. 2009;2:356–64.
38. Lee JM, Okumura MJ, Davis MM, Herman WH, Gurney JG. Prevalence and determinants of insulin resistance among U.S. adolescents: a population-based study. Diabetes Care. 2006;29:2427–32.
39. Phillips RA, Krakoff LR, Dunaif A, Finegood DT, Gorlin R, Shimabukuro S. Relation among left ventricular mass, insulin resistance, and blood pressure in nonobese subjects. J Clin Endocrinol Metab. 1998;83:4284–8.
40. Fu Q, Xu B, Liu Y, Parikh D, Li J, Li Y, Zhang Y, Riehle C, Zhu Y, Rawlings T, Shi Q, Clark RB, Chen X, Abel ED, Xiang YK. Insulin inhibits cardiac contractility by inducing a Gi-biased β2-adrenergic signaling in hearts. Diabetes. 2014;63:2676–89.
41. Aurigemma GP, de Simone G, Fitzgibbons TP. Cardiac remodeling in obesity. Circ Cardiovasc Imaging. 2013;6:142–52.
42. Tadic M, Cuspidi C. Childhood obesity and cardiac remodeling. J Cardiovasc Med. 2015;16:538–46.

11

Hyperpolarized ^{13}C urea myocardial first-pass perfusion imaging using velocity-selective excitation

Maximilian Fuetterer[1], Julia Busch[1], Sophie M. Peereboom[1], Constantin von Deuster[1], Lukas Wissmann[1], Miriam Lipiski[2], Thea Fleischmann[2], Nikola Cesarovic[2], Christian T. Stoeck[1] and Sebastian Kozerke[1*]

Abstract

Background: A velocity-selective binomial excitation scheme for myocardial first-pass perfusion measurements with hyperpolarized ^{13}C substrates, which preserves bolus magnetization inside the blood pool, is presented. The proposed method is evaluated against gadolinium-enhanced ^{1}H measurements in-vivo.

Methods: The proposed excitation with an echo-planar imaging readout was implemented on a clinical CMR system. Dynamic myocardial stress perfusion images were acquired in six healthy pigs after bolus injection of hyperpolarized ^{13}C urea with the velocity-selective vs. conventional excitation, as well as standard ^{1}H gadolinium-enhanced images. Signal-to-noise, contrast-to-noise (CNR) and homogeneity of semi-quantitative perfusion measures were compared between methods based on first-pass signal-intensity time curves extracted from a mid-ventricular slice. Diagnostic feasibility is demonstrated in a case of septal infarction.

Results: Velocity-selective excitation provides over three-fold reduction in blood pool signal with a two-fold increase in myocardial CNR. Extracted first-pass perfusion curves reveal a significantly reduced variability of semi-quantitative first-pass perfusion measures (12–20%) for velocity-selective excitation compared to conventional excitation (28–93%), comparable to that of reference ^{1}H gadolinium data (9–15%). Overall image quality appears comparable between the velocity-selective hyperpolarized and gadolinium-enhanced imaging.

Conclusion: The feasibility of hyperpolarized ^{13}C first-pass perfusion CMR has been demonstrated in swine. Comparison with reference ^{1}H gadolinium data revealed sufficient data quality and indicates the potential of hyperpolarized perfusion imaging for human applications.

Keywords: Myocardial perfusion, First-pass perfusion, Hyperpolarization, 13C urea, Dynamic imaging

Background

Cardiovascular Magnetic Resonance (CMR) perfusion imaging is widely used for the clinical assessment of myocardial ischemia and has proven its excellent diagnostic value [1]. To increase the sensitivity and specificity of detecting perfusion defects, imaging under pharmacologically induced stress is performed, followed by an optional measurement under rest condition [2]. In a clinical setting, stress is typically induced by administration of adenosine [3] or dobutamine [4].

* Correspondence: kozerke@biomed.ee.ethz.ch
[1]Institute for Biomedical Engineering, University and ETH Zurich, Gloriastrasse 35, 8092 Zurich, Switzerland
Full list of author information is available at the end of the article

Conventional first-pass perfusion CMR [5] is based on dynamic contrast enhancement (DCE) of saturation recovery [6] in response to bolus administration of a chelated gadolinium based contrast agent. Due to the exponential nature of spin-lattice relaxation and partial saturation effects of the image sequence itself, the relationship between signal and contrast agent concentration is non-linear, which renders the determination of actual contrast agent concentration non-trivial [7]. Using dual-bolus [8] or dual-sequences approaches [9] this issue can be addressed, but adds to complexity of data acquisition and analysis.

Despite a long history of safe use of gadolinium contrast agents in patients with normal kidney function, linear gadolinium based contrast agents have recently come under scrutiny in the wake of reports of gadolinium accumulation after repeated administration of certain types of agents [10–12]. To this end, alternative methods to assess tissue perfusion have attracted attention. Arterial spin labelling (ASL) has been applied to the heart in experimental and clinical settings [13]. Also, intra voxel incoherent motion (IVIM) measurements have allowed assessing perfusion fractions without the use of contrast agents [14–16]. However, both approaches provide limited contrast-to-noise ratios (CNR) compared to contrast-enhanced first-pass perfusion imaging and further research is required to translate these methods into clinical use.

Dissolution dynamic nuclear polarization (DNP) allows to produce solutions of highly polarized ^{13}C–labeled molecules with >10′000-fold enhancement [17] relative to thermal signal. To compensate for the low abundance of carbon containing molecules in-vivo, a variety of endogenous ^{13}C–labeled DNP substrates have been used for in-vivo imaging and spectroscopy studies, mostly probing metabolic pathways and their pathologic alterations in various organs and animal models [18]. Recently, first results of the application of hyperpolarized [1–^{13}C] pyruvate to measure cardiac metabolism in humans have been reported [19].

Metabolically inert hyperpolarized substrates have been suggested as alternative contrast agents for perfusion measurements using DNP. HP001, a customized non-endogenous substrate has been shown to enable hyperpolarized perfusion assessment in rats [20]. Endogenous alternatives include the freely diffusible pre-deuterated 2-methylpropan-2ol (tert-butanol) [21], as well as α-trideuteromethyl [^{15}N] glutamine with a particularly long T1 in-vivo [22]. Most prominently, ^{13}C- labeled urea has been used to study perfusion in kidneys [23–26], liver [27, 28] and tumors [20, 28] in rodent and porcine models. In addition to qualitative assessments, the linear dependency of signal intensity on substrate concentration can simplify absolute blood flow quantification under certain assumptions [29]. Simultaneous probing of metabolism and perfusion with co-polarization of metabolically active and inert substrates may also improve diagnostic value by differentiation of metabolic and perfusion defects [30].

The feasibility of myocardial perfusion imaging using hyperpolarized ^{13}C urea has recently been demonstrated in rodents [31]. The particular anatomy of the heart poses a major challenge: the close proximity of the myocardium to the left ventricular (LV) and right ventricular (RV) blood pools with comparatively high signal intensities causes signal contamination at practically achievable spatial resolutions. Accordingly, meaningful signal-intensity time curves are only obtainable if the blood pool signal is suppressed. To this end, flow-sensitizing gradients have been proposed to spoil signal contributions from the non-stationary blood pool [31]. This approach, however, depletes magnetization inside the blood pool, which in turn limits the achievable signal-to-noise ratio (SNR) inside the myocardium.

Dynamic metabolic imaging of hyperpolarized substrates in the heart typically relies on spectral-spatial excitation schemes, in which metabolites are excited depending on their chemical shift [32, 33]. Downstream metabolites are selectively excited with high flip angles, while the input substrate in the blood pool experiences reduced excitation angles. However, this approach is not applicable for metabolically inert substrates with a single resonance frequency, such as ^{13}C urea.

In this work a velocity-selective tip-back excitation that mitigates polarization saturation inside the blood pool whilst retaining the suppression of blood pool signal is proposed. By integration of a bipolar velocity-encoding gradient into slice selection of a binomial excitation pulse, a velocity dependent phase shift in the blood pool signal is introduced, which can be utilized to preserve longitudinal magnetization in the blood pool. The method is validated using phantom measurements and the in-vivo applicability is demonstrated in swine. Myocardial signal-intensity time curves obtained with the proposed method are compared to conventional excitation and clinically used gadolinium enhanced perfusion CMR.

Methods

Sequence design

The accumulated phase ϕ of spins moving with velocity $\vec{v}$ subject to a bipolar gradient pair with amplitude $\vec{G}^{(t)}$ is dependent on the first gradient moment $\vec{m_1}$:

$$\phi = \gamma\left(\vec{m_1}\cdot\vec{v}\right) \tag{1}$$

With

$$\vec{m_1} = \int \vec{G}(t)t\,dt \tag{2}$$

As phase encoding only occurs along the gradient direction $\hat{e}_G$, a scalar notation of velocities as projections of $v = \vec{v}\cdot\hat{e}_G$ is used in this manuscript.

When combined with a binomial 1–1 excitation separated by the bipolar gradient pair, motion induced phase accrual can be exploited to tip back the magnetization of spins moving along the gradient direction by adjusting the excitation phase of the second radio-frequency (RF) pulse.

Alternatively, the accumulated phase between excitations for a given velocity v_{enc} can be set to π by scaling amplitude $G(t)$ and duration T of the bipolar gradients such that:

$$\gamma\, v_{enc} \int_0^T G(t)t\, dt = \pi \tag{3}$$

This approach does not require adjustments of the excitation phase for the second RF pulse with the additional benefit of being relatively robust towards small deviations from the nominal velocity v_{enc}. Stationary spins inside the myocardium that do not accumulate motion-dependent phase effectively undergo two excitations, while the magnetization of moving spins inside the left ventricular blood pool is retained by tipping it back to the longitudinal axis by the second RF excitation. This excitation can be combined with any single-shot readout, such as echo-planar (EPI) or spiral imaging.

For through-plane motion, which is predominant for the left ventricular blood pool in short axis acquisitions, the bipolar gradients can be efficiently integrated into the slice selection scheme as illustrated in Fig. 1. Velocity components along other directions than through-plane will not be affected by the velocity-selective excitation and experience full excitation instead. In cases where the predominating direction of blood flow is not perpendicular to the slice orientation, the encoding gradients could be separated from the slice selection gradients and applied to different gradient axes at the cost of prolonged echo times.

The effective excitation pattern for various v_{enc} encodings as a function of through-plane velocity over the imaging slice is illustrated in Fig. 2. For a given v_{enc} encoding, the relative signal amplitude s in dependency of the through-plane velocity v can be determined as:

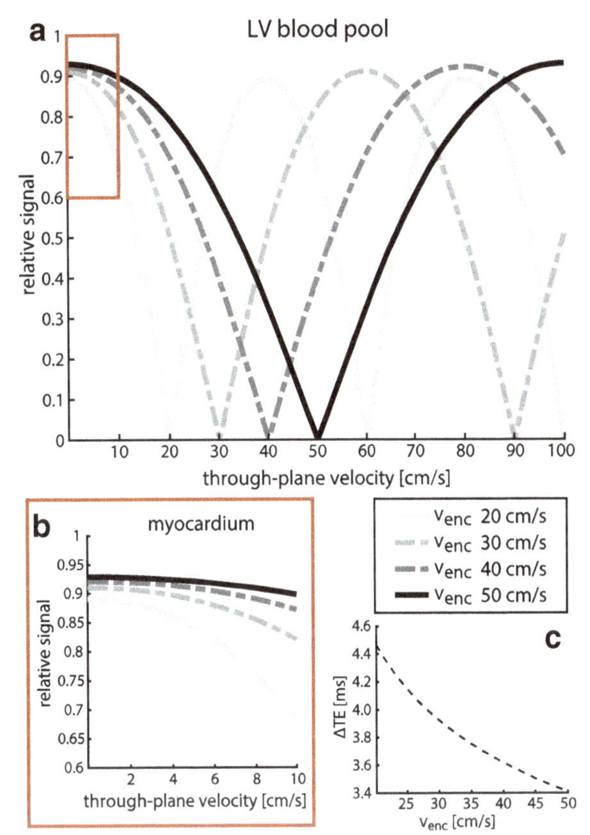

Fig. 2 Calculated excitation patterns for velocity-selective excitation, relative to conventional single-pulse excitation. (**a**) effective excitation patterns for various encoding strengths inside the LV blood pool. Encoding of higher velocities yields a wider suppression band around the nominal values. (**b**) zoomed-in view for velocity range typically observed inside the myocardium (*red box, a*). For encoding strengths >30 cm/s the myocardial signal is hardly affected (<10%). (**c**) echo-time prolongation for velocity-selective excitation with respect to conventional single-pulse excitation for various encoding strengths

$$s(v) = \left| \sin\left(\frac{(v_{enc}-v)}{v_{enc}}\frac{\pi}{2}\right) \right| \tag{4}$$

Conversely, the amount of preserved magnetization M_z in the blood pool can be estimated as:

$$M_z(v) = \left| \cos\left(\frac{(v_{enc}-v)}{v_{enc}}\frac{\pi}{2}\right) \right| \tag{5}$$

As the phase evolution is symmetric, the sign of the velocity and encoding gradients can be neglected. For the encoding velocity, the magnetization will be fully restored, while deviations due to spatial flow variations or missetting of the encoding velocity will result in imperfect

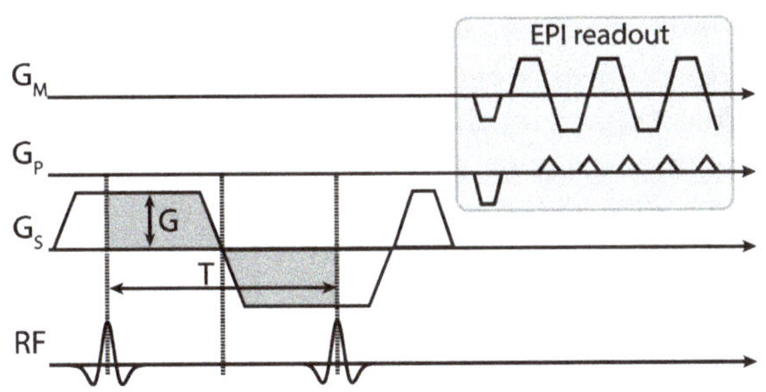

Fig. 1 Velocity-selective excitation scheme: Bipolar velocity encoding gradients (*dark grey*) are incorporated into the slice selection gradients of a 1–1 binomial excitation. The accumulated phase of moving spins between the two RF pulses can be used to tip-back magnetization into the longitudinal axis with the second RF pulse. The approach is similar to spectrally selective binomial excitation, with the key difference that phase is induced by velocity encoding gradients instead of chemical shift variations of different molecules. The proposed excitation can be combined with arbitrary single-shot sampling approaches, such as echo-planar or spiral imaging

tip-back and residual signal according to Eqs. 4 and 5 (see Fig. 2a). It is therefore crucial that encoding velocities are set to the specific mean systolic or diastolic velocity for each subject, which can be obtained from phase contrast pre-scans. Higher through-plane velocities in the LV blood pool, with higher respective v_{enc} encodings, benefit from a wider stop band around the target velocities (see Fig. 2a), whilst reducing unwanted signal dampening inside the slowly moving myocardium (see Fig. 2b). This makes the proposed excitation especially suited for stress perfusion measurements with increased blood velocities as presented in this work, but poses challenges for measurements under rest conditions. Additionally, echo time (TE) increases towards lower v_{enc} encodings, which limits the maximum attainable signal due to T_2* decay (see Fig. 2c). The gap between the two RF pulses depends on encoding strength and gradient hardware and ranged from 6.8 ms (v_{enc}: 50 cm/s) to 8.4 ms (v_{enc}: 25 cm/s) on the clinical CMR system used in this study.

CMR setup

All measurements were performed on a clinical 3 T Ingenia wide-bore scanner (Philips, Best, The Netherlands) equipped with a gradient system delivering 30 mT/m maximum amplitude at 200 T/m/s slew rate. Data on ^{13}C were acquired using a custom-made 4-channel transmit/receive coil array (Clinical MR Solutions, Shadybrook, WI, USA) while the 2-channel body coil was utilized to sample on the ^{1}H frequency. Animals were placed in right recumbency inside the scanner bore to allow for optimal placement of the coil arrays. A peripheral pulse oximeter unit was used for cardiac synchronization.

Hyperpolarization

A 6.4 M ^{13}C urea glycerol solution was prepared and doped with 18.5 mM AH111501 trityl radical. 1 mL samples were polarized for 4 h in a commercial 5 T SpinLab Polarizer (General Electric Healthcare, Waukesha, Wisconsin, USA) before dissolution using a buffer consisting of 30 mL 0.1% EDTA dissolved in water. Upon sample collection, the prepared solution was further diluted and cooled down with additional 4.5 mL of buffer at 0 °C to achieve body temperature for injection. 20 mL of the final 200 mM ^{13}C urea solution were transferred to the scanner using an electromagnetic carrier device [34] built in-house, ensuring a magnetic field >7 mT over the whole syringe volume and transport period (15–20 s).

Polarization levels were established in separate experiments and amounted to 48 ± 5% at time of dissolution and 29 ± 3% at time of injection. T_1 relaxation times inside the 3 T magnet were measured for the neat solutions (58 ± 1 s, n = 5) and after dilution in porcine heparinized venous blood samples within 15 min after sampling. Two urea concentrations (n = 5, each) were measured: 10% and 33%, with an observed T1 of 25 ± 2 s and 34 ± 0.5 s, respectively.

Phantom validation

The proposed excitation scheme was validated using ^{1}H imaging of a water tube embedded in a solid gel phantom. Water flow was adjusted to ~50 cm/s, which is in accordance with LV velocities typically observed in-vivo. A single 2D slice perpendicular to the direction of flow was acquired using a single-shot EPI readout. Signals inside the water tube as well as the stationary gel region were compared to simulations for the conventional single-pulse and the proposed tip-back excitation with varying v_{enc} encodings. All measurements were normalized to the water signal of the conventional excitation.

Animal handling

Seven healthy female swine (Edelschwein, weight 30–35 kg) were used for the experiments. All swine were premedicated, intubated and sheaths (5 F) were introduced into both femoral arteries and veins. 100 IU/kgBW Heparin was given intravenously and repeated every hour. General anesthesia was maintained with isoflurane (2% - 3%) by positive pressure ventilation with 100% oxygen. Heart rate and rhythm and variability (ECG), inspiratory and expiratory gases (CO_2, O_2, isoflurane), pulse oximetry, temperature, direct arterial blood pressure, urine output, and arterial and venous blood gases were monitored continuously throughout the procedure. Hyperpolarized ^{13}C urea and ^{1}H gadolinium were administered through separate catheters in the femoral veins.

Cardiac stress was pharmacologically induced by intravenous administration of dobutamine (Dobutrex, TEVA Pharma AG, Basel, Switzerland) at increasing infusion rates until the target heart rate of 120 bpm was reached. Upon reaching the target heart rate, infusion rates were kept constant during all imaging experiments. 20 mL of hyperpolarized ^{13}C urea solution was injected as a bolus at a rate of 10 mL/s. No adverse effects were observed as a result of ^{13}C urea injections.

In one animal, acute myocardial infarction in the apical septum was induced by permanent distal ligation of the left anterior descending coronary artery (LAD). Corresponding data was not included in the main analysis of this study, but used as demonstration of sensitivity of the proposed excitation scheme to detect ischemic myocardium. After the procedure, all animals were euthanized in deep anesthesia by lethal injection of pentobarbital.

In-vivo measurements

Prior to each ^{13}C measurement, ^{1}H phase-contrast images were acquired using a 2D short-axis cine sequence under stress condition. Sequence parameters were: FOV = 250 × 220 mm^2, slice thickness 8 mm, in-plane resolution 2.5 × 2.5 mm^2, TR = 4.8 ms, TE = 2.8 ms, FA = 7°, cardiac phases = 35, v_{enc} = 100 cm/s. These short-axis cine images were used to determine through-plane velocities and trigger delays for subsequent ^{13}C perfusion CMR.

Anatomical reference 2D cine short-axis CMR was performed using a balanced steady-state free precession gradient echo sequence with the following parameters: FOV = 350 × 280 mm^2, slice thickness 8 mm, in-plane resolution 1.9 × 1.9 mm^2, TR = 2.7 ms, TE = 1.35 ms, FA = 45°, cardiac phases = 60.

Dynamic series of ^{13}C perfusion images were acquired with cardiac triggering starting seven heart beats after the start of injection to minimize bolus saturation in the RV blood pool. Ventilation was suspended for the first 45 s of imaging to avoid misregistration between individual time frames. The proposed 1–1 binomial tip-back excitation (FA: 2 × 30°) was compared to single-pulse excitation (FA: 60°) in each animal under maintained stress condition with two hyperpolarized bolus injections, separated by 10 min. Identical single-shot echo planar imaging readouts were employed in both cases with following parameters: FOV = 110 × 110 mm^2, slice thickness 15 mm, in-plane resolution 3.0 × 3.0 mm^2, TR = 1 heartbeat, partial Fourier factor 0.65, readout duration 32 ms. Effective echo times for the proposed excitation increased from TE = 10.2 ms (conventional) to TE = 13.3–14.2 ms in dependence of flow encoding as illustrated in Fig. 2c. Encoding strengths (v_{enc}) between 25 cm/s and 52 cm/s (mean ± std.: 38 ± 7 cm/s) for the velocity-selective excitation were used based on measured through-plane velocities.

Conventional ^{1}H gadolinium contrast-enhanced perfusion CMR under stress was performed as a reference method in each animal. A dose of 0.1 mmol/kg gadolinium (Gadovist 1.0, Bayer, Zurich, Switzerland), followed by a 30 mL saline flush was injected at a rate of 4 mL/s using a power injector (Medrad, Indianola, PA, USA). Dynamic image series were acquired every heart beat using a saturation-recovery spoiled gradient echo sequence with parameters: FOV = 220 × 210 mm^2, slice thickness 10 mm, in-plane resolution 3.0 × 3.0 mm^2, TR = 1.9 ms, TE = 0.7 ms, FA = 15°, WET saturation [35] delay = 100 ms. A total of 100 dynamics were acquired during suspended ventilation.

Image reconstruction

All in-vivo images were reconstructed from raw data using MRecon (GyroTools LLC, Zurich, Switzerland) and zero-filled to a common resolution of 1 × 1 mm^2. ^{1}H images were then rotated, aligned and cropped to the FOV of the ^{13}C images. Nyquist-ghosts of the EPI readout were removed by first order phase correction maximizing signal intensity in a predefined region of interest (e.g. LV blood pool). ^{13}C coil combination was implemented as root of weighted sum of squares [36].

Post-processing

Left ventricular myocardium and LV blood pool were manually segmented on overlays of ^{13}C perfusion and ^{1}H reference images. The myocardium was subsequently divided into six segments corresponding to the basal/mid-ventricular slices in the 16 segment AHA model [37].

Coil sensitivities were estimated and corrected by fitting a plane over the myocardial signal at a time frame prior to and after bolus passage for ^{1}H and ^{13}C scans, respectively.

^{13}C urea signal intensities were calculated as mean values over each segment and the LV blood pool. Global magnitude offsets were corrected for by subtraction of mean noise levels of the last 10 time frames in the image series.

Three-parameter gamma-variate functions

$$s(t) = a\, t^b\, e^{-\frac{t}{c}} \tag{6}$$

were fitted to the signal time curves $s(t)$ for further data analysis of ^{13}C urea data. ^{1}H gadolinium time curves were fitted with fourth order polynomials respectively. Area under the curve (AUC), peak myocardial contrast-to-noise ratio (pCNR) and up-slope were extracted from the fitted curves as semi-quantitative perfusion measures for ^{13}C urea and ^{1}H contrast-enhanced scans [7]. Signal-to-noise ratio (SNR) was calculated as mean signal intensities divided by the standard deviation over the difference of two noise frames pre (^{1}H) or post (^{13}C) bolus [38]. CNR was calculated as differences of peak contrast-enhanced SNR and mean baseline SNR as described in [39].

Absolute values and variability over the six myocardial segments were compared between conventional and the proposed tip-back excitation, as well as to ^{1}H gadolinium based measurements. Analysis was restricted to first-pass signal contributions in all cases. Coefficients of variance (CoV) were calculated as standard deviation divided by mean values. A paired, two-sided Wilcoxon signed rank test was employed for statistical comparisons. A p-value <0.05 was considered significant.

Results

Phantom experiments

Figure 3 illustrates measured signal intensities of the proposed and conventional excitation in a phantom with constant flow of 48 cm/s in comparison to simulations. Variations in v_{enc} encoding strength show good agreement with the predicted signal overall. Encoding with the nominal velocity (48 cm/s) yields a > 80% reduction in water signal. Residual signal is observed at the tube boundary, where velocities deviate from the nominal value. Encoding with approximately half the nominal velocity (25 cm/s),

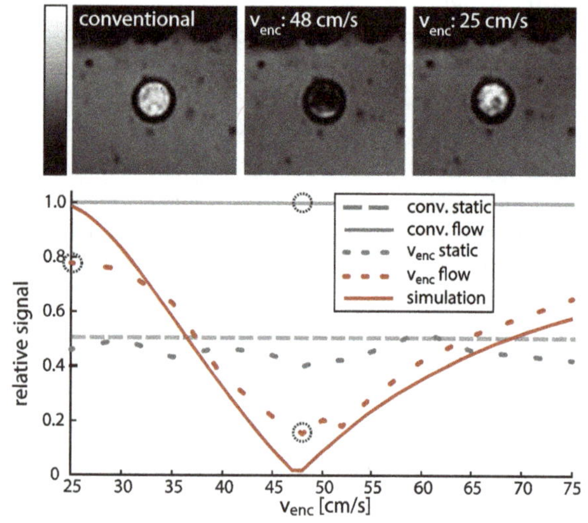

Fig. 3 Phantom validation in ^{1}H gel phantom around water pipe with mean flow velocity of 48 cm/s. (*top row*) Images acquired using a conventional single-pulse excitation (*left*), the proposed velocity-selective binomial excitation at nominal encoding strength (*center*) and half the nominal encoding velocity (*right*). (*bottom*) Measured vs. simulated signal intensities in static and flow compartments for varying velocity encodings. Data points corresponding to the *top images* are highlighted in *dashed circles*. Measured signal intensities overall match the predictions with maximum deviations of 20%. At nominal velocity encoding, residual signal stems from the low velocity regime at the boundary of the tube (see also Fig. 4). Encoding with half the nominal velocity restores most of the signal due to an accumulated phase of 2π. Deviations from nominal velocity and stronger T_2* weighting for smaller v_{enc} values prohibit perfect recovery of magnetization in measurements

which results in an accumulated phase of 2π, recovers 78% of the signal as expected due to inflow effects, stronger T_2* weighting of the prolonged excitation and finite sharpness of the velocity distribution.

In-vivo experiments

Figure 4a shows measured through-plane velocities over the cardiac cycle in short axis orientation under dobutamine stress. Variability of blood velocities between ejection phase (35 cm/s) and filling phase (− 42 cm/s) is observed in contrast to minor variations inside the myocardium (≤ 7 cm/s). The velocity difference between LV blood pool and myocardium is particularly pronounced in early systole and early diastole. Figure 4b illustrates the distributions of measured through-plane velocities of myocardium (−0.82 ± 5.2 cm/s) and LV blood pool (33.4 ± 6.2 cm/s) in early systole with the overlaid excitation pattern. Myocardial tissue gets excited with a relative amplitude >0.9, the LV blood pool with a relative amplitude <0.4 (within one standard deviation of the respective mean velocities). Preserved magnetization in the LV blood pool was estimated as 93 ± 4% over all subjects, based on spatial integration of Eq. 5. Saturation from sideband effects and blood exchange during excitation were considered negligible under in-vivo conditions.

In Fig. 5, a comparison of dynamic image series of myocardial bolus passage for ^{13}C urea conventional excitation, ^{13}C urea velocity-selective excitation and ^{1}H gadolinium based contrast agent is shown. During LV bolus peak at 2 s (second column), blood pool signal suppression is apparent for the velocity-selective in contrast to conventional excitation. Residual LV signal stems from low blood flow near the trabeculae. Myocardial bolus signal (4–6 s) is significantly enhanced for the proposed method, with a clear distinction of right and left ventricular myocardium.

Figure 6 provides representative signal-time curves extracted from a six-sector AHA segmentation for ^{1}H gadolinium (Gd), ^{13}C velocity-selective (VS) and ^{13}C conventional (C) measurements. Mean myocardial SNR averaged over each sector was 18.4 ± 1.5 (Gd), 25.7 ± 2.6 (VS) and 15.1 ± 2.5 (C), respectively.

For conventional excitation, blood pool spillover in the septal sectors 1 and 2, as well as the lateral sector 5 is observed. Myocardial peak signal appears at an unphysiologically early time point with respect to the LV peak bolus. Velocity-selective excitation yields uncontaminated myocardial response curves with good homogeneity over the six sectors. Myocardial peak signal is observed at the physiologically expected time point 2–3 s after the LV blood pool signal peak. Up-slope, timing and homogeneity are comparable with signal curves obtained from gadolinium-enhanced measurements.

Intramyocardial coefficients of variance of semi-quantitative perfusion measures over six animals are evaluated for six animals in Fig. 7a. The variability of peak myocardial CNR is ≤20% for the three sequences (9 ± 5% (Gd), 12 ± 3% (VS), 20 ± 5% (C)). AUC variability is significantly (P = 0.03) higher for conventional excitation (47 ± 53%) compared to ^{1}H gadolinium (12 ± 6%) and velocity-selective excitation (14 ± 4%). Upslope variability shows the largest inter-sequence discrepancy: 15 ± 5% (Gd), 20 ± 9% (VS), 93 ± 61% (C).

Peak SNR of LV blood pool is significantly (P = 0.03) lower for velocity-selective excitation (149 ± 117) compared to conventional excitation (473 ± 125), as illustrated in Fig. 7b.

Absolute myocardial peak CNR values are shown in Fig. 7c. The proposed excitation scheme shows a more than two-fold CNR increase compared to ^{1}H gadolinium (19.2 ± 3.7 vs. 9.6 ± 3.9), and a significant (P = 0.03) increase compared to conventional excitation (9.5 ± 3.5).

Acute infarction

In Fig. 8 the feasibility of the proposed method to detect perfusion defects is demonstrated. In this case reduced septal perfusion is seen in both ^{13}C velocity-selective

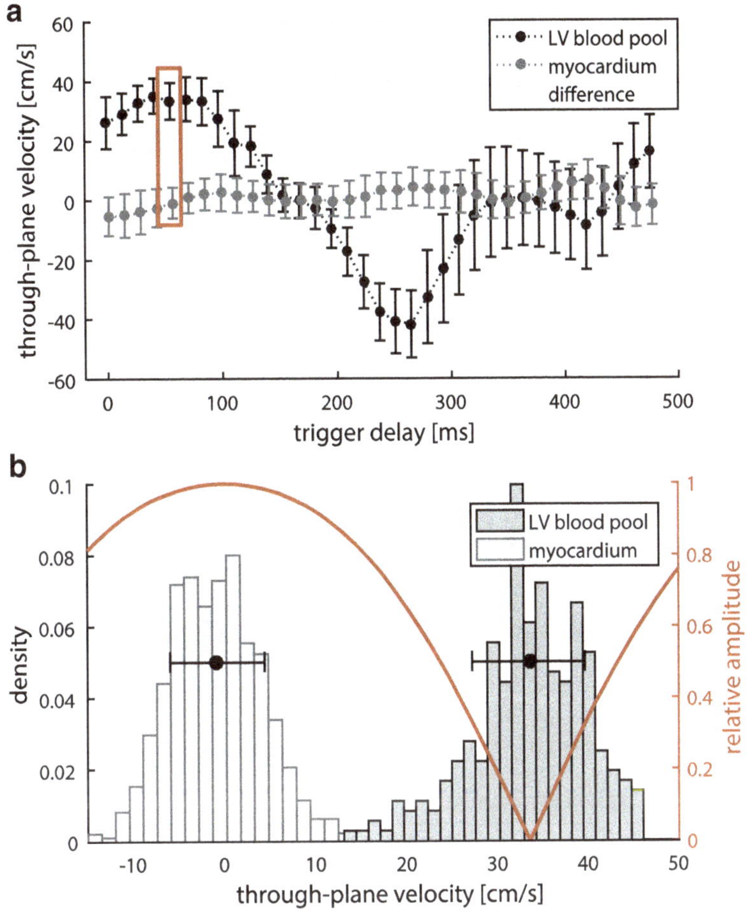

Fig. 4 (**a**) measured through-plane velocities under dobutamine stress (120 bpm) over the cardiac cycle for *left* ventricular myocardium and blood pool. Mean and standard deviation over the respectively segmented areas are presented. Contrast of the proposed excitation is based on velocity differences between tissue and blood as highlighted in *grey*. Early systole (*red box*) and early diastole are therefore especially suited heart phases for the proposed method. (**b**) histogram of velocity distributions inside LV myocardium and blood pool in early systole (*red box, top plot*). Mean and standard deviation over both compartments are overlaid in *black*. Relative excitation amplitudes for encoding with the mean velocity inside the LV blood pool are shown in *red*. Blood pool signal is strongly suppressed whilst myocardial signal is largely retained

and ^{1}H gadolinium-enhanced images. Extracted myocardial perfusion curves confirm the perfusion defect in AHA sector 2 in both datasets. Increased LV signal spill-over is detected for the urea measurement.

Discussion

In this study, the feasibility of hyperpolarized myocardial first-pass perfusion CMR using velocity-selective excitation was demonstrated. Significantly enhanced SNR and CNR compared to conventional excitation ($P < 0.05$), as well as good discrimination of LV blood pool signal have been shown. Direct comparison with ^{1}H gadolinium data indicates that the proposed method can produce sufficient data quality for diagnostic purposes in large subjects.

Comparison of velocity-selective ^{13}C urea and ^{1}H gadolinium measurements revealed good agreement between both methods. The signal enhancement during the myocardial first-pass showed similar patterns with respect to relative timing and signal amplitudes. Differences in signal-time curves were associated with differences in contrast agent characteristics. While gadolinium based agents showed a second bolus pass, the hyperpolarized signal vanished after the first-pass due to polarization decay and quenching by excitation. Accordingly, there was no baseline signal enhancement remaining at the end of the measurement, hence allowing individual hyperpolarized measurements to be performed in rapid succession, whereas gadolinium based contrast agents require a washout period. CNR and signal homogeneity of ^{13}C urea imaging appeared to be sufficient for detecting perfusion defects as demonstrated in the ischemia example.

^{1}H gadolinium measurements were performed using a relatively high contrast agent dose of 0.1 mmol/kg,

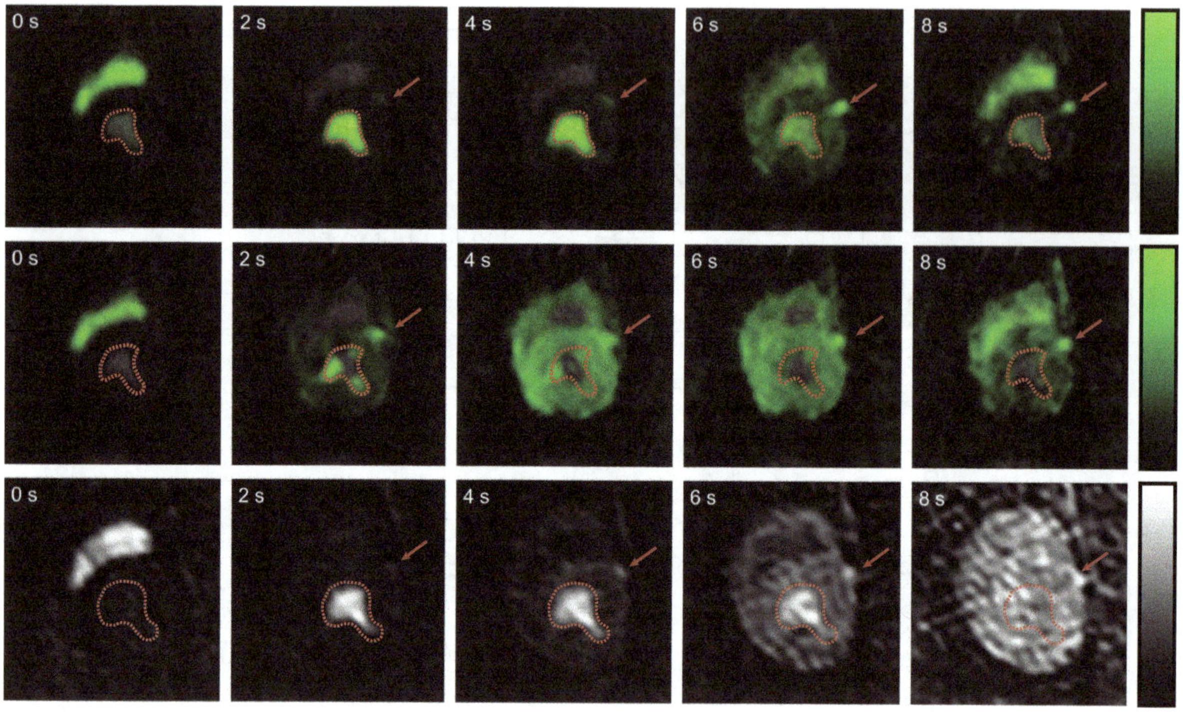

Fig. 5 Dynamically enhanced cardiac perfusion imaging series covering bolus passage in LV blood pool and myocardium. (**a**) ^{13}C urea conventional excitation. (**b**) ^{13}C urea velocity-selective excitation. (**c**) ^{1}H gadolinium based contrast agent. Image series were sequentially acquired in one animal under maintained stress conditioning. Myocardial bolus peak occurs between 4 and 6 s after injection (see Fig. 6). Left anterior descending coronary artery (LAD) is indicated by *red arrow*. LV blood pool is visualized by the *red contour*

which is at the upper end of clinical administration for qualitative and quantitative perfusion CMR. Despite this CNR-optimal dose, the average peak myocardial CNR was 50% lower than in velocity-selective ^{13}C urea measurements.

Perfusion CMR in this study was limited to acquisitions under stress condition, while clinical protocols often include an optional reference measurement under rest condition. Precursor stages of coronary artery disease, however, are only detectable under increased myocardial workload [4], which gives stress perfusion a higher diagnostic value. Nonetheless, rest perfusion is required for the calculation of perfusion reserve as a semi-quantitative marker for myocardial ischemia that is widely used in clinical diagnostics [40]. Absolute quantification of myocardial blood flow (MBF) is a way of mitigating the need for additional measurements under rest conditions, whilst providing quantitative physiological parameters.

Due to limitations in scanner hardware, ^{1}H gadolinium measurements had to be performed with the 2-channel body coil as a receiver, while a 4-channel surface coil was used for ^{13}C urea detection. Consequently, image quality of ^{1}H gadolinium data in this work was lower than in a standard perfusion CMR setup. A two-fold increase in SNR and 1.5-fold increase in CNR is estimated for measurements with a dedicated 28 channel cardiac coil array based on previous experiments. To this end, a dedicated $^{1}H/^{13}C$ receiver array will be commissioned to allow for improved $^{1}H/^{13}C$ signal detection in the future.

With the velocity-selective excitation scheme, the encoding gradients can in principle be scaled to any blood velocity. However, excitation profiles become narrower with lower velocities (see Fig. 2a), while measured velocity distributions remain relatively broad. This effect leads to a reduced effectiveness of the method under rest condition. Higher order velocity encoding could be used to broaden the suppression band of the excitation patterns in these cases. The efficacy of this approach given the necessary echo time prolongation needs to be investigated. During rest, the imaging window is meanwhile restricted to diastole, where rapid inflow of blood at >20 cm/s occurs. Preliminary acquired diastolic images appear sufficient for visual assessment of perfusion defects, however, the extraction of signal-intensity time curves is challenging due to the relatively thin myocardium (see Additional file 1: Figure S1).

Given a minimum TR < 50 ms, multiple slices within one cardiac cycle can be acquired. Depending on the number of slices and their distribution over the cardiac cycle, velocity encoding needs to be adjusted for each slice based on flow measurements at the respective heart phase (see Fig. 4b). While basal

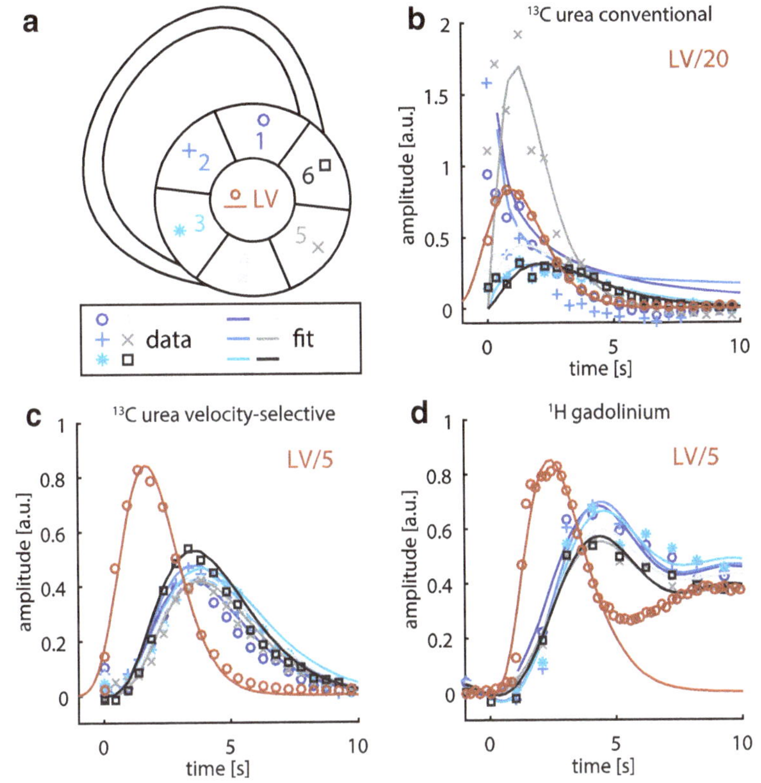

Fig. 6 Representative comparison of perfusion curves extracted from a 6 sector AHA segmentation (**a**). Measurements were obtained within the same maintained dobutamine administration in the same animal for: (**b**) ^{13}C urea conventional excitation. (**c**) ^{13}C urea velocity selective excitation. (**d**) ^{1}H gadolinium. Myocardial response data is presented as measured (*markers*) and fitted (*lines*). Arterial input data (*red*) is downscaled by factors 5 or 20 for better visualization. Gamma-variate fitting was employed for input curves and ^{13}C urea response, 4th order polynomials were used for ^{1}H gadolinium response

and mid-ventricular slices are well suited for velocity-selective excitation, acquisitions of apical slices remain challenging due to low through-plane velocities of blood in the apex. In order to utilize the radial blood flow pattern in the apical region, encoding along lateral directions might prove beneficial in this case. Encoding along directions orthogonal to the slice selection direction however results in additional echo time prolongation, as the encoding gradients must be separated from the slice selection gradients.

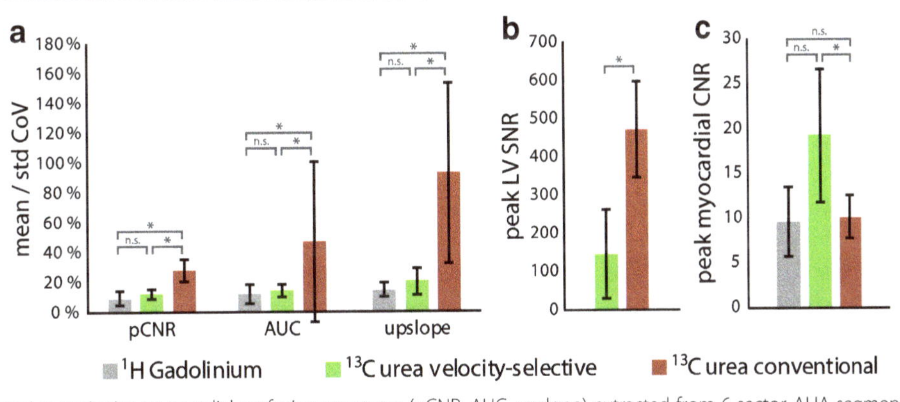

Fig. 7 Analysis of semi-quantitative myocardial perfusion measures (pCNR, AUC, upslope) extracted from 6 sector AHA segmentation in six animals. ^{1}H gadolinium, ^{13}C urea velocity-selective excitation and ^{13}C urea conventional excitation measurements were performed for each animal during maintained dobutamine administration. (**a**) Coefficient of Variance of semi-quantitative perfusion measures over the 6 myocardial AHA sectors (mean +/− std). (**b**) Absolute peak SNR of LV blood pool signal. (**c**) Absolute peak myocardial contrast-to-noise ratio for each modality (mean +/− std). n.s.: not significant, *: $P < 0.05$

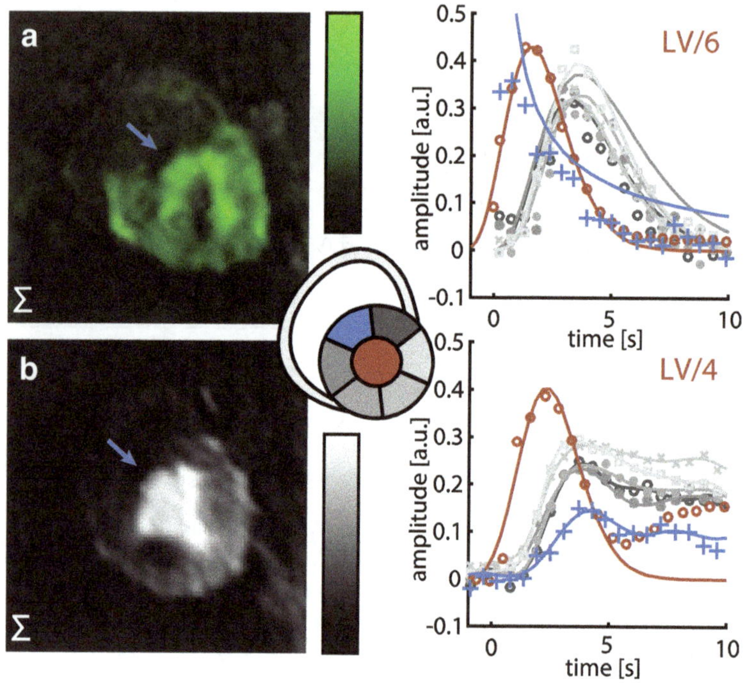

Fig. 8 Stress perfusion measurements with septal infarction induced by permanent ligation of the distal anterior descending coronary artery. (*left*) Sum over three time frames at myocardial bolus peak. (*right*) corresponding perfusion curves for six AHA segments. Perfusion defect is visually observed in septal wall (*blue arrow*) and time curves of sector 2 (*blue curve*) for both modalities. LV signal spillover in the ^{13}C urea perfusion curves stems from thinned myocardium in the infarct region. At myocardial bolus passage, the infarcted region shows strongly reduced signal. LAD is not detectable in either modality due to ligation. (**a**) ^{13}C urea velocity-selective excitation. (**b**) ^{1}H gadolinium based contrast agent

Alternatively, encoding gradients may be adjusted to encode acceleration [41] in conjunction with a higher order binomial excitation. Despite the apparent echo time penalty, this approach could enable imaging in more heart phases and regions with non-uniform flow patterns such as the apex.

To maximize the efficacy of the proposed method, the bipolar gradient pair should be aligned with the predominant flow direction within the LV blood pool (basal to apical). Short axis acquisitions are therefore especially suited, as the encoding gradients can be partly integrated into slice selection gradients without echo time penalty. Nevertheless, the encoding gradients can be applied along directions other than the slice selection direction for applications where different slice orientations (e.g. long axis) are required. In addition to an echo time penalty from temporal gradient separation, this approach would also require an additional bipolar gradient along the slice selection direction to compensate for the phase accrual generated by the binomial excitation. The feasibility and efficacy of such an approach remain to be investigated.

Related to our work, the use of flow sensitizing gradients for the suppression of LV blood pool signal has previously been proposed [31]. In contrast to the signal dephasing of moving spins as in [31], the velocity-selective excitation proposed here has several advantages. Firstly, the magnetization inside the blood pool is preserved, which prevents pre-saturation of the hyperpolarized substrate bolus before its arrival in the myocardium. Consequently, large flip angles >45° can be applied to maximize signal in the first bolus passage. Secondly, dephasing the blood pool signal by means of bipolar gradients requires large first gradient moments, which also compromise myocardial signal.

As an alternative to the single-shot EPI readout used in this work, spiral k-space trajectories may be employed [30, 31, 42, 43]. However, the limited gradient performance of typical clinical systems renders sufficient in-plane resolution at reasonable field of views in large animals and humans challenging.

Qualitative and semi-quantitative perfusion CMR, as covered by this work, is diagnostically valuable for the detection of local ischemia. To reduce operator dependence during analysis and to enable the detection of absolute changes in perfusion, myocardial blood flow (MBF) quantification is preferred [7]. However, the determination of accurate arterial input functions from measured signals requires models of varying complexity [40, 44] and appropriate treatment of baseline signals. Hyperpolarized metabolically inactive substrates may present an advantage as the agent concentration is directly proportional to the measured signal upon correction for T_1 decay and flip angle. Absolute perfusion quantification using hyperpolarized ^{13}C substrates has been demonstrated in cancer, brain and kidneys [20, 28, 45]. These approaches are, however, not directly applicable to MBF quantification, as the myocardial response is affected by bolus saturation inside the blood pool. Future studies will combine velocity-selective imaging of the heart with interleaved sampling of the arterial input to address these issues.

Conclusion

A velocity-selective excitation scheme for first-pass myocardial perfusion measurements using hyperpolarized ^{13}C urea has been presented. Direct comparison with ^1H gadolinium measurements showed very good agreement, indicating the potential of hyperpolarized ^{13}C urea perfusion imaging for diagnostic purposes.

Additional file

Additional file 1: Figure S1. Dynamically enhanced cardiac perfusion imaging series acquired under rest condition (heart rate = 90 bpm) in diastole using hyperpolarized ^{13}C urea and velocity-selective excitation (v_{enc} = 25 cm/s). Myocardial bolus peak under rest condition is delayed by approximately 2 s compared with stress measurements due to lower heart rates.

Abbreviations

AHA: American Heart Association (segmentation); ASL: Arterial spin labelling; AUC: Area under the curve; CMR: Cardiovascular magnetic resonance; CNR: Contrast-to-noise ratio; CoV: Coefficient of variance; DCE: Dynamic contrast enhancement; DNP: Dissolution dynamic nuclear polarization; EPI: Echo planar imaging; FA: Flip angle; FOV: Field-of-view; IVIM: Intra voxel incoherent motion; LAD: Left anterior descending coronary artery; LV: Left ventricular; MBF: Myocardial blood flow; pCNR: Peak contrast-to-noise ratio; RF: Radiofrequency; RV: Right ventricular; SNR: Signal-to-noise ratio; TE: Echo time; TR: Repetition time

Funding

This research was funded in parts by the Clinical Research Priority Program for Molecular Imaging of the University of Zurich (MINZ) and the Swiss National Science Foundation, grant SNF 320030_153014.

Author's contributions

MF, JB: study design, CMR sequence programming. MF: phantom measurements, image reconstruction and post-processing, manuscript drafting. MF, JB, SMP, CVD, CTS: in-vivo measurements, participation in animal preparation. MF, JB, SMP: preparation of hyperpolarized ^{13}C urea solution. MF, JB, SMP, LW, CVD, ML, TF, NC, CTS, SK: manuscript revision. LW: guidance for gadolinium CMR, advice on post-processing. ML, TF, NC: preparation and monitoring of animals, ethics approval. CTS, SK: study coordination, study design. All authors read and approved the final manuscript.

Competing interests

The authors declare that they have no competing interests.

Author details

[1]Institute for Biomedical Engineering, University and ETH Zurich, Gloriastrasse 35, 8092 Zurich, Switzerland. [2]Division of Surgical Research, University Hospital Zurich, Sternwartstrasse 14, 8091 Zurich, Switzerland.

References

1. Schwitter J, Wacker CM, Wilke N, Al-Saadi N, Sauer E, Huettle K, et al. MR-IMPACT II: magnetic resonance imaging for myocardial perfusion assessment in coronary artery disease trial: perfusion-cardiac magnetic resonance vs. single-photon emission computed tomography for the detection of coronary artery disease: a comparative. Eur Heart J. 2013;34:775–81.
2. Hendel RC, Friedrich MG, Schulz-Menger J, Zemmrich C, Bengel F, Berman DS, et al. CMR first-pass perfusion for suspected inducible myocardial ischemia. JACC Cardiovasc Imaging. 2016;9:1338–48.
3. Nagel E. Magnetic resonance perfusion measurements for the noninvasive detection of coronary artery disease. Circulation. 2003;108:432–7.
4. Gebker R, Jahnke C, Manka R, Hamdan A, Schnackenburg B, Fleck E, et al. Additional value of myocardial perfusion imaging during dobutamine stress magnetic resonance for the assessment of coronary artery disease. Circ Cardiovasc Imaging. 2008;1:122–30.
5. Gerber BL, Raman SV, Nayak K, Epstein FH, Ferreira P, Axel L, et al. Myocardial first-pass perfusion cardiovascular magnetic resonance: history, theory, and current state of the art. J Cardiovasc Magn Reson. 2008;10:18.
6. Kellman P, Arai AE. Imaging sequences for first pass perfusion—a review. J Cardiovasc Magn Reson. 2007;9:525–37.
7. Jerosch-Herold M. Quantification of myocardial perfusion by cardiovascular magnetic resonance. J Cardiovasc Magn Reson. 2010;12:57.
8. Köstler H, Ritter C, Lipp M, Beer M, Hahn D, Sandstede J. Prebolus quantitative MR heart perfusion imaging. Magn Reson Med. 2004;52:296–9.
9. Gatehouse PD, Elkington AG, Ablitt NA, Yang G-Z, Pennell DJ, Firmin DN. Accurate assessment of the arterial input function during high-dose myocardial perfusion cardiovascular magnetic resonance. J Magn Reson Imaging. 2004;20:39–45.
10. Kanda I, Ishii K, Kawaguchi H, Kitajima K, Takenaka D. High signal intensity in the dentate nucleus and globus pallidus on unenhanced T1-weighted MR images: relationship with increasing cumulative dose of a gadolinium-based contrast material. Radiology. 2014;270:834–41.
11. McDonald RJ, McDonald JS, Kallmes DF, Jentoft ME, Murray DL, Thielen KR, et al. Intracranial gadolinium deposition after contrast-enhanced MR imaging. Radiology. 2015;0:150025.
12. Murata N, Murata K, Gonzalez-Cuyar LF, Maravilla K. Gadolinium tissue deposition in brain and bone. Magn Reson Imaging. 2016;34:1359–65.
13. Kober F, Jao T, Troalen T, Nayak KS. Myocardial arterial spin labeling. J Cardiovasc Magn Reson. 2016;18:22.
14. Delattre BM, Viallon M, Wei H, Zhu Y, Pai VM, Wen H, et al. Intravoxel incoherent motion applied to cardiac diffusion weighted MRI using breath-hold acquisitions in healthy volunteers. J Cardiovasc Magn Reson. 2012; 14(Suppl 1):P261.
15. Froeling M, Strijkers GJ, Nederveen AJ, Chamuleau SA, Luijten PR. Feasibility of in vivo whole heart DTI and IVIM with a 15 minute acquisition protocol. J Cardiovasc Magn Reson. 2014;16(Suppl 1):O15.
16. Moulin K, Croisille P, Feiweier T, Delattre BMA, Wei H, Robert B, et al. In vivo free-breathing DTI and IVIM of the whole human heart using a real-time slice-followed SE-EPI navigator-based sequence: a reproducibility study in healthy volunteers. Magn Reson Med. 2016;76:70–82.
17. Ardenkjaer-Larsen JH, Fridlund B, Gram A, Hansson G, Hansson L, Lerche MH, et al. Increase in signal-to-noise ratio of > 10,000 times in liquid-state NMR. Proc Natl Acad Sci U S A. 2003;100:10158–63.
18. Golman K, Petersson JS, Magnusson P, Johansson E, Akeson P, Chai C-M, et al. Cardiac metabolism measured noninvasively by hyperpolarized 13C MRI. Magn Reson Med. 2008;59:1005–13.
19. Cunningham CH, Lau JYC, Chen AP, Geraghty BJ, Perks WJ, Roifman I, et al. Hyperpolarized 13C metabolic MRI of the human heart: initial experience. Circ Res. 2016;119:1177–82.
20. Von Morze C, Larson PEZ, Hu S, Yoshihara HAI, Bok RA, Goga A, et al. Investigating tumor perfusion and metabolism using multiple hyperpolarized 13C compounds: HP001, pyruvate and urea. Magn Reson Imaging. 2012;30:305–11.
21. Grant AK, Vinogradov E, Wang X, Lenkinski RE, Alsop DC. Perfusion imaging with a freely diffusible hyperpolarized contrast agent. Magn Reson Med. 2011;66:746–55.

22. Durst M, Chiavazza E, Haase A, Aime S, Schwaiger M, Schulte RF. α-trideuteromethyl [15N] glutamine: a long-lived hyperpolarized perfusion marker. Magn Reson Med. 2016;76:1900–4.
23. Reed GD, von Morze C, Bok R, Koelsch BL, Van Criekinge M, Smith KJ, et al. High resolution 13 C MRI with hyperpolarized urea: in vivo T2 mapping and 15 N labeling effects. IEEE Trans Med Imaging. 2014;33:362–71.
24. Laustsen C, Stokholm Nørlinger T, Christoffer Hansen D, Qi H, Mose Nielsen P, Bonde Bertelsen L, et al. Hyperpolarized 13 C urea relaxation mechanism reveals renal changes in diabetic nephropathy. Magn Reson Med. 2016;75:515–8.
25. Nielsen PM, Szocska Hansen ES, Nørlinger TS, Nørregaard R, Bonde Bertelsen L, Stødkilde Jørgensen H, et al. Renal ischemia and reperfusion assessment with three-dimensional hyperpolarized 13 C, 15 N2-urea. Magn Reson Med. 2016;0:1–7.
26. Hansen ESS, Stewart NJ, Wild JM, Stødkilde-Jørgensen H, Laustsen C. Hyperpolarized (13) C,(15) N2-urea MRI for assessment of the urea gradient in the porcine kidney. Magn Reson Med. 2016;76:1895–9.
27. Bahrami N, Swisher CL, Von Morze C, Vigneron DB, Larson PEZ. Kinetic and perfusion modeling of hyperpolarized (13) C pyruvate and urea in cancer with arbitrary RF flip angles. Quant Imaging Med Surg. 2014;4: 24–32.
28. Von Morze C, Larson PEZ, Hu S, Keshari K, Wilson DM, Ardenkjaer-Larsen JH, et al. Imaging of blood flow using hyperpolarized [13C] urea in preclinical cancer models. J Magn Reson Imaging. 2011;33:692–7.
29. Johansson E, Månsson S, Wirestam R, Svensson J, Petersson JS, Golman K, et al. Cerebral perfusion assessment by bolus tracking using hyperpolarized 13C. Magn Reson Med. 2004;51:464–72.
30. Lau AZ, Miller JJ, Robson MD, Tyler DJ. Simultaneous assessment of cardiac metabolism and perfusion using copolarized [1-13 C] pyruvate and 13 C-urea. Magn Reson Med. 2017;77:151–8.
31. Lau AZ, Miller JJ, Robson MD, Tyler DJ. Cardiac perfusion imaging using hyperpolarized 13 c urea using flow sensitizing gradients. Magn Reson Med. 2016;75:1474–83.
32. Lau AZ, Chen AP, Hurd RE, Cunningham CH. Spectral-spatial excitation for rapid imaging of DNP compounds. NMR Biomed. 2011;24:988–96.
33. Sigfridsson A, Weiss K, Wissmann L, Busch J, Krajewski M, Batel M, et al. Hybrid multiband excitation multiecho acquisition for hyperpolarized ^{13}C spectroscopic imaging. Magn Reson Med. 2015;73:1713–7.
34. Shang H, Skloss T, von Morze C, Carvajal L, Van Criekinge M, Milshteyn E, et al. Handheld electromagnet carrier for transfer of hyperpolarized carbon-13 samples. Magn Reson Med. 2016;75:917–22.
35. Ogg RJ, Kingsley PB, Taylor JS. WET, a T1- and B1-insensitive water-suppression method for in vivo localized 1H NMR spectroscopy. J Magn Reson B. 1994;104:1–10.
36. Roemer PB, Edelstein WA, Hayes CE, Souza SP, Mueller OM. The NMR phased array. Magn Reson Med. 1990;16:192–225.
37. Cerqueira MD. Standardized myocardial segmentation and nomenclature for tomographic imaging of the heart: a statement for healthcare professionals from the cardiac imaging Committee of the Council on Clinical Cardiology of the American Heart Association. Circulation. 2002;105:539–42.
38. Firbank MJ, Coulthard A, Harrison RM, Williams ED. A comparison of two methods for measuring the signal to noise ratio on MR images. Phys Med Biol. 1999;44:N261–4.
39. Li X, Huang W, Rooney WD. Signal-to-noise ratio, contrast-to-noise ratio and pharmacokinetic modeling considerations in dynamic contrast-enhanced magnetic resonance imaging. Magn Reson Imaging. 2012;30:1313–22.
40. Jerosch-Herold M, Stillman AE, Wilke N. Magnetic resonance quantification of the myocardial perfusion reserve with a fermi function model for constrained deconvolution. Med Phys. 1998;25:73–84.
41. Forster J, Sieverding L, Breuer J, Lutz O, Schick F. Fast acceleration-encoded magnetic resonance imaging. Med Phys. 2001;28:28–35.
42. Wiesinger F, Weidl E, Menzel MI, Janich MA, Khegai O, Glaser SJ, et al. IDEAL spiral CSI for dynamic metabolic MR imaging of hyperpolarized [1-13C] pyruvate. Magn Reson Med. 2012;68:8–16.
43. Durst M, Koellisch U, Frank A, Rancan G, Gringeri CV, Karas V, et al. Comparison of acquisition schemes for hyperpolarised 13 C imaging. NMR Biomed. 2015;28:715–25.
44. Wissmann L, Niemann M, Gotschy A, Manka R, Kozerke S. Quantitative three-dimensional myocardial perfusion cardiovascular magnetic resonance with accurate two-dimensional arterial input function assessment. J Cardiovasc Magn Reson. 2015;17:108.
45. Johansson E, Olsson LE, Månsson S, Petersson JS, Golman K, Ståhlberg F, et al. Perfusion assessment with bolus differentiation: a technique applicable to hyperpolarized tracers. Magn Reson Med. 2004;52:1043–51.

12

Cardiovascular magnetic resonance in an adult human population: serial observations from the multi-ethnic study of atherosclerosis

Kihei Yoneyama[1,4], Bharath A. Venkatesh[1], David A. Bluemke[2], Robyn L. McClelland[3] and João A.C. Lima[1,5*]

Abstract

The Multi-Ethnic Study of Atherosclerosis (MESA) is the first large-scale multi-ethnic population study in the U.S. to use advanced cardiovascular magnetic resonance (CMR) imaging. MESA participants were free of cardiovascular disease at baseline between 2000 and 2002, and were followed up between 2009 and 2011 with repeated CMR examinations as part of MESA. CMR allows the clinician to visualize and accurately quantify volume and dimensions of all four cardiac chambers; measure systolic and diastolic ventricular function; assess myocardial fibrosis; assess vessel lumen size, vessel wall morphology, and vessel stiffness. CMR has a number of advantages over other imaging modalities such as echocardiography, computed tomography, and invasive angiography, and has been proposed as a diagnostic strategy for high-risk populations. MESA has been extensively evaluating CMR imaging biomarkers, as markers of subclinical disease, in the last 15 years for low-risk populations. On a more practical level, some of the imaging biomarkers developed and studied are translatable to at-risk populations. In this review, we discuss the progression of subclinical cardiovascular disease and the mechanisms responsible for the transition to symptomatic clinical outcomes based on our findings from MESA.

Keywords: Ageing, Fibrosis, Heart failure, Cardiovascular disease, Torsion

Background

The Multi-Ethnic Study of Atherosclerosis (MESA) is a prospective study sponsored by the National Heart, Lung, and Blood Institute (NHLBI) of the National Institutes of Health. The major objective of MESA was to evaluate the mechanisms that underlie the development and progression of subclinical cardiovascular disease (CVD) among asymptomatic individuals in the general population. MESA was primarily designed to study the progression of subclinical CVD and the mechanisms responsible for the transition to symptomatic clinical outcomes [1]. In brief, between July 2000 and August 2002, 6814 men and women, 45 to 84 years of age—who identified themselves as Caucasian, African American, Hispanic, or Chinese, and who were free of clinically apparent CVD were recruited. Cardiovascular magnetic resonance imaging (CMR) was performed on 5004 participants as part of the baseline examination and 3015 underwent a follow-up CMR between 2010 and 2012 (year-10).

CMR is a noninvasive medical test that creates detailed pictures of the beating heart and vessels to look at their structure and function. In MESA, CMR was used to accurately quantify volume and dimensions of all four cardiac chambers, systolic and diastolic ventricular and atrial function, assess extent of replacement and interstitial fibrosis, and measure aortic structure and function, to evaluate patterns of cardiac structural remodeling and the prevalence of myocardial fibrosis across the life course, identify the myocardial mechanical consequences of remodeling, explore ventricular-arterial coupling and the role of arterial stiffness in CVD, and to study the prognostic importance of CMR biomarkers.

* Correspondence: jlima@jhmi.edu
[1]Department of Cardiology, Johns Hopkins University, Baltimore, MD, USA
[5]Professor of Medicine, Radiology and Epidemiology, Johns Hopkins Hospital, Johns Hopkins University, Blalock 524D1, 600 North Wolfe Street, Baltimore, MD 21287, USA
Full list of author information is available at the end of the article

In this review, we discuss the progression of subclinical CVD and the mechanisms responsible for the transition to symptomatic clinical outcomes based on our findings from MESA.

Left ventricular (LV) remodeling across the life course

The observed variations in the structure of the left ventricle might be attributable to differences in demographic variables (e.g., age, gender, and race), traditional risk factors (e.g., LV overload by blood pressure or atherosclerosis), other medical conditions, socioeconomic status, and genetic influences in general populations. In MESA, LV wall thickness by CMR was associated with gender, race, body size, and LV function [2]. Chinese participants had lower volumes and mass than other ethnic groups among normal participants without known CVD risk factors [3]. LV volumes and mass were significantly greater for men than women, and, more spherical shape of LV was seen in women as compared to men [4–6].

The average age of populations around the globe is increasing; as a result, an increasing number of older individuals become afflicted by CVD [7]. While age is one of the most powerful risk factors for CVD, it is important to understand the LV adaptation mechanisms that function against the altered cardiovascular system during aging in human adult life. The findings of MESA CMR related to aging are summarized in Fig. 1. The MESA serial longitudinal study confirmed that a pattern of LV remodeling across the life course is concentric remodeling with progressively reduced LV volumes resulting in an increased LV mass-to-volume ratio. Specifically, we see a significant age-related longitudinal increase in LV mass in men and a slight longitudinal decrease in women over 9 years follow-up; additionally, longitudinal decreases in LV end-diastolic volume and stroke volume were seen in both men and women, leading to significant increases in adverse LV concentric remodeling (increased mass-to-volume ratio) in both men and women [8]. The LV ejection fraction (LVEF), however, was maintained with age due to a progressive decline in LV end-diastolic volume (Fig. 1) [5].

Aging prolongs exposure to CVD risk factors, therefore, understanding the influences of adverse LV remodeling by risk factors in the general population is important. In cross-sectional studies, CVD risk factors were associated with LV concentric remodeling (i.e., increased blood pressure, body mass index, body fat, insulin resistance, and presence of hypertension and diabetes), even though variants of LV remodeling patterns were observed with

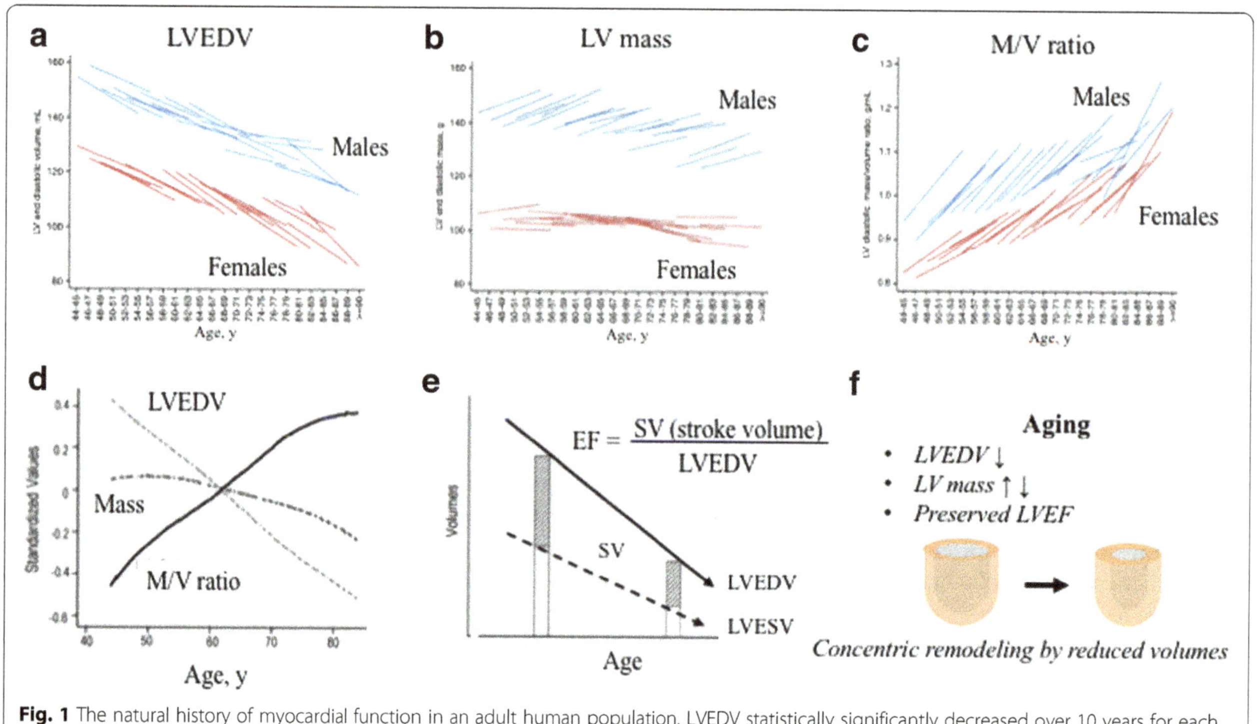

Fig. 1 The natural history of myocardial function in an adult human population. LVEDV statistically significantly decreased over 10 years for each age category **a** and LV mass increased in Men **b** and M/V ratio increased **c** despite LV mass did not progressively increase **b** and **d**. Although SV progressively falls, LVEF maintains due to progressive decline in LV volumes **e**. Aging is associated with the development of a concentric remodeling pattern secondary to a progressive decline in LV volume **f**. LV = left ventricular; LVEF = left ventricular ejection fraction; LVEDV = Left ventricular end diastolic volume; LVESV = Left ventricular end systolic volume; M/V = mass-to-volume ratio Figures prepared based on data from Eng et al. [8], and Cheng et al. [5]

each CVD risk factor (i.e, hypertensive participants had concentric remodeling with greater LV volumes, whereas diabetic participants had concentric remodeling with lower volumes) [4, 6, 9–12]. In addition, a higher ankle-brachial index, traffic exposure, and genetic variation were associated with higher LV mass [13–15]. Higher physical activity was associated with higher LV mass but not with concentric remodeling, and higher activity was associated with lower heart rate [16]. MESA longitudinal studies confirmed some of the findings of the cross-sectional studies by showing that changes in CVD risk factors are associated with changes in LV remodeling, e.g., weight loss, reduced blood pressure, and reduced heart rate were associated with a smaller increase in age-related concentric remodeling [11, 12].

LV remodeling and cardiac events

Progressive LV remodeling may identify individuals at high risk for cardiac events in the general population. For example, in contrast to the natural history of concentric remodeling, the risk of incident CVD is greater for those individuals who develop concentric remodeling at a younger age (Fig. 2a). This pattern of ventricular remodeling appears to confer significant CVD risk, especially when present earlier in life [5].

Heart failure (HF) is an important contributor to the burden and cost of national healthcare expenditures, and with the aging of worldwide populations, the estimated prevalence and cost of care for HF will increase markedly for all sex and racial/ethnic subgroups [7, 17]. The pattern of hypertrophy is related to pressure overload leading to concentric hypertrophy and volume overload leading to eccentric hypertrophy.

The Framingham study has suggested that early identification of LV hypertrophy by electrocardiogram (ECG) or echocardiography may provide an opportunity to prevent the development of cardiac events, however, the MESA CMR study found that ECG had low sensitivity (10% to 26%) for detecting CMR-defined hypertrophy [18], and that CMR is highly accurate using 3-dimensional ventricular size and shape compared to conventional echocardiography [19]. The predictive value of CMR for heart failure (HF) events exceeded that of coronary artery calcium (CAC) and carotid intima-medial thickness (IMT) for both men and women [20].

In MESA, higher LV mass at baseline (≥95th percentile compared to the reference group of the <50% percentile) is strongly associated with incident HF with a hazard ratio of 8.6 (95% confidence interval: 3.9 to 19.9) (Fig. 2b) [21]. The addition of N-terminal pro b-type natriuretic peptide (NT-pro BNP) with LV mass produced the largest increase in the c-statistic over the basic traditional risk assessment for predicting HF (Fig. 2c) [22]. Extreme LV sphericity was associated with higher incidence of HF and atrial fibrillation [23]. The strengths of MESA include high-quality assessments of multiple risk factors for HF including traditional risk factors and biomarkers, which are responsible for the high predictive value of the MESA HF score [22].

LV replacement fibrosis in the general population

Late gadolinium-enhancement imaging (LGE) can be used to detect replacement or focal myocardial fibrosis (scar) with a high degree of accuracy [24, 25]. CMR LGE represents end-organ damage and worse cardiac prognosis among patients with cardiomyopathy [26, 27]; identification of LGE might significantly improve risk stratification in the general population.

From a community-based cohort in Iceland with a median age of 76 years, the prevalence of unrecognized

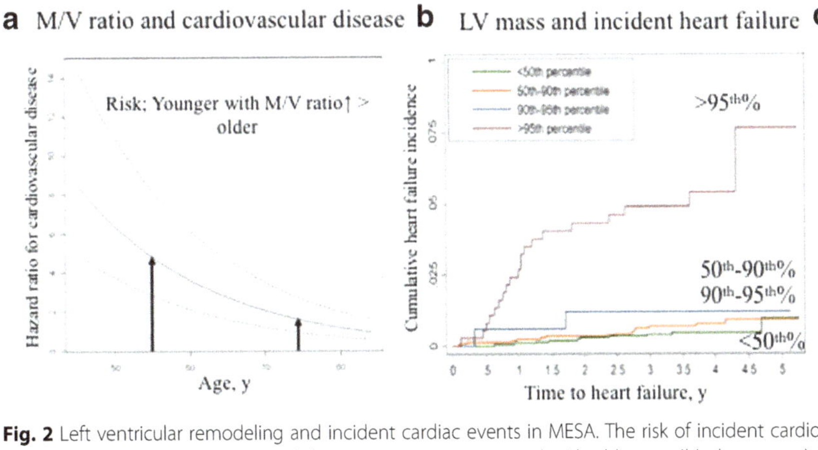

c Heart failure prediction from MESA

Models	C-statistic	NRI (p value)
Traditional risk	0.80	
(Risk)+LV mass	0.85	0.25 (<0.001)
(Risk+LV mass)+logNT-proBNP	0.89	0.15 (0.018)

NRI = net reclassification improvement, NT-proBNP = N-terminal pro-B-type natriuretic peptide.

Fig. 2 Left ventricular remodeling and incident cardiac events in MESA. The risk of incident cardiovascular disease is greater for those individuals who develop the concentric remodeling at a younger compared with older age (*black arrows*, **a**). Higher LV mass (hypertrophy) is associated with incident heart failure **b**. Additional LV mass and log NT-pro BNP produces the largest increased in c-statistic and improves the NRI beyond traditional risk factors **c**. Figures prepared based on data from Cheng et al. [5], Bluemke et al. [21], and Chahal et al. [22]. Abbreviations as in Fig. 1

myocardial infarction (MI) detected by CMR with LGE was 17% (157/936), and was associated with increased mortality similar to recognized MI, compared to individuals with no MI [28]. In MESA, of 1840 participants with a mean age of 68 years, 7.9% had myocardial scars defined by focal LGE, of which 78% (114/146) were undetected by ECG or by clinical adjudication [29]. The following individual risk factors were associated with higher odds of myocardial scar: age, male sex, body mass index, current smoking, and hypertension at baseline in 2000 to 2002 [29]. Importantly, CAC score by CT at baseline was associated with a typical ischemic scar pattern in 2009 to 2011 [29]. These suggest that unrecognized MI appears to represent a phenotype of coronary heart disease related to atherosclerosis risk factors.

From a clinical longitudinal study of patients with idiopathic, dilated cardiomyopathy (non-ischemic) receiving optimal medical therapy, LV systolic function decreased during a 24-month follow-up in patients with myocardial scar at baseline, while reverse remodeling was observed in patients without myocardial scar [30]. MESA reported results similar to that in a high-risk population, namely that asymptomatic individuals with prevalent LGE had an enlarged left ventricle (concentric hypertrophy in women and LV dilatation in men) with progressively declining LVEF; conversely, individuals without myocardial scar maintained LV function [31]. Therefore, the presence of replacement fibrosis was associated with changing LV volumes and reduced function over time even in individuals in lower-risk populations, and who may be at risk to develop asymptomatic HF regardless of whether fibrosis was ischemic or atypical.

LV interstitial fibrosis in a general population

Although LGE CMR allows for the assessment of replacement myocardial fibrosis, it is limited in the evaluation of diffuse interstitial fibrosis. T1 myocardial mapping—a fairly new technique that can be used to identify the exact T1 value of tissue—enables direct myocardial signal quantification, characterization of myocardial tissue composition and assessment of interstitial fibrosis, and correlates with interstitial fibrosis as assessed by means of invasive biopsy [24, 25].

Our study, using contrast T1 found the following two main results: First, the age-related remodeling pattern of left ventricule—which is a progressive decline in LV volumes leading to concentric remodeling—is seen with progressive LV diffuse fibrosis. In other words, persions with either greater LV mass or without concentric remodeling are likely to have less interstitial fibrosis on average [31, 32]. Cardiac aging, characterized by shrinking LV volume with diffuse interstitial fibrosis, can support the pathological finding of an age-related increase in myocyte deaths accompanied with reductions in coronary vasculature through the cardiac life course [31, 33]. Second, hypertension contributed to interstitial fibrosis [31, 32]. This also supports the pathological findings of increases in the extracellular matrix by accumulation of perivascular fibrosis and fibrosis of the endomysium and perimysium in hypertensive heart disease [34].

In MESA, both replacement and interstitial fibrosis are important determinants of LV function, as shown in Fig. 3. Interestingly, men had a linear decline in LV systolic function with interstitial fibrosis, whereas women had a progressive decline in LV diastolic (not systolic) function with fibrosis [31, 35]. Perhaps restrictive filling with eventual diastolic dysfunction—due to progressive diffuse myocardial fibrosis with fewer myocytes (related to aging)—could progress to a stiffer left ventricule. In addition, men had progressively increased interstitial fibrosis with burden of CVD risk factors, while women were likely to have more interstitial fibrosis than men independent of CVD risk factors [32, 36]. Of note, these results concur with a previous epidemiology study finding that diastolic HF is more common in elderly men and women than in younger patients [37].

Cardiac deformation imaging using tagged CMR

CMR tissue tagging provides precise quantification of incipient myocardial dysfunction through the assessment of myocardial strain and torsion, and has been used as the reference standard to validate two-dimensional speckle tracking echocardiography.

In the MESA population, reduced regional peak systolic circumferential strain was associated with impaired regional myocardial perfusion in participants who did not have relevant coronary artery stenosis (Fig. 4a) [38]. This suggests that impaired myocardial shortening enhances the ability to identify early subendocardial ischemia and has a potential role in risk stratification beyond traditional LVEF. For example, worse circumferential myocardial strain has been observed to be associated with LV hypertrophy, concentric remodeling, subclinical atherosclerosis, older age, male sex, hypertension, resting higher heart rate, smoking, and metabolic syndrome [5, 6, 39–44], and has been shown to have incremental predictive value for HF events beyond the traditional LVEF (Fig. 4b) [45]. Diastolic function from circumferential strain curves showed a powerful independent ability for the prediction of HF and atrial fibrillation over an 8-year follow-up period [46]. In addition, tagged CMR provides further insight into the depth of the cardiac pump mechanism in humans. For example, it has been noted that perhaps the discrepancy between the age-associated increase in LVEF and the decline in circumferential shortening can be explained by the

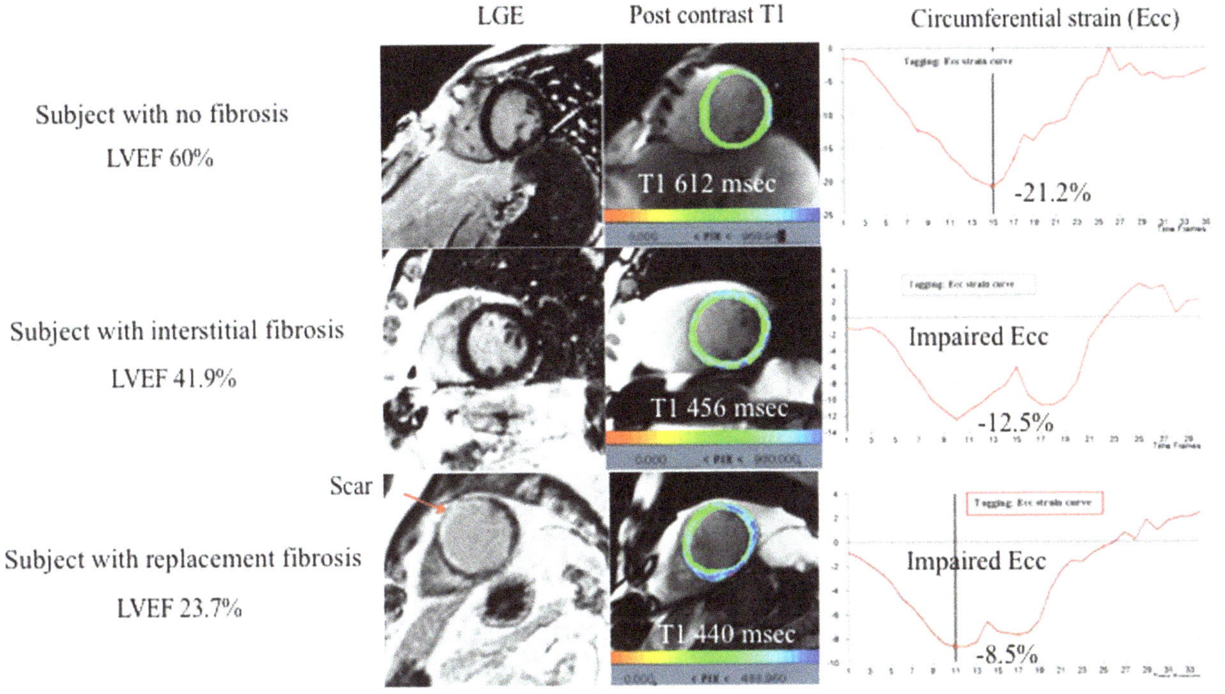

Fig. 3 Fibrosis and left ventricular function in MESA. The subject without a LGE-defined scar had a relatively lower post contrast T1 time at 25 min with altered regional myocardial shortening and LVEF compared to the subject without an LGE-defined myocardial scar and no evidence of extra-cellular expansion. The subject with a LGE-defined replacement fibrosis had a progressively reduced systolic function. Figures prepared based on data from Donekal et al. [35]. LGE = late gadolinium-enhanced image; LVEF = left ventricular ejection fraction

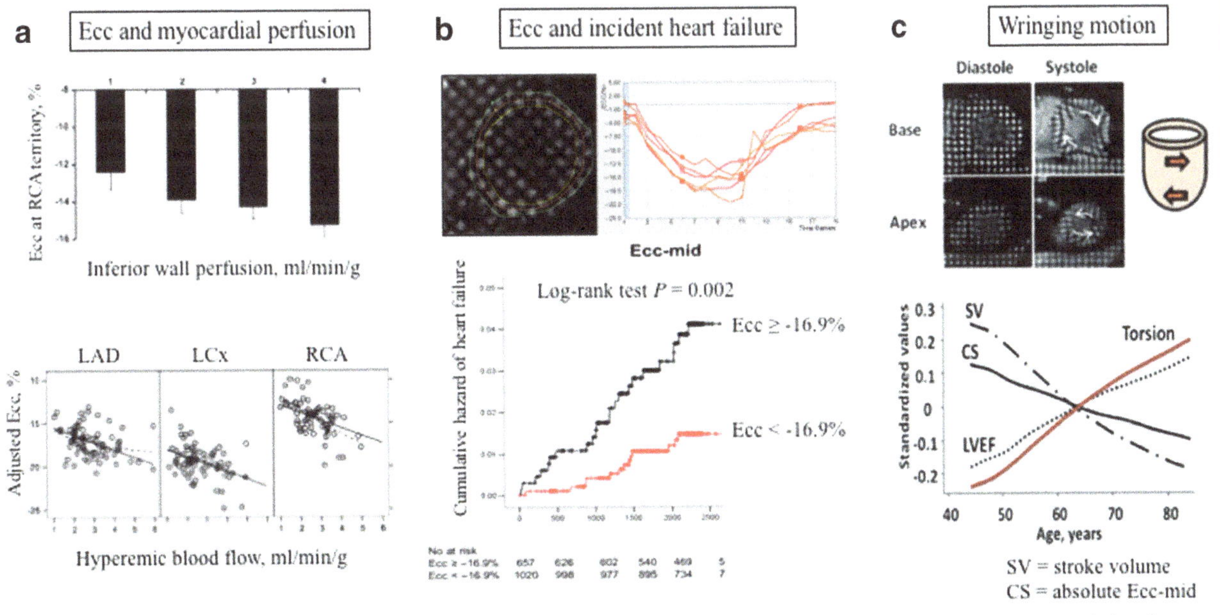

Fig. 4 Cardiac deformation imaging using tagged CMR in asymptomatic individuals. Impaired Ecc is associated with lower myocardial perfusion and blood flow **a** Impaired LV circumferential shortening (Ecc) provides predictive value for incident heart failure during 5.5 years follow-up **b** LV torsion, however, is greater with older age despite lower stroke volume and myocardial shortening **c**. LV wringing motion might represents a compensatory mechanism for systolic dysfunction to maintain LVEF. Figures prepared based on date from Rosen et al. [38], Choi et al. [45], and Yoneyama et al. [6]. LAD = left anterior descending artery; LCx = left circumflex artery; RCA = right coronary artery. Abbreviations as in Fig. 1

enhanced wringing motion of the left ventricule assessed by tagged CMR (Fig. 4c) [6], which represents a human compensatory mechanism to maintain LVEF in age-related concentric remodeling.

Finally, progression of symptomatic events from asymptomatic individuals is summarized in Fig. 5.

A novel CMR marker for LV trabeculation

Clinically, LV noncompaction is a myocardial disorder characterized by excessive LV trabeculae. Although a high degree of noncompacted (trabeculated) myocardium in relationship to compact myocardium (trabeculated to compact myocardium [T/M] ratio > 2.3) has been associated with a diagnosis of LV noncompaction, MESA found that 43% of subjects without cardiac disease or hypertension had a T/M ratio > 2.3 in at least 1 myocardial segment [47]. Using fractal dimension, which is an automated assessment for trabecular quantification that is relatively insensitive to compacted myocardium wall thickness, the LV was more trabeculated in African-American and Hispanic participants than white participants, and smoothest in Chinese-American participants [48]. MESA also confirmed in a longitudinal observation study that a greater extent of LV trabeculation was not associated with an absolute decline in LVEF during the approximately 10 years of the MESA study. Our findings suggest that in subjects with a low pre-test probability for cardiomyopathy and marked trabeculation, greater trabeculation is not related to ejection fraction in asymptomatic subjects [49]. However, the relationship of high degrees of trabeculations to regional function and other remodeling mechanisms has not yet been determined [50].

Right ventricle in a general population

CMR is the preferred method for evaluating right ventricular structure and function due to its crescent-shape in cross-sectional images. In MESA, older age was associated with lower RV (right ventricular) mass and higher RV ejection fraction; men had greater RV mass and larger RV volumes than women, but had lower RV ejection fraction; African-Americans had lower RV mass than whites, whereas Hispanics had higher RV mass [51]. Traffic exposure was associated with higher RV mass, i.e., participants who lived in the same neighborhood for several years had the strongest associations

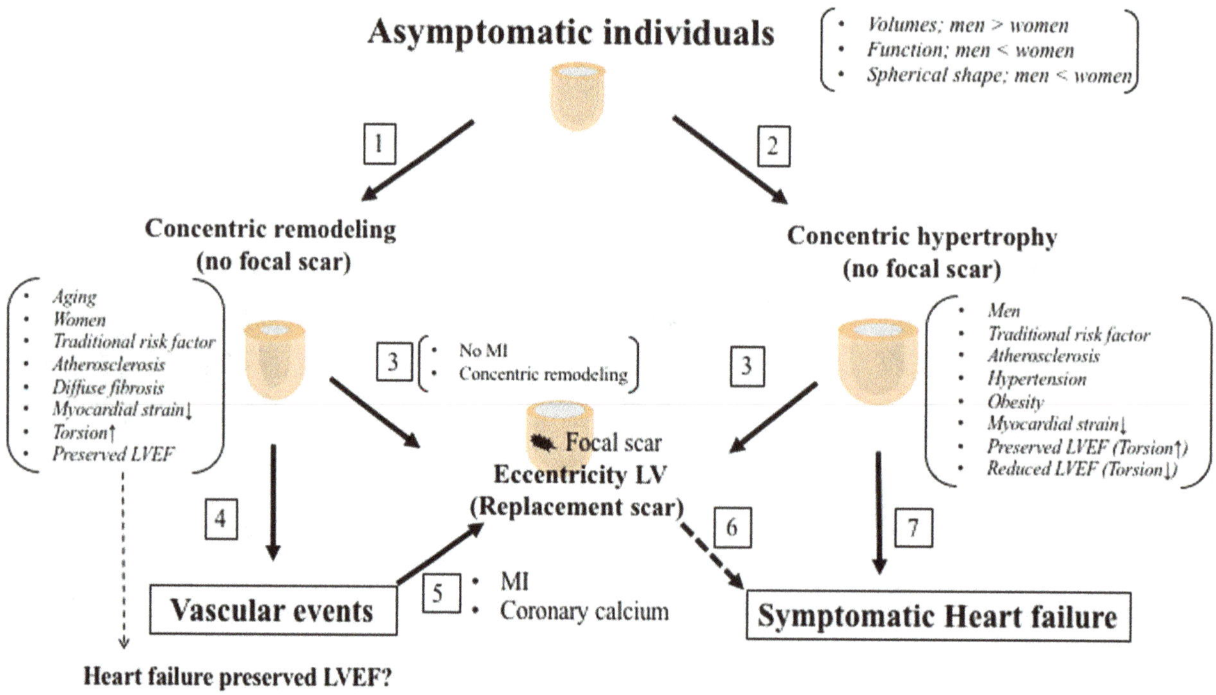

Fig. 5 Potential pathways in the progression from asymptomatic to symptomatic cardiovascular events from MESA CMR remodeling and fibrosis data. Aging leads to concentric remodeling (higher M/V ratio and maintained LV mass) without no focal scar (pathway 1) [5, 6, 69]. Typically hypertension progresses to concentric hypertrophy (higher M/V ratio and LV mass) without focal scar (pathway 2) [6, 31]. The pathway from concentric remodeling and hypertrophy to replacement fibrosis without MI (pathway 3) [31]. Individuals with concentric remodeling can develop vascular events with preserved LVEF (pathway 4) [5, 21]. Individuals with concentric remodeling with MI or severe coronary calcification can contribute to replacement fibrosis (pathway 5) [29]. Individuals with concentric hypertrophy can develop symptomatic vascular events either with replacement scar (pathway 6) [28] or without (pathway 7) [21, 22]. Black arrows depict MESA CMR results, and thicker dot arrow, a known pathway. MI = myocardial infarction. Abbreviations as in Fig. 1

between nitrogen dioxide and RV mass [52]. Participants with RV hypertrophy had a significant increase in the risk of HF or death that was independent of LV mass, and had a stronger association with the outcome in the setting of lower LV mass [53].

Left atrial (LA) measurements by tissue-tracking CMR in asymptomatic individuals

In normal sinus rhythm, LA performance is characterized by a complex of three basic functions: reservoir function (collection of pulmonary venous flow during LV systole), conduit function (passage of blood to the LV during early diastole), and active booster pump function (augments LV filling during LV late diastole) [54, 55]. Hoit's review of clinical studies examining LA size and function found that LA ejection fraction, which is volume assessment, is a promising measure for predicting CVD in a patient population [56].

Tissue-tracking on LA wall from cine CMR can provide an alternative and additional assessment of risk

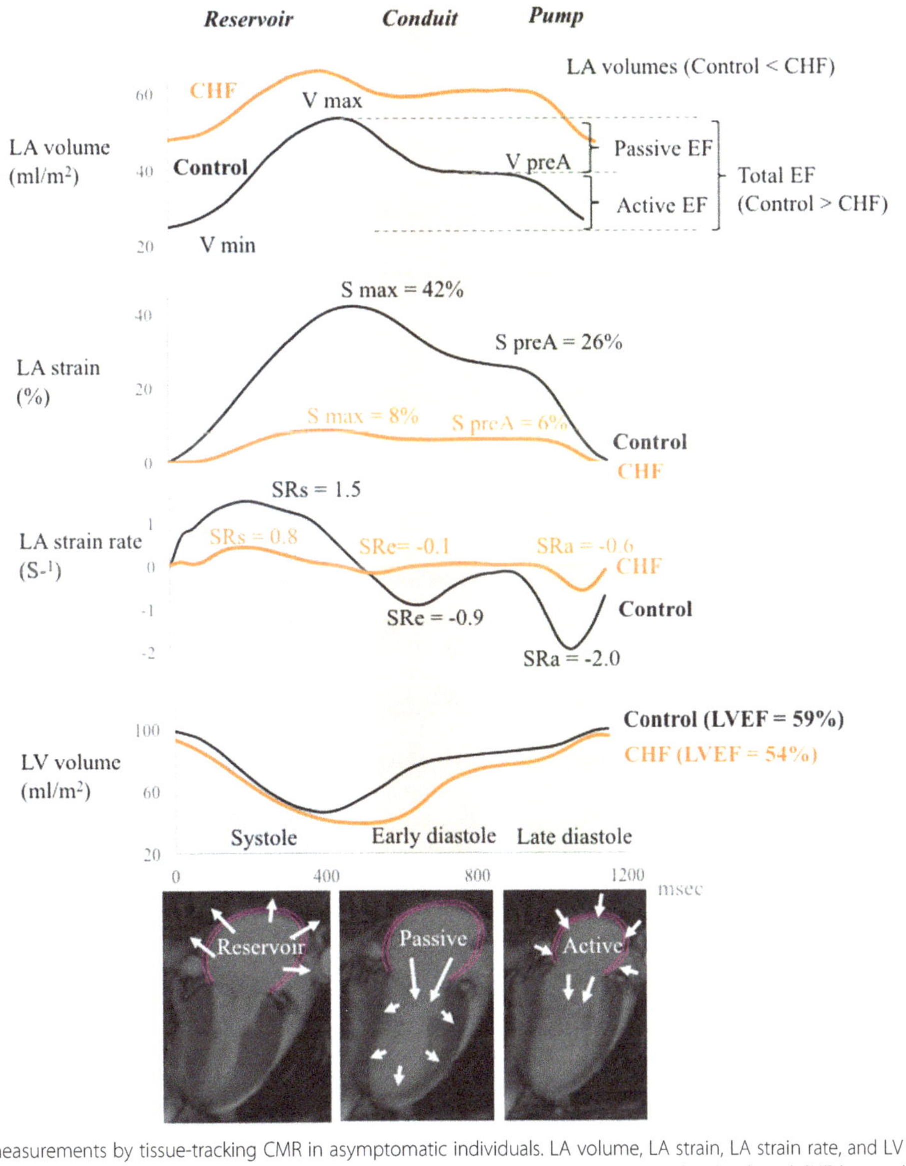

Fig. 6 Left atrial measurements by tissue-tracking CMR in asymptomatic individuals. LA volume, LA strain, LA strain rate, and LV volume in a asymptomatic participant free of cardiovascular daises as a control (*block line*) and a MESA participant who developed CHF (*orange line*). A case of CHF had a relatively greater LA volumes with impaired LA strains (S max and S preA) and LA strain rates (SRs, SRe, and SRa) than a control. Volumes are index to body surface area. LA function was analyzed by using a tissue-tracking method with semiauto mated software (multimodality tissue tracking [MTT] version 5.0; Toshiba, Tochigi, Japan). CHF; congestive heart failure; LA = left atrial; LV = left ventricular; S max = maximum strain; S preA = pre atrial contraction strain; SRa = strain rate at atrial contraction; SRe = strain rate at LV early diastole; SRs = maximum strain rate, V max = maximum indexed volume; V min = minimum indexed volume; V pre A = pre-atrial contraction indexed volume

stratification or diastolic function beyond LA volume assessment. Data from a clinical study using this technique on 169 patients with a history of atrial fibrillation indicated that lower LA strain and strain rate during LV diastole (impaired LA reservoir function) is significantly associated with a prior history of stroke, and that the incremental value of LA strain for diagnosis of stroke is further increased by adding LA global strain to LA volume [55]. Similarly, in the MESA population, asymptomatic individuals who developed HF had a lower LA strain during LV diastole (impaired LA reservoir function) and a higher minimum LA volume (impaired pump function and volume) than those without HF events. The deteriorations in LA performance appeared to robustly predict HF events independent of LV mass and NT-pro BNP [57].

Our study also reported the following: first, a presence of replacement scar on LV was associated with all three basic LA performance functions including an impaired reservoir function (lower maximum LA strain and strain rate), a conduit function (lower absolute strain rate), and a pump function (lower absolute strain rate), but was not significantly associated with total LAEF. Second, LV diffuse myocardial fibrosis assessed by contrast T1 was associated with an impaired reservoir function (lower LA strain) and a pump function (lower LA strain rate) but was not significantly associated with LA volumes [58]. These findings suggests that tissue-tracking on the LA wall can be a more sensitive marker to detect early myocardial disease among asymptomatic individuals despite the fact that LAEF might decrease, as documented in advanced decompensated cardiac disease (Fig. 6).

Vascular imaging using CMR in MESA

CMR has a distinct advantage over ultrasound in that three-dimensional visualization of the vessel wall and identification of components on the atherosclerotic plaque are possible. CMR has the unique ability to assess aortic geometry and function, representing vascular stiffness by vessel distensibility and pulse wave velocity with high reproducibility [59, 60].

Of over 3500 MESA participants with a mean age of 61 years, ascending aorta diameter was increased with age; higher aortic stiffness as measured by aortic distensibility was associated with hypertension, larger left ventricle, and incident CVD events (Fig. 7a) [60–63]. Individuals with high aortic stiffness had an almost 4-fold increase in risk of incident CVD compared to individuals with preserved aortic distensibility if they had a low-to-intermediate-risk CVD profile [62].

In a longitudinal MESA study over 10 years of follow-up, aortic stiffness was associated with wall thickness of the aorta, which increases by 0.032 mm/year [63]. Age, smoking, and increased blood pressure were associated with increases in aortic stiffness, but reduction in blood pressure was associated with less increase in the stiffness [64]. The loss of proximal aortic function was a robust

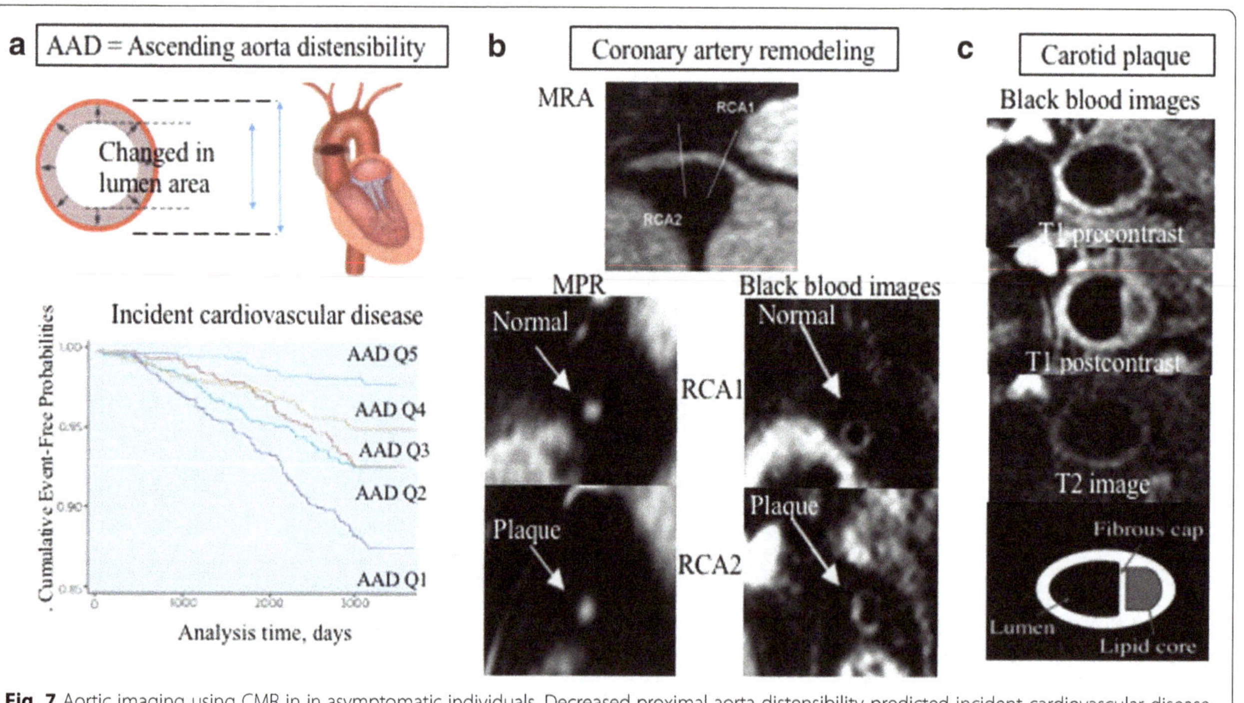

Fig. 7 Aortic imaging using CMR in in asymptomatic individuals. Decreased proximal aorta distensibility predicted incident cardiovascular disease **a** MRA without contrast shows no significant stenosis in the proximal RCA, and black blood images shows normal wall and eccentric plaque **b** Black blood images obtained the carotid artery, and identify lipid core **c**. Figures prepared based on date from Redheuil et al. [62], Miao et al. [66] and Wasserman et al. [67]

marker of vascular alteration, particularly in individuals with a lower traditional CVD risk profile as compared to those with a higher risk profile.

Atherosclerotic coronary artery plaque rupture is a key event leading to acute coronary syndromes. Black-blood coronary arterial wall CMR provides a unique new method to nonivasively image and assess the morphological features of the coronary arteries (Fig. 7b). MESA has reported the ability of CMR to identify coronary artery remodeling as an early marker of subclinical coronary atherosclerosis among participants with zero CAC score by computed tomography. The spatial resolution of CMR, however, needs improvement [65, 66].

MESA also has used black-blood sequences to noninvasively characterize carotid-artery atheroma composition (Fig. 7c). Using this technique, a lipid core was seen in 71% as selected from this asymptomatic population who had thickened carotid walls (>1.5 mm by CMR), and plasma total cholesterol rather than other CVD risk factors, was strongly associated with lipid core presence by CMR [67]. In addition, carotid artery remodeling and lipid core presence were independent predictors of incident CVD events in MESA [68]. Consequently, vascular imaging features by CMR might be important predictors of cardiovascular risk in asymptomatic individuals.

Conclusion

MESA is one of the first large-scale population studies to use advanced CMR imaging techniques among asymptomatic individuals, and to follow up with repeated CMR examinations as part of a large multi-ethnic population study. A dominant pattern of LV remodeling across the life course is concentric remodeling by progressively reduced LV volumes. Progressively increased LV concentric remodeling is associated with interstitial fibrosis and is a marker of CVD events. Abnormal remodeling with LV hypertrophy is associated with replacement fibrosis, and a high risk for developing HF. Replacement scar, however, in more than half of the participants with scar by CMR LGE is undetected by ECG or by clinical adjudication.

Assessing LA and vascular geometry and function can be alternative tools to detect early stage subclinical disease. These CMR markers may significantly improve risk stratification in the general population. Finally, further advances in imaging are required to understand the role of risk factors and the progression of symptomatic disease pathways in the asymptomatic.

Abbreviations

CAC: Coronary artery calcium; CMR: Cardiovascular magnetic resonance; CVD: Cardiovascular diseases; HF: Heart failure; LA: Left atrial; LGE: Late gadolinium enhancement; LV: Left ventricular; MESA: Multi-Ethnic Study of Atherosclerosis; MI: myocardial infarction; RV: Right ventricular

Acknowledgements

The authors thank the other investigators, staff, and participants of the MESA study for their valuable contributions. A full list of participating MESA investigators and institutions can be found at http://www.mesa-nhlbi.org.

Funding

This research was supported by contracts N01-HC-95159, N01-HC-95160, N01-HC-95161, N01-HC-95162, N01-HC-95163, N01-HC-95164, N01-HC-95165, N01-HC-95166, N01-HC-95167, N01-HC-95168, and N01-HC-95169 from the National Heart, Lung, and Blood Institute and by grants UL1-TR-000040 and UL1-TR-001079 from NCRR.

Authors' contribution

KY, manuscript design, drafting, and revision, literature review, coordination among co-authors, final revisions. BAV, literature review, manuscript drafting and revision. DAB, literature review, manuscript drafting and revision. RLM, literature review, manuscript drafting and revision. JL, manuscript design, drafting, and revision, literature review, coordination among co-authors. All authors read and approved the manuscript.

Competing interests

The authors declare that they have no competing interests.

Author details

[1]Department of Cardiology, Johns Hopkins University, Baltimore, MD, USA. [2]Radiology and Imaging Sciences, National Institutes of Health Clinical Center, Bethesda, MD, USA. [3]Department of Biostatistics, University of Washington, Seattle, WA, USA. [4]St. Marianna University School of Medicine, Kawasaki, Japan. [5]Professor of Medicine, Radiology and Epidemiology, Johns Hopkins Hospital, Johns Hopkins University, Blalock 524D1, 600 North Wolfe Street, Baltimore, MD 21287, USA.

References

1. Bild DE, Bluemke DA, Burke GL, Detrano R, Diez Roux AV, Folsom AR, et al. Multi-ethnic study of atherosclerosis: objectives and design. Am J Epidemiol. 2002;156:871–81.
2. Kawel N, Turkbey EB, Carr JJ, Eng J, Gomes AS, Hundley WG, et al. Normal left ventricular myocardial thickness for middle-aged and older subjects with steady-state free precession cardiac magnetic resonance: the multi-ethnic study of atherosclerosis. Circ Cardiovasc Imaging. 2012;5:500–8.
3. Natori S, Lai S, Finn JP, Gomes AS, Hundley WG, Jerosch-Herold M, et al. Cardiovascular function in multi-ethnic study of atherosclerosis: normal values by age, sex, and ethnicity. AJR Am J Roentgenol. 2006;186:S357–65.
4. Heckbert SR, Post W, Pearson GD, Arnett DK, Gomes AS, Jerosch-Herold M, et al. Traditional cardiovascular risk factors in relation to left ventricular mass, volume, and systolic function by cardiac magnetic resonance imaging: the multiethnic study of atherosclerosis. J Am Coll Cardiol. 2006;48:2285–92.
5. Cheng S, Fernandes VR, Bluemke DA, McClelland RL, Kronmal RA, Lima JA. Age-related left ventricular remodeling and associated risk for cardiovascular outcomes: the multi-ethnic study of atherosclerosis. Circ Cardiovasc Imaging. 2009;2:191–8.
6. Yoneyama K, Gjesdal O, Choi EY, Wu CO, Hundley WG, Gomes AS, et al. Age, sex, and hypertension-related remodeling influences left ventricular torsion assessed by tagged cardiac magnetic resonance in asymptomatic individuals: the multi-ethnic study of atherosclerosis. Circulation. 2012;126:2481–90.

7. Roth GA, Forouzanfar MH, Moran AE, Barber R, Nguyen G, Feigin VL, et al. Demographic and epidemiologic drivers of global cardiovascular mortality. N Engl J Med. 2015;372:1333–41.
8. Eng J, McClelland RL, Gomes AS, Hundley WG, Cheng S, Wu CO, et al. Adverse Left Ventricular Remodeling and Age Assessed with Cardiac MR Imaging: The Multi-Ethnic Study of Atherosclerosis. Radiology. 2016:278:714–22.
9. Turkbey EB, McClelland RL, Kronmal RA, Burke GL, Bild DE, Tracy RP, et al. The impact of obesity on the left ventricle: the multi-ethnic study of atherosclerosis (MESA). JACC Cardiovasc Imaging. 2010;3:266–74.
10. Shah RV, Abbasi SA, Heydari B, Rickers C, Jacobs DR Jr, Wang L, et al. Insulin resistance, subclinical left ventricular remodeling, and the obesity paradox: MESA (multi-ethnic study of atherosclerosis). J Am Coll Cardiol. 2013;61:1698–706.
11. Shah RV, Murthy VL, Abbasi SA, Eng J, Wu C, Ouyang P, et al. Weight loss and progressive left ventricular remodelling: the multi-ethnic study of atherosclerosis (MESA). Eur J Prev Cardiol. 2015;22:1408–18.
12. Yoneyama K, Donekal S, Venkatesh BA, Wu CO, Liu CY, Souto Nacif M, et al. Natural history of myocardial function in an adult human population: serial longitudinal observations from MESA. JACC Cardiovasc Imaging. 2016;9:1164–73.
13. Van Hee VC, Adar SD, Szpiro AA, Barr RG, Bluemke DA, Diez Roux AV, et al. Exposure to traffic and left ventricular mass and function: the multi-ethnic study of atherosclerosis. Am J Respir Crit Care Med. 2009;179:827–34.
14. Ix JH, Katz R, Peralta CA, de Boer IH, Allison MA, Bluemke DA, et al. A high ankle brachial index is associated with greater left ventricular mass MESA (multi-ethnic study of atherosclerosis). J Am Coll Cardiol. 2010;55:342–9.
15. Van Hee VC, Adar SD, Szpiro AA, Barr RG, Diez Roux A, Bluemke DA, et al. Common genetic variation, residential proximity to traffic exposure, and left ventricular mass: the multi-ethnic study of atherosclerosis. Environ Health Perspect. 2010;118:962–9.
16. Turkbey EB, Jorgensen NW, Johnson WC, Bertoni AG, Polak JF, Diez Roux AV, et al. Physical activity and physiological cardiac remodelling in a community setting: the multi-ethnic study of atherosclerosis (MESA). Heart. 2010;96:42–8.
17. Heidenreich PA, Albert NM, Allen LA, Bluemke DA, Butler J, Fonarow GC, et al. Forecasting the impact of heart failure in the United States: a policy statement from the American Heart Association. Circ Heart Fail. 2013;6:606–19.
18. Jain A, Tandri H, Dalal D, Chahal H, Soliman EZ, Prineas RJ, et al. Diagnostic and prognostic utility of electrocardiography for left ventricular hypertrophy defined by magnetic resonance imaging in relationship to ethnicity: the multi-ethnic study of atherosclerosis (MESA). Am Heart J. 2010;159:652–8.
19. Armstrong AC, Gidding S, Gjesdal O, Wu C, Bluemke DA, Lima JA. LV mass assessed by echocardiography and CMR, cardiovascular outcomes, and medical practice. JACC Cardiovasc Imaging. 2012;5:837–48.
20. Jain A, McClelland RL, Polak JF, Shea S, Burke GL, Bild DE, et al. Cardiovascular imaging for assessing cardiovascular risk in asymptomatic men versus women: the multi-ethnic study of atherosclerosis (MESA). Circ Cardiovasc Imaging. 2011;4:8–15.
21. Bluemke DA, Kronmal RA, Lima JA, Liu K, Olson J, Burke GL, et al. The relationship of left ventricular mass and geometry to incident cardiovascular events: the MESA (multi-ethnic study of atherosclerosis) study. J Am Coll Cardiol. 2008;52:2148–55.
22. Chahal H, Bluemke DA, Wu CO, McClelland R, Liu K, Shea SJ, et al. Heart failure risk prediction in the multi-ethnic study of atherosclerosis. Heart. 2015;101:58–64.
23. Ambale-Venkatesh B, Yoneyama K, Sharma RK, Ohyama Y, Wu CO, Burke GL, et al. Left ventricular shape predicts different types of cardiovascular events in the general population. Heart. 2017;103:499–507.
24. Sibley CT, Noureldin RA, Gai N, Nacif MS, Liu S, Turkbey EB, et al. T1 mapping in cardiomyopathy at cardiac MR: comparison with endomyocardial biopsy. Radiology. 2012;265:724–32.
25. Ambale-Venkatesh B, Lima JA. Cardiac MRI: a central prognostic tool in myocardial fibrosis. Nat Rev Cardiol. 2015;12:18–29.
26. Wu KC, Weiss RG, Thiemann DR, Kitagawa K, Schmidt A, Dalal D, et al. Late gadolinium enhancement by cardiovascular magnetic resonance heralds an adverse prognosis in nonischemic cardiomyopathy. J Am Coll Cardiol. 2008;51:2414–21.
27. Briasoulis A, Mallikethi-Reddy S, Palla M, Alesh I, Afonso L. Myocardial fibrosis on cardiac magnetic resonance and cardiac outcomes in hypertrophic cardiomyopathy: a meta-analysis. Heart. 2015;101:1406–11.
28. Schelbert EB, Cao JJ, Sigurdsson S, Aspelund T, Kellman P, Aletras AH, et al. Prevalence and prognosis of unrecognized myocardial infarction determined by cardiac magnetic resonance in older adults. JAMA. 2012; 308:890–6.
29. Turkbey EB, Nacif MS, Guo M, McClelland RL, Teixeira PB, Bild DE, et al. Prevalence and correlates of myocardial scar in a US cohort. JAMA. 2015;314:1945–54.
30. Masci PG, Schuurman R, Andrea B, Ripoli A, Coceani M, Chiappino S, et al. Myocardial fibrosis as a key determinant of left ventricular remodeling in idiopathic dilated Cardiomyopathy a contrast-enhanced cardiovascular magnetic study. Circulation-Cardiovascular Imaging. 2013; 6:790–9.
31. Ambale Venkatesh B, Volpe GJ, Donekal S, Mewton N, Liu CY, Shea S, et al. Association of longitudinal changes in left ventricular structure and function with myocardial fibrosis: the multi-ethnic study of atherosclerosis study. Hypertension. 2014;64:508–15.
32. Liu CY, Liu YC, Wu C, Armstrong A, Volpe GJ, van der Geest RJ, et al. Evaluation of age-related interstitial myocardial fibrosis with cardiac magnetic resonance contrast-enhanced T1 mapping: MESA (multi-ethnic study of atherosclerosis). J Am Coll Cardiol. 2013;62:1280–7.
33. Anversa P, Nadal-Ginard B. Myocyte renewal and ventricular remodelling. Nature. 2002;415:240–3.
34. Berk BC, Fujiwara K, Lehoux S. ECM remodeling in hypertensive heart disease. J Clin Invest. 2007;117:568–75.
35. Donekal S, Venkatesh BA, Liu YC, Liu CY, Yoneyama K, Wu CO, et al. Interstitial fibrosis, left ventricular remodeling, and myocardial mechanical behavior in a population-based multiethnic cohort: the multi-ethnic study of atherosclerosis (MESA) study. Circ Cardiovasc Imaging. 2014;7:292–302.
36. Yi CJ, Wu CO, Tee M, Liu CY, Volpe GJ, Prince MR, et al. The association between cardiovascular risk and cardiovascular magnetic resonance measures of fibrosis: the multi-ethnic study of atherosclerosis (MESA). J Cardiovasc Magn Reson. 2015;17:15.
37. Bursi F, Weston SA, Redfield MM, Jacobsen SJ, Pakhomov S, Nkomo VT, et al. Systolic and diastolic heart failure in the community. JAMA. 2006;296:2209–16.
38. Rosen BD, Lima JA, Nasir K, Edvardsen T, Folsom AR, Lai S, et al. Lower myocardial perfusion reserve is associated with decreased regional left ventricular function in asymptomatic participants of the multi-ethnic study of atherosclerosis. Circulation. 2006;114:289–97.
39. Edvardsen T, Rosen BD, Pan L, Jerosch-Herold M, Lai S, Hundley WG, et al. Regional diastolic dysfunction in individuals with left ventricular hypertrophy measured by tagged magnetic resonance imaging–the multi-ethnic study of atherosclerosis (MESA). Am Heart J. 2006;151:109–14.
40. Rosen BD, Edvardsen T, Lai S, Castillo E, Pan L, Jerosch-Herold M, et al. Left ventricular concentric remodeling is associated with decreased global and regional systolic function: the multi-ethnic study of atherosclerosis. Circulation. 2005;112:984–91.
41. Rosen BD, Saad MF, Shea S, Nasir K, Edvardsen T, Burke G, et al. Hypertension and smoking are associated with reduced regional left ventricular function in asymptomatic: individuals the multi-ethnic study of atherosclerosis. J Am Coll Cardiol. 2006;47:1150–8.
42. Fernandes VR, Polak JF, Edvardsen T, Carvalho B, Gomes A, Bluemke DA, et al. Subclinical atherosclerosis and incipient regional myocardial dysfunction in asymptomatic individuals: the multi-ethnic study of atherosclerosis (MESA). J Am Coll Cardiol. 2006;47:2420–8.
43. Almeida AL, Teixido-Tura G, Choi EY, Opdahl A, Fernandes VR, Wu CO, et al. Metabolic syndrome, strain, and reduced myocardial function: multi-ethnic study of atherosclerosis. Arq Bras Cardiol. 2014;102:327–35.
44. Opdahl A, Ambale Venkatesh B, Fernandes VR, Wu CO, Nasir K, Choi EY, et al. Resting heart rate as predictor for left ventricular dysfunction and heart failure: MESA (multi-ethnic study of atherosclerosis). J Am Coll Cardiol. 2014; 63:1182–9.
45. Choi EY, Rosen BD, Fernandes VR, Yan RT, Yoneyama K, Donekal S, et al. Prognostic value of myocardial circumferential strain for incident heart failure and cardiovascular events in asymptomatic individuals: the multi-ethnic study of atherosclerosis. Eur Heart J. 2013;34:2354–61.
46. Ambale-Venkatesh B, Armstrong AC, Liu CY, Donekal S, Yoneyama K, Wu CO, et al. Diastolic function assessed from tagged MRI predicts heart failure and atrial fibrillation over an 8-year follow-up period: the multi-ethnic study of atherosclerosis. Eur Heart J Cardiovasc Imaging. 2014;15:442–9.
47. Kawel N, Nacif M, Arai AE, Gomes AS, Hundley WG, Johnson WC, et al. Trabeculated (noncompacted) and compact myocardium in adults: the multi-ethnic study of atherosclerosis. Circ Cardiovasc Imaging. 2012;5:357–66.
48. Captur G, Zemrak F, Muthurangu V, Petersen SE, Li C, Bassett P, et al. Fractal analysis of myocardial Trabeculations in 2547 study participants: multi-ethnic study of atherosclerosis. Radiology. 2015;277:707–15.

49. Zemrak F, Ahlman MA, Captur G, Mohiddin SA, Kawel-Boehm N, Prince MR, et al. The relationship of left ventricular trabeculation to ventricular function and structure over a 9.5-year follow-up: the MESA study. J Am Coll Cardiol. 2014;64:1971–80.
50. Arbustini E, Weidemann F, Hall JL. Left ventricular noncompaction: a distinct cardiomyopathy or a trait shared by different cardiac diseases? J Am Coll Cardiol. 2014;64:1840–50.
51. Kawut SM, Lima JA, Barr RG, Chahal H, Jain A, Tandri H, et al. Sex and race differences in right ventricular structure and function: the multi-ethnic study of atherosclerosis-right ventricle study. Circulation. 2011;123:2542–51.
52. Leary PJ, Kaufman JD, Barr RG, Bluemke DA, Curl CL, Hough CL, et al. Traffic-related air pollution and the right ventricle. The multi-ethnic study of atherosclerosis. Am J Respir Crit Care Med. 2014;189:1093–100.
53. Kawut SM, Barr RG, Lima JA, Praestgaard A, Johnson WC, Chahal H, et al. Right ventricular structure is associated with the risk of heart failure and cardiovascular death: the multi-ethnic study of atherosclerosis (MESA)–right ventricle study. Circulation. 2012;126:1681–8.
54. Vieira MJ, Teixeira R, Goncalves L, Gersh BJ. Left atrial mechanics: echocardiographic assessment and clinical implications. J Am Soc Echocardiogr. 2014;27:463–78.
55. Inoue YY, Alissa A, Khurram IM, Fukumoto K, Habibi M, Venkatesh BA, et al. Quantitative tissue-tracking cardiac magnetic resonance (CMR) of left atrial deformation and the risk of stroke in patients with atrial fibrillation. J Am Heart Assoc. 2015;4
56. Hoit BD. Left atrial size and function: role in prognosis. J Am Coll Cardiol. 2014;63:493–505.
57. Habibi M, Chahal H, Opdahl A, Gjesdal O, Helle-Valle TM, Heckbert SR, et al. Association of CMR-measured LA function with heart failure development: results from the MESA study. JACC Cardiovasc Imaging. 2014;7:570–9.
58. Imai M, Ambale Venkatesh B, Samiei S, Donekal S, Habibi M, Armstrong AC, et al. Multi-ethnic study of atherosclerosis: association between left atrial function using tissue tracking from cine MR imaging and myocardial fibrosis. Radiology. 2014;273:703–13.
59. Noda C, Ambale Venkatesh B, Ohyama Y, Liu CY, Chamera E, Redheuil A, et al. Reproducibility of functional aortic analysis using magnetic resonance imaging: the MESA. Eur Heart J Cardiovasc Imaging. 2016;17:909–17.
60. Turkbey EB, Jain A, Johnson C, Redheuil A, Arai AE, Gomes AS, et al. Determinants and normal values of ascending aortic diameter by age, gender, and race/ethnicity in the multi-ethnic study of atherosclerosis (MESA). J Magn Reson Imaging. 2014;39:360–8.
61. Al-Mallah MH, Nasir K, Katz R, Lima JA, Bluemke DA, Blumenthal RS, et al. Relation of thoracic aortic distensibility to left ventricular area (from the multi-ethnic study of atherosclerosis [MESA]). Am J Cardiol. 2014;113:178–82.
62. Redheuil A, Wu CO, Kachenoura N, Ohyama Y, Yan RT, Bertoni AG, et al. Proximal aortic distensibility is an independent predictor of all-cause mortality and incident CV events: the MESA study. J Am Coll Cardiol. 2014;64:2619–29.
63. Liu CY, Chen D, Bluemke DA, Wu CO, Teixido-Tura G, Chugh A, et al. Evolution of aortic wall thickness and stiffness with atherosclerosis: long-term follow up from the multi-ethnic study of atherosclerosis. Hypertension. 2015;65:1015–9.
64. Ohyama Y, Teixido-Tura G, Ambale-Venkatesh B, Noda C, Chugh AR, Liu CY, et al. Ten-year longitudinal change in aortic stiffness assessed by cardiac MRI in the second half of the human lifespan: the multi-ethnic study of atherosclerosis. Eur Heart J Cardiovasc Imaging. 2016;17:1044–53.
65. Macedo R, Chen S, Lai S, Shea S, Malayeri AA, Szklo M, et al. MRI detects increased coronary wall thickness in asymptomatic individuals: the multi-ethnic study of atherosclerosis (MESA). J Magn Reson Imaging. 2008;28:1108–15.
66. Miao C, Chen S, Macedo R, Lai S, Liu K, Li D, et al. Positive remodeling of the coronary arteries detected by magnetic resonance imaging in an asymptomatic population: MESA (multi-ethnic study of atherosclerosis). J Am Coll Cardiol. 2009;53:1708–15.
67. Wasserman BA, Sharrett AR, Lai S, Gomes AS, Cushman M, Folsom AR, et al. Risk factor associations with the presence of a lipid core in carotid plaque of asymptomatic individuals using high-resolution MRI: the multi-ethnic study of atherosclerosis (MESA). Stroke. 2008;39:329–35.
68. Zavodni AE, Wasserman BA, McClelland RL, Gomes AS, Folsom AR, Polak JF, et al. Carotid artery plaque morphology and composition in relation to incident cardiovascular events: the multi-ethnic study of atherosclerosis (MESA). Radiology. 2014;271:381–9.
69. Ebong IA, Watson KE, Goff DC Jr, Bluemke DA, Srikanthan P, Horwich T, et al. Age at menopause and incident heart failure: the multi-ethnic study of atherosclerosis. Menopause. 2014;21:585–91.

13

Fully quantitative cardiovascular magnetic resonance myocardial perfusion ready for clinical use: a comparison between cardiovascular magnetic resonance imaging and positron emission tomography

Henrik Engblom[1], Hui Xue[2], Shahnaz Akil[1], Marcus Carlsson[1], Cecilia Hindorf[3], Jenny Oddstig[3], Fredrik Hedeer[1], Michael S. Hansen[2], Anthony H. Aletras[1,4], Peter Kellman[2] and Håkan Arheden[1*]

Abstract

Background: Recent studies have shown that quantification of myocardial perfusion (MP) at stress and myocardial perfusion reserve (MPR) offer additional diagnostic and prognostic information compared to qualitative and semi-quantitative assessment of myocardial perfusion distribution in patients with coronary artery disease (CAD). Technical advancements have enabled fully automatic quantification of MP using cardiovascular magnetic resonance (CMR) to be performed in-line in a clinical workflow. The aim of this study was to validate the use of the automated CMR perfusion mapping technique for quantification of MP using 13N–NH3 cardiac positron emission tomography (PET) as the reference method.

Methods: Twenty-one patients with stable CAD were included in the study. All patients underwent adenosine stress and rest perfusion imaging with 13N–NH3 PET and a dual sequence, single contrast bolus CMR on the same day. Global and regional MP were quantified both at stress and rest using PET and CMR.

Results: There was good agreement between global MP quantified by PET and CMR both at stress (−0.1 ± 0.5 ml/min/g) and at rest (0 ± 0.2 ml/min/g) with a strong correlation ($r = 0.92$, $p < 0.001$; $y = 0.94x + 0.14$). Furthermore, there was strong correlation between CMR and PET with regards to regional MP ($r = 0.83$, $p < 0.001$; $y = 0.87x + 0.26$) with a good agreement (−0.1 ± 0.6 ml/min/g). There was also a significant correlation between CMR and PET with regard to global and regional MPR ($r = 0.69$, $p = 0.001$ and $r = 0.57$, $p < 0.001$, respectively).

Conclusions: There is good agreement between MP quantified by 13N–NH3 PET and dual sequence, single contrast bolus CMR in patients with stable CAD. Thus, CMR is viable in clinical practice for quantification of MP.

Keywords: Myocardial perfusion, Cardiac magnetic resonance, Positron emission tomography, Myocardial perfusion reserve

* Correspondence: hakan.arheden@med.lu.se
[1]Department of Clinical Physiology, Clinical Sciences, Lund University and Lund University Hospital, Lund, Sweden
Full list of author information is available at the end of the article

Background

Ischemic heart disease (IHD) is the most common cause of mortality and morbidity in the western world. Obstructive coronary artery disease (CAD) compromising myocardial perfusion is the main pathophysiological mechanism underlying stress-induced myocardial ischemia. The extent of stress-induced ischemia due to CAD has been shown to be of important prognostic value [1, 2]. Significant advances in both diagnosing and treating epicardial CAD have improved survival and reduced morbidity during the last decades in patients suffering from this disease [3–5]. Most clinical methods used for diagnosing stress-induced myocardial ischemia focus on epicardial obstructive CAD and rely on qualitative or semi-quantitative assessment of the relative spatial perfusion distribution i.e. myocardial perfusion single photon emission computed tomography (SPECT), first-pass perfusion cardiac magnetic resonance (CMR) and non-dynamic cardiac positron emission tomography (PET). There are, however, data suggesting that the use of qualitative or semi-quantitative methods for assessing stress-induced ischemia have limited ability to depict the full extent of the atherosclerotic coronary disease [6]. Furthermore, recent studies have shown that full quantification of myocardial perfusion (MP) expressed in terms of ml/min/g myocardial tissue offers independent prognostic information in patients with CAD [7–9].

Cardiovascular magnetic resonance (CMR) with a dual sequence, single contrast bolus approach has been shown to enable quantitative assessment of MP [10]. However, there have been challenges associated with this technique such as the non-linear relationship between signal intensity and gadolinium concentration, respiratory motion correction and gadolinium kinetic modelling. Recent technical developments have shown promising results to overcome these challenges [11]. The proposed CMR perfusion mapping method is implemented in-line, is fully automatic and is readily integrated into the clinical workflow via the Gadgetron framework [12]. Thus, this technique seems to be ready for clinical implementation, making quantitative perfusion available as a routine examination in patients with suspected or established ischemic heart disease. Even though this is a promising technique, clinical validation against an independent reference standard is still lacking.

Cardiac positron emission tomography (PET) with dynamic image acquisition during bolus injection of a radioactive perfusion tracer at rest and stress is currently considered to be the clinical reference method for quantitative assessment of MP. However, cardiac PET is of limited use as a wide spread routine clinical examination due to its limited availability and sometimes challenging logistics as well as due to the ionizing radiation associated with this technique.

Therefore, the aim of this study was to validate MP by a fully automatic, in-line, dual sequence, single contrast bolus CMR perfusion mapping sequence using cardiac 13N–NH3 PET as the reference method in stable CAD patients.

Methods

Study population and study design

The study protocol was approved by the regional ethical committee and all subjects gave written informed consent prior to participation. Patients eligible for inclusion had all been clinically evaluated and a decision to perform an elective coronary angiography with preparedness for percutaneous coronary intervention (PCI) had been made, with or without prior stress imaging. Patients were excluded if they had contraindications for CMR such as pacemaker or other CMR-incompatible devices or claustrophobia. The patients were recruited between September 2016 and February 2017 and examined at Lund University Hospital, Lund, Sweden. All patients underwent both adenosine stress/rest CMR with dual sequence, single contrast bolus approach as well as adenosine stress/rest 13N–NH3 PET on the same day (4–5 h apart) for assessment of MP. Rate pressure products (heart rate x systolic blood pressure) were calculated both at rest and stress as a measure of the hemodynamic response to adenosine during PET and CMR, respectively. For 12 patients the CMR and PET examination was performed within a month prior to the angiography. For 9 patients, the CMR and PET examinations were performed as a follow-up approximately 6 months after the angiography.

Dual sequence, single contrast bolus CMR for MP quantification

Image acquisition

All images were acquired on a Magnetom Aera 1.5 T system (Siemens Healthcare, Erlangen, Germany). A basal, a mid-ventricular and an apical short-axis image were acquired both at rest and at stress. The stress images were acquired during 90 heart beats, starting three minutes after initiation of intravenous adenosine infusion (140 μg/kg/min). The arterial input function was calculated using the left ventricular (LV) blood pool which was automatically segmented from low resolution images optimized for the high gadolinium concentration. Higher spatial resolution images were used for estimating myocardial perfusion. In order to achieve a linear relationship between the LV blood signal used as an input function and the gadolinium contrast agent concentration a number of steps were taken in the design of the sequence protocol and image reconstruction as previously described [11]. The sequence uses a low flip angle FLASH low resolution protocol with 2 echoes such that the echo times were short to minimize T2* losses at high concentration, and so that remaining T2* losses could be estimated and corrected. The non-linearity of saturation recovery was minimized by using a short saturation delay achieved using a small matrix and parallel imaging to reduce the number of phase encode lines. The remaining non-linear response is corrected by converting to gadolinium concentration units.

Late gadolinium enhancement (LGE) imaging was performed to assess regions of myocardial infarction.

Image reconstruction & perfusion mapping

The input function and myocardial images are converted to units of gadolinium contrast agent concentration (mmol/L) which were input to the tissue model used in quantification [11]. Conversion to gadolinium units effectively addresses the non-linearity between the measured saturation recovery signal and actual gadolinium concentration. Conversion to contrast concentration was accomplished by means of a look-up-table that is calculated by a Bloch simulation of the specific protocol. This look-up-table is recalculated for each scan as part of the image reconstruction. The input to the look-up-table is the measured saturation recovery signal which is normalized by a proton density used as a reference. MP was calculated using a blood tissue exchange model originally developed by Bassingthwaighte [13], which is a distributed model described by partial differential equations. In addition to myocardial blood flow, the model estimates the permeability surface area product for the capillaries which determines the extraction fraction and the intracapillary plasma and interstitial fluid volumes.

Image analysis

All images were analyzed using the software Segment (v2.0 R5378) [14]. The endo- and epicardial borders for the basal, mid-ventricular and apical short-axis images were manually delineated both at stress and rest. To avoid inclusion of blood pool or extracardiac structures within the regions of interest where MP was quantified, the delineations were kept approximately 1 pixel away from the endo- and epicardial borders. Obvious image artifacts and coronary arteries were excluded from the regions of interest. Myocardial perfusion in ml/min/g was assessed regionally according to the 17-segment model [15], excluding the apical segment, resulting in 16 segments per patient. MP was assessed globally (average MP for all 16 segments). Myocardial perfusion reserve (MPR) was also calculated, defined as the ratio between MP at stress over rest and was expressed both regionally and globally. Both regional and global MP were compared to corresponding measures by PET. Infarct size was assessed from the LGE short-axis images by the use of the recently described EWA (expectation maximization weighted intensity A priori information*)* algorithm for infarct quantification [16]. In short, the EWA algorithm is based on combining an intensity classification by Expectation Maximization with a pixel intensity weighting approach to account for partial volume effects. Furthermore, a priori information on coronary artery supply territory is taken into consideration for the automatic infarct size quantification.

Cardiac 13NH$_3$-PET for MP quantification

Image acquisition and reconstruction

All patients underwent a standard clinical cardiac 13N–NH3 PET at rest and stress, with a minimum of 50 min between the examinations to allow for physical decay of the radiopharmaceutical. All images were acquired with a Discovery 690 PET/CT scanner (General Electric Healthcare, Waukesha, Wisconsin, USA). A CT localization image over the chest was acquired to enable accurate patient positioning, followed by a low-dose computed tomography (CT) used for attenuation correction (120 kV; 10 mAs, 10; rotation time 0.5 s). Thereafter, the patients received an intravenous injection of 430–600 MBq of 13N–NH3 at rest. An ECG-gated PET acquisition with a total duration of 15 min was started simultaneously with the tracer injection. For the stress image acquisition, the patient was injected with the same amount of 13N–NH3 after 3 min of adenosine infusion (140 µg/kg/min) which continued, with continuous ECG monitoring, for 4 min after the injection of the radiopharmaceutical during which the images for quantitative perfusion were acquired.

The 0-4 min PET acquisition data were reconstructed into dynamic images, with 21 time frames (12x5s, 4x10s, 4x20s and 1x60s). The images were reconstructed according to recommendations from the vendor, with OSEM without time-of-flight (TOF), and with point spread function (PSF) modelling, with 3 iterations, 12 subsets and a 5 mm post filter. Static images were reconstructed from the data acquired 4–15 min after start of injection to depict the relative spatial myocardial perfusion using the following reconstruction parameters: OSEM with TOF and PSF modelling with 5 iterations and 18 subsets and a 3 mm post filter. The PET and the CT images were checked for patient motion before reconstruction.

Analysis of the quantitative myocardial perfusion

All PET images were analyzed using the software Carimas (version 2.7, Turku, Finland), developed for quantitative perfusion assessment by cardiac PET, including 13N–NH3 [17, 18]. The LV endo-and epicardial borders were automatically segmented with manual adjustment when needed. The arterial input function was derived from a blood pool volume of interest which was placed in the basal part of the LV cavity. The activity in the blood and the myocardial wall as a function of time served as input function for the deGrado compartment model for 13N–NH3 [19] implemented in the Carimas correcting the input function for extraction fraction of 13N–NH3 (approximately 90%). Myocardial perfusion was calculated at rest and stress, both globally and in each of the corresponding 16 segments of the left ventricle used for CMR.

Statistics

Data are expressed as mean ± standard deviation (SD). The relationship between MP by PET and CMR, both global and regional, as well as MPR was assessed with Pearson's correlation coefficient. The agreement between the MP by PET and CMR was expressed as bias ± SD and graphically shown as difference plots according to Bland and Altman [20]. The difference in rate pressure products between PET and CMR was assessed by Student's t-test. All statistical analyses were performed using Excel 2013 (Microsoft Corporation, Redmond, Washington, USA). Results with a p value < 0.05 was considered to be statistically significant.

Results

Patient characteristics are shown in Table 1. Typical images obtained by PET and CMR in a patient with right coronary artery (RCA) disease and stress-induced ischemia in the inferior LV wall are shown in Fig. 1. Myocardial infarction was detected in 4 of 21 patients. Infarct size in these 4 patients was 8 ± 5%. Of the 12 patients that underwent CMR and PET before angiography, 4 patients had signs of stenosis in left anterior descending coronary artery (LAD) of whom 3 underwent revascularization, 3 patients had stenosis in RCA of whom 2 underwent revascularization, 1 patient had stenosis in the left circumflex coronary artery (LCX) who underwent revascularization and 6 patients had no significant stenosis. Of the patients with CMR and PET 6 months after angiography 4 patients had stenosis in LAD of whom 3 had been revascularized, 2 had stenosis in RCA of whom 1 had been revascularized, 2 patients had stenosis in LCX of whom 1 had been revascularized and 2 patients had no significant stenosis. Complete records of the PET and CMR rate pressure products at both rest and stress were available for 12 patients. There were similar mean rate pressure products for PET and CMR both at rest (8932 ± 1563 vs 9189 ± 1756, p = 0.37) and at stress (10,945 ± 2170 vs 11,351 ± 2463, p = 0.53). Furthermore, the difference between stress and rest rate pressure products did not differ between PET and CMR (2014 ± 2554 vs 2162 ± 2120, p = 0.75) indicating similar hemodynamic responses to adenosine stress.

Table 1 Patient characteristics

Age (years)	68 ± 9
Female	4 (19%)
Smoking	3 (14%)
Prior CABG	0 (0%)
Prior PCI	5 (24%)
Prior MI	3 (14%)
Diabetes	4 (19%)
Hypertension	14 (67%)
Hyperlipidemia	12 (57%)
MI by LGE	4 (19%)
Beta-blockers	12 (60%)
Statins	20 (95%)
ACE-inhibitors/ARB	9 (43%)
Anti-coagulants	17 (81%)

ACE angiotensin converting enzyme, *ARB* angiotensin receptor blocker, *CABG* coronary artery bypass grafting, *LGE* late gadolinium enhancement, *MI* myocardial infarction, *PCI* percutaneous coronary intervention

Global MP

The global MP at rest and stress ranged from 0.6–4.0 ml/min/g and 0.6–3.8 ml/min/g for PET and CMR, respectively. Figure 2a shows that there was a strong correlation (r = 0.92 $p < 0.001$; y = 0.94x + 0.14) between MP quantified by PET and CMR. There was a good agreement between PET and CMR both at stress (−0.1 ± 0.5 ml/min/g) and at rest (0 ± 0.2 ml/min/g) (Fig. 2b). Furthermore, there was a significant correlation between global MPR by PET and CMR (r = 0.69, p = 0.001; y = 0.83x + 0.53) and a good agreement (−0.1 ± 0.6 ml/min/g).

Regional MP

The regional MP at rest and stress ranged from 0.4–4.6 ml/min/g and 0.5–5.3 ml/min/g for PET and CMR, respectively. Figure 3a shows the correlation between regional MP by PET and CMR (r = 0.83, $p <$ 0.001; y = 0.87x + 0.26). There was a good agreement between PET and CMR both at stress (−0.1 ± 0.7 ml/min/g) and at rest (0 ± 0.3 ml/min/g) (Fig. 3b). The correlation between MPR by PET and CMR was r = 0.57, $p < 0.001$ (y = 0.68x + 1.02) with a good agreement (0 ± 1.1 ml/min/g). Table 2 shows what the angiographer evaluated as significant stenosis by angiography in relation to regional stress MP < 2.0 ml/min/g as recently suggested as optimal cut-off for 13N–NH3 PET for detection of significant coronary stenosis [21].

Global MP reduction

Absolute quantification of MP is particularly important in cases exhibiting a global reduction in stress flow which arises in multi-vessel disease or microvascular disease. Figure 4 shows an example of a patient with a

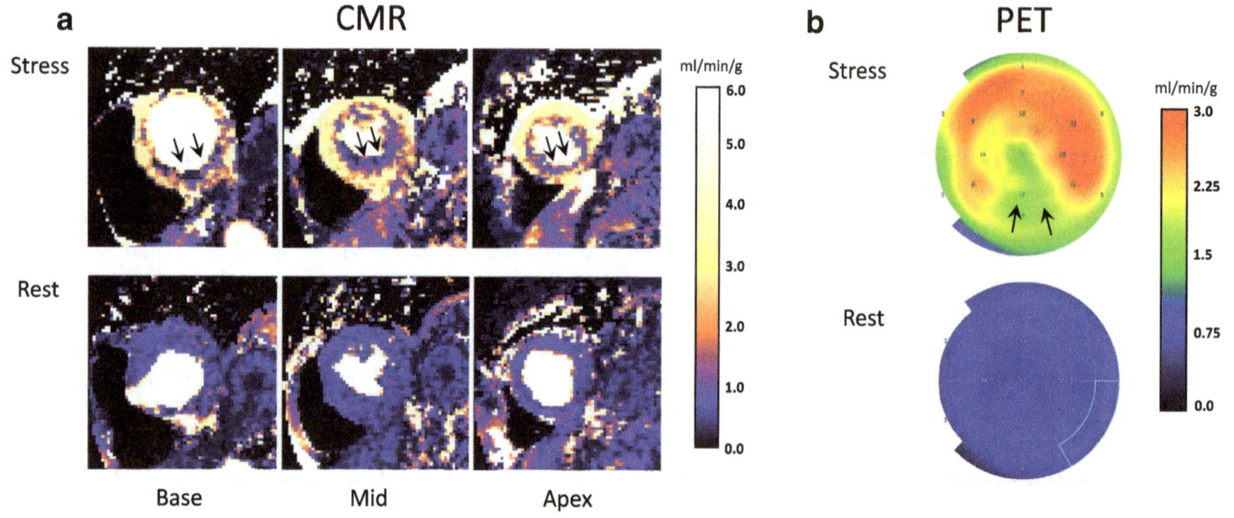

Fig. 1 A patient with stress-induced ischemia in the inferior LV wall with a significant stenosis in the right coronary artery. **a** Rest and stress perfusion maps in basal, mid-ventricular and apical short-axis image of the left ventricle acquired using the dual sequence, single contrast bolus CMR perfusion mapping approach, showing stress-induced ischemia in the inferior LV wall (arrows). **b** Rest and stress polar plot PET perfusion maps obtained by dynamic 13N–NH3 imaging showing stress-induced ischemia in the inferior LV wall (arrows) corresponding well with the CMR findings. The central part of the polar plot represents the LV apex and the periphery represents the basal parts of the LV. Of note, the colors for PET and CMR perfusion maps are different and in concordance with colors typically used for each method. Furthermore, the color scales in this case are different for the two methods to optimize visualization of regional pathology. CMR = cardiovascularmagnetic resonance, LV = left ventricle/left ventricular, MP = myocardial perfusion, PET = positron emission tomography

deceased global MP without regional ischemia on qualitative assessment of perfusion distribution. The MP appears to be normal in the raw first-pass CMR perfusion images (Fig. 4b) and in the non-dynamic, non-quantitative PET images (Fig. 4d), used in routine clinical practice for CMR and nuclear cardiology, respectively. Absolute quantification of MP (Fig. 4 a,c), however, clearly shows a significant reduction in flow and corresponding low flow reserve which could be attributed to either microvascular disease or multi-vessel disease. In this case, multi-vessel disease was confirmed by invasive angiography.

Discussion

The present study shows that fully quantitative CMR MP mapping is ready for clinical use by validating the

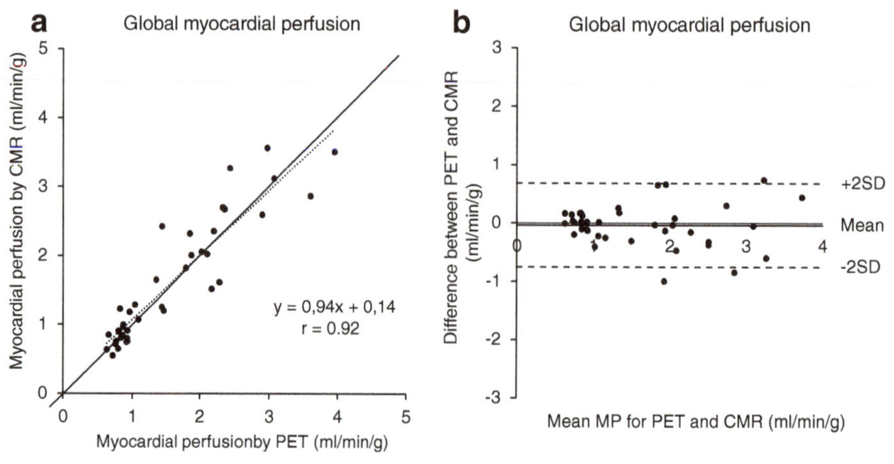

Fig. 2 The relationship between PET and CMR for global myocardial perfusion rest and stress included, **a**). The dashed line represents the line of regression. The solid line indicates the line of identity. **b** Bland-Altman plots for the difference between PET and CMR for global MP. The solid line represents the mean difference between the two methods and the dashed lines indicate +2SD and -2SD, respectively. There is strong correlation and small bias between PET and CMR for assessing global MP. CMR = cardiovascular magnetic resonance, MP = myocardial perfusion, PET = positron emission tomography

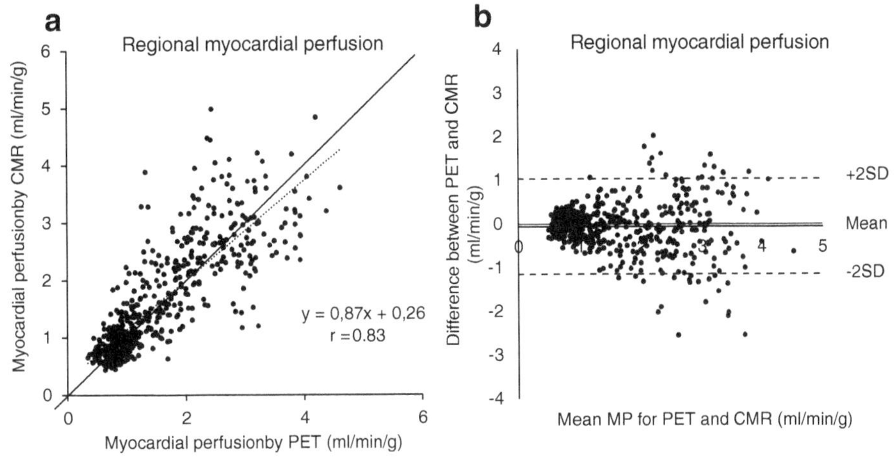

Fig. 3 The relationship between PET and CMR for regional myocardial perfusion (rest and stress included, **a**). The dashed line represents the line of regression. The solid line indicates the line of identity. **b** Bland-Altman plots for the difference between PET and CMR for regional MP. The solid line represents the mean difference between the two methods. The dashed lines indicate +2SD and -2SD, respectively. There is significant correlation and small bias between PET and CMR for assessing regional MP in 16 of the 17 segments of the left ventricle. CMR = cardiovascular magnetic resonance, MP = myocardial perfusion, PET = positron emission tomography

method against 13N–NH3 PET, which was used as the independent reference standard. There was strong correlation between the two methods with negligible bias for both global and regional MP. Thus, using CMR for quantifying MP is an attractive alternative to PET in the clinic. However, routine clinical implementation of quantitative CMR MP will rely on its importance on therapeutic decision making, which needs to be proven by large clinical outcome trials that use MP as an endpoint.

Quantification of MP and MPR in routine clinical practice will have important implications on the management of patients with established or suspected CAD. Even though a normal perfusion scan with qualitative or semi-quantitative evaluation of first-pass perfusion has been shown to predict low risk of future coronary events [22–24], there remain patients in this group with adverse prognosis due to multi-vessel disease or non-obstructive CAD [25–27]. Thus, even in the absence of obstructive CAD, such as for 3 of 12 patients in Table 2, patients with pathologic MP at stress and low MPR are most likely in need of medical attention. The pathophysiological mechanisms explaining a decreased MP in the absence of obstructive coronary artery disease are likely

Table 2 Comparison between angiography and regional myocardial stress perfusion < 2.0 ml/min/g for the 12 patients with PET (A) and CMR (B) before angiography

A		Angiography		B		Angiography	
		+	–			+	–
PET	+	6	3	CMR	+	4	2
	–	0	3		–	2	4

related to disease states shown to affect the coronary microvascular function, such as dyslipidemia [28, 29], hypertension [30], diabetes [31, 32], and smoking [33]. Significant vascular dysfunction related to these diseases may precede development of obstructive CAD [34], which makes quantification of MP and MPR potential diagnostic methods for identifying patients at risk of developing coronary stenosis. Furthermore, there are currently patients being treated with PCI in coronaries supplying myocardium with normal MPR [35]. Thus, these patients are put at risk associated with invasive treatment (endothelial injury, bleeding complications, risk of coronary artery dissection etc.) with little or no benefit to be gained from the procedure.

Using relative perfusion distribution, typically applied in routine clinical practice of nuclear cardiology, for diagnosing ischemic heart disease means that the counts in the perfusion maps are normalized to the highest regional counts. Thus, there might be variability in counts within normal myocardium due to variability of perfusion within the normal range. Hence, parts of the normal myocardium might have lower counts, potentially interpreted as ischemia and therefore compromising the diagnostic accuracy as recently shown by Kajander et al. [36]. They showed that the positive and negative predictive values for detecting or excluding invasively diagnosed fractional flow reserve (FFR)-positive coronary stenoses decreased significantly when using relative spatial perfusion distribution instead of quantitative MP.

One major challenge with quantitative perfusion imaging, including both CMR and PET in the present study, is to find a perfusion tracer with uptake kinetics that reflects the actual myocardial perfusion over a wide

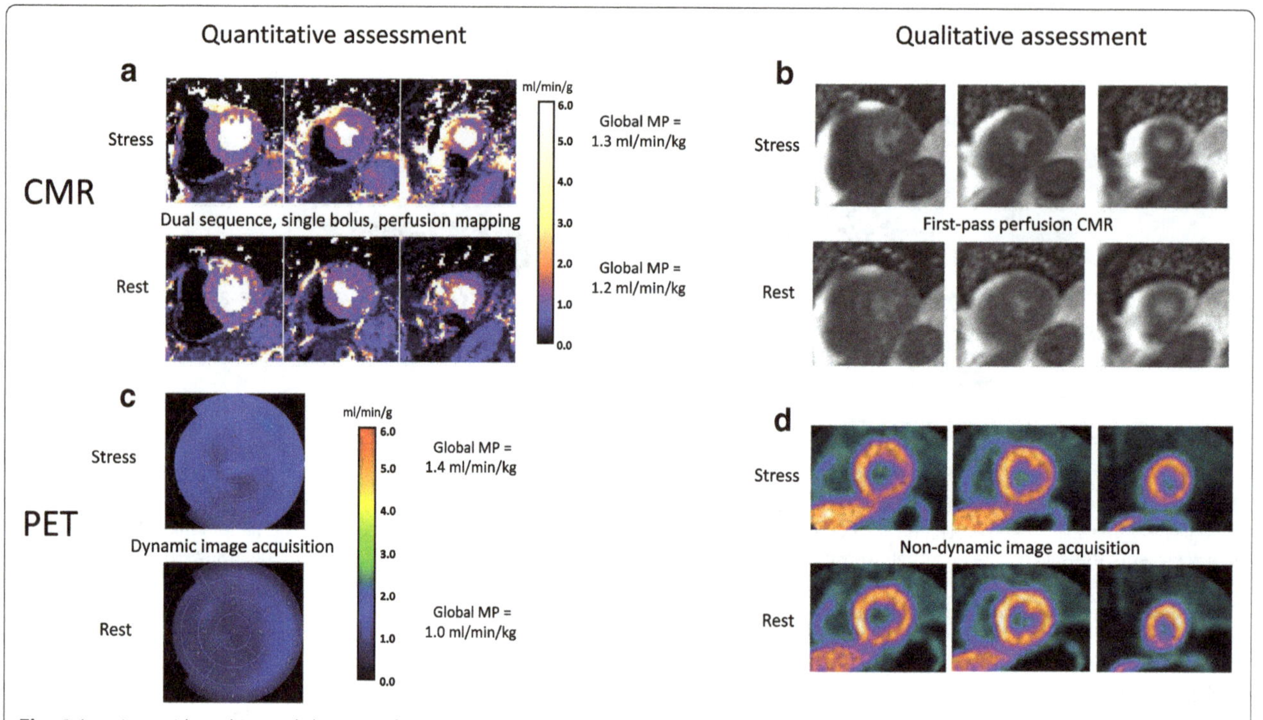

Fig. 4 A patient with multi-vessel disease. **a** CMR MP maps at rest and stress, **b** first-pass perfusion images at rest and stress, **c** PET polar plot MP maps from dynamic 13 N-NH3 PET acquisition at rest and stress and **d** non-dynamic 13 N-NH3 PET images at rest and stress. Note the absence of any regional perfusion defect in any of (**a-d**). For the quantitative assessment of MP (**a**, **c**), the patient had signs of a global decrease in myocardial perfusion reserve with only a slight increase of MP during stress as assessed both with PET and CMR. However, for the qualitative assessment of relative perfusion distribution (**b**, **d**), the patient was evaluated as having normal distribution and no stress-induced ischemia. The angiography for this patient showed signs of stenosis in all three main coronary arteries. CMR = cardiovascular magnetic resonance, MP = myocardial perfusion, PET = positron emission tomography

range of blood flows. It has previously been shown that 13N–NH3 uptake is approximately linearly proportional to flow at low MPs but that there is an underestimation of actual blood flow at high flows, which was compensated for by correcting for ammonia extraction [37]. The same underestimation has been shown for CMR and gadolinium-based extracellular contrast agents [38]. In the current approach [11], however, the gadolinium extraction fraction is estimated and used in calculating MP to avoid this underestimation of MP for CMR.

Imaging for both PET and CMR was initiated at the same time point (3 min) following the start of adenosine infusion. However, the duration for PET imaging and adenosine administration for the PET examination was significantly longer than for CMR. Thus, the adenosine response may differ somewhat [39] affecting the validation to some extent.

The results in the present study indicate that a dual sequence, single contrast bolus CMR perfusion imaging and 13N–NH3 PET have similar abilities in terms of quantifying myocardial blood flow over a wide range of flows. Thus, these techniques should be interchangeable and could therefore be used in accordance with local experience and expertise on the method of choice. A major limitation with 13N–NH3 PET is the cumbersome logistics with producing the tracer, requiring a cyclotron close to the imaging facility. Given the short half-life of 13N–NH3 (< 10 min) the tracer has to be produced and transported to the PET scanner within a limited time window. This requires advanced logistics and significant manpower, which also affects the cost per examination. With dual sequence, single contrast bolus CMR there are no such limitations. CMR offers superior characterization of myocardial morphology and function compared to 13N–NH3 PET due to its excellent spatial resolution. Furthermore, PET imaging is associated with ionizing radiation which CMR is not, making CMR the method of choice in younger patients and in situations where serial follow-up examinations is expected to be necessary, such as monitoring of treatment effects.

For wide spread clinical use of quantification of CMR-based MP, image acquisition, reconstruction and post-processing need to be both automated and standardized. The CMR technique described in the present study is highly automated and standardized with regards to imaging protocol, image reconstruction and post-processing of the data. The same requirements regarding automation and standardization is true for cardiac PET involving different perfusion tracers and different mathematical data modeling for quantification of MP built into different imaging software. The use of 13N–NH3 for quantification of MP and MPR has recently been shown to be stable across different software implementations [40].

Quantification requires knowledge of the amount of contrast agent in the myocardial tissue and the arterial input function (AIF) driving the delivery of this contrast agent. Accurate quantification is challenged by the lack of linearity between the measured signal and contrast agent concentration. The main sources of non-linearity and bias are: spatial signal variations caused by the sensitivity profiles of the surface coils, imperfect saturation of magnetization during contrast bolus passage, T2* decay (and signal loss) caused by high contrast agent concentrations in the blood pool, and the non-linear signal response inherent due to saturation recovery that depends on the parameters of the imaging protocol. The proposed dual sequence [11] is designed to address all of these issues. It has been proposed that some of the non-linearity of the AIF response curve can be mitigated by imaging the AIF during a separate injection of a bolus with lower concentration (the dual bolus approach) [41], but this approach has some practical drawbacks as it requires multiple injections and a longer overall acquisition time. Moreover, there are other potential bias sources with this approach, since changes in breathing, etc. between the two measurements may introduce new sources of variation. Consequently, it is desirable to acquire the AIF curve simultaneously with the tissue response curve.

Conclusions

There is a good agreement between MP quantified by CMR with inline perfusion flow mapping and 13N–NH3 PET in patients with suspected stable CAD. Thus, CMR is a viable alternative in clinical practice for quantification of MP.

Abbreviations

ACE: Angiotensin converting enzyme; ARB: Angiotensin receptor blocker; CABG: Coronary artery bypass grafting; CAD: Coronary artery disease; CMR: Cardiovascular magnetic resonance; CT: Computed tomography; ECG: Electrocardiography; EWA: Expectation maximization, weighted intensity A priori information; FFR: Fractional flow reserve; IHD: Ischemic heart disease; LGE: Late gadolinium enhancement; LV: Left ventricle/left ventricular; MI: Myocardial infarction; MP: Myocardial perfusion; MPR: Myocardial perfusion reserve; OSEM: Ordered subsets expectation maximization; PCI: Percutaneous coronary intervention; PET: Positron emission tomography; PSF: Point spread function; SD: Standard deviation; SPECT: Single photon emission computed tomography; TOF: Time-of-flight

Acknowledgements

The authors acknowledge the technologists at the Department Clinical Physiology and Nuclear Imaging for their excellent skills and support in acquiring the CMR and PET data. Furthermore, the authors acknowledge Dr. Christos Xanthis for his engineering skills making the data acquisition possible.

Funding

This study was supported by Swedish Heart and Lund Foundation, Region of Scania, Lund University Medical Faculty.

Authors' contributions

HE took part of designing the study, analyzing and interpreting all patient data and was a major contributor in writing the manuscript. HX took part of designing the study, processing of CMR raw data, generating CMR perfusion maps for analysis as well as for the manuscript illustrations and critically drafting the manuscript. SA was responsible for all data inclusion, analyzing the PET data and critically drafting the manuscript. MC took part of designing the study, interpreting data and critically drafting the manuscript. CH and JO was responsible for the technical aspects of the PET acquisition, participating in all PET data inclusion, participating in PET data analysis and critically drafting the manuscript. FH took part of the data inclusion, analysis of PET data and critically drafting the manuscript. MSH provided the technical foundation for all CMR data post-processing and critically drafting the manuscript. AA took part of designing the study, interpreting data and critically drafting the manuscript. PK took part of designing the study, post-processing of the CMR data, interpreting data and critically drafting the manuscript. HA took part of designing the study, interpreting data and critically drafting the manuscript. All authors have read and approved the final manuscript.

Competing interests

The authors declare that they have no competing interests.

Author details

[1]Department of Clinical Physiology, Clinical Sciences, Lund University and Lund University Hospital, Lund, Sweden. [2]National Heart, Lung, and Blood Institute, National Institutes of Health, DHHS, 10 Center Drive, Bethesda, MD 20892, USA. [3]Department of Radiation Physics, Lund University Hospital, Lund, Sweden. [4]Laboratory of Computing, Medical Informatics and Biomedical – Imaging Technologies, School of Medicine, Aristotle University of Thessaloniki, Thessaloniki, Greece.

References

1. Hachamovitch R, Berman DS, Shaw LJ, et al. Incremental prognostic value of myocardial perfusion single photon emission computed tomography for the prediction of cardiac death: differential stratification for risk of cardiac death and myocardial infarction. Circulation. 1998;97: 535–43.
2. Shaw LJ, Hachamovitch R, Berman DS, et al. The economic consequences of available diagnostic and prognostic strategies for the evaluation of stable angina patients: an observational assessment of the value of precatheterization ischemia. Economics of Noninvasive Diagnosis (END) Multicenter Study Group. J Am Coll Cardiol. 1999;33:661–9.
3. Ford ES, Ajani UA, Croft JB, et al. Explaining the decrease in U.S. deaths from coronary disease, 1980-2000. N Engl J Med. 2007;356:2388–98.
4. Roger VL, Go AS, Lloyd-Jones DM, et al. Heart disease and stroke statistics–2012 update: a report from the American Heart Association. Circulation. 2012;125:e2–e220.
5. Smith SC Jr, Benjamin EJ, Bonow RO, et al. AHA/ACCF Secondary prevention and risk reduction therapy for patients with coronary and other atherosclerotic vascular disease: 2011 update: a guideline from the American Heart Association and American College of Cardiology Foundation. Circulation. 2011;124:2458–73.
6. Salerno M, Beller GA. Noninvasive assessment of myocardial perfusion. Circ Cardiovasc Imaging. 2009;2:412–24.
7. Murthy VL, Naya M, Foster CR, et al. Improved cardiac risk assessment with noninvasive measures of coronary flow reserve. Circulation. 2011;124:2215–24.
8. Herzog BA, Husmann L, Valenta I, et al. Long-term prognostic value of 13N-ammonia myocardial perfusion positron emission tomography added value of coronary flow reserve. J Am Coll Cardiol. 2009;54:150–6.

9. Tio RA, Dabeshlim A, Siebelink HM, et al. Comparison between the prognostic value of left ventricular function and myocardial perfusion reserve in patients with ischemic heart disease. J Nucl Med. 2009;50:214–9.
10. Gatehouse PD, Elkington AG, Ablitt NA, Yang GZ, Pennell DJ, Firmin DN. Accurate assessment of the arterial input function during high-dose myocardial perfusion cardiovascular magnetic resonance. J Magn Reson Imaging. 2004;20:39–45.
11. Kellman P, Hansen MS, Nielles-Vallespin S, et al. Myocardial perfusion cardiovascular magnetic resonance: optimized dual sequence and reconstruction for quantification. J Cardiovasc Magn Reson. 2017;19:43.
12. Hansen MS, Sorensen TS. Gadgetron: an open source framework for medical image reconstruction. Magn Reson Med. 2013;69:1768–76.
13. Bassingthwaighte JB, Wang CY, Chan IS. Blood-tissue exchange via transport and transformation by capillary endothelial cells. Circ Res. 1989;65:997–1020.
14. Heiberg E, Sjogren J, Ugander M, Carlsson M, Engblom H, Arheden H. Design and validation of Segment–freely available software for cardiovascular image analysis. BMC Med Imaging. 2010;10:1.
15. Cerqueira MD, Weissman NJ, Dilsizian V, et al. Standardized myocardial segmentation and nomenclature for tomographic imaging of the heart: a statement for healthcare professionals from the Cardiac Imaging Committee of the Council on Clinical Cardiology of the American Heart Association. Circulation. 2002;105:539–42.
16. Engblom H, Tufvesson J, Jablonowski R, et al. A new automatic algorithm for quantification of myocardial infarction imaged by late gadolinium enhancement cardiovascular magnetic resonance: experimental validation and comparison to expert delineations in multi-center, multi-vendor patient data. J Cardiovasc Magn Reson. 2016;18:27.
17. Nesterov SV, Deshayes E, Sciagra R, et al. Quantification of myocardial blood flow in absolute terms using (82)Rb PET imaging: the RUBY-10 Study. JACC Cardiovasc Imaging. 2014;7:1119–27.
18. Nesterov SV, Settimo L, Mäki M et al. Imaging analysis systems—Carimas, FlowQuant and PMOD—agree well on myocardial perfusion quantification of 13N–ammonia PET: a cross-comparison study. Abstract, EANM 2012, Milan, Italy 2012.
19. DeGrado TR, Hanson MW, Turkington TG, et al. Estimation of myocardial blood flow for longitudinal studies with 13N-labeled ammonia and positron emission tomography. J Nucl Cardiol. 1996;3:494–507.
20. Bland JM, Altman DG. Statistical methods for assessing agreement between two methods of clinical measurement. Lancet. 1986;1:307–10.
21. Lee JM, Kim CH, Koo BK, et al. Integrated myocardial perfusion imaging diagnostics improve detection of functionally significant coronary artery stenosis by 13N-ammonia positron emission tomography. Circ Cardiovasc Imaging. 2016;9
22. Ingkanisorn WP, Kwong RY, Bohme NS, et al. Prognosis of negative adenosine stress magnetic resonance in patients presenting to an emergency department with chest pain. J Am Coll Cardiol. 2006;47:1427–32.
23. Lerakis S, McLean DS, Anadiotis AV, et al. Prognostic value of adenosine stress cardiovascular magnetic resonance in patients with low-risk chest pain. J Cardiovasc Magn Reson. 2009;11:37.
24. Pilz G, Eierle S, Heer T, et al. Negative predictive value of normal adenosine-stress cardiac MRI in the assessment of coronary artery disease and correlation with semiquantitative perfusion analysis. J Magn Reson Imaging. 2010;32:615–21.
25. Uren NG, Crake T, Lefroy DC, de Silva R, Davies GJ, Maseri A. Reduced coronary vasodilator function in infarcted and normal myocardium after myocardial infarction. N Engl J Med. 1994;331:222–7.
26. Fujiwara M, Tamura T, Yoshida K, et al. Coronary flow reserve in angiographically normal coronary arteries with one-vessel coronary artery disease without traditional risk factors. Eur Heart J. 2001;22:479–87.
27. De Bruyne B, Hersbach F, Pijls NH, et al. Abnormal epicardial coronary resistance in patients with diffuse atherosclerosis but "Normal" coronary angiography. Circulation. 2001;104:2401–6.
28. Dayanikli F, Grambow D, Muzik O, Mosca L, Rubenfire M, Schwaiger M. Early detection of abnormal coronary flow reserve in asymptomatic men at high risk for coronary artery disease using positron emission tomography. Circulation. 1994;90:808–17.
29. Kaufmann PA, Gnecchi-Ruscone T, Schafers KP, Luscher TF, Camici PG. Low density lipoprotein cholesterol and coronary microvascular dysfunction in hypercholesterolemia. J Am Coll Cardiol. 2000;36:103–9.
30. Laine H, Raitakari OT, Niinikoski H, et al. Early impairment of coronary flow reserve in young men with borderline hypertension. J Am Coll Cardiol. 1998;32:147–53.

30. Laine H, Raitakari OT, Niinikoski H, et al. Early impairment of coronary flow reserve in young men with borderline hypertension. J Am Coll Cardiol. 1998;32:147–53.

31. Di Carli MF, Afonso L, Campisi R, et al. Coronary vascular dysfunction in premenopausal women with diabetes mellitus. Am Heart J. 2002;144:711–8.
32. Yokoyama I, Momomura S, Ohtake T, et al. Reduced myocardial flow reserve in non-insulin-dependent diabetes mellitus. J Am Coll Cardiol. 1997;30:1472–7.
33. Campisi R, Czernin J, Schoder H, et al. Effects of long-term smoking on myocardial blood flow, coronary vasomotion, and vasodilator capacity. Circulation. 1998;98:119–25.
34. Zeiher AM, Drexler H, Wollschlager H, Just H. Endothelial dysfunction of the coronary microvasculature is associated with coronary blood flow regulation in patients with early atherosclerosis. Circulation. 1991;84:1984–92.
35. Akil S, Hedeer F, Carlsson M, Arheden H, Hindorf C, Engblom H. Qualitative perfusion assessment by cardiac magnetic resonance imaging and invasive coronary angiography is not enough when evaluating patients with coronary artery disease - a cardiac positron emission tomography study. Abstract 2017;SCMR Scientific Sessions. Washington.
36. Kajander SA, Joutsiniemi E, Saraste M, et al. Clinical value of absolute quantification of myocardial perfusion with (15)O-water in coronary artery disease. Circ Cardiovasc Imaging. 2011;4:678–84.
37. Schelbert HR, Phelps ME, Huang SC, et al. N-13 ammonia as an indicator of myocardial blood flow. Circulation. 1981;63:1259–72.
38. Larsson HB, Fritz-Hansen T, Rostrup E, Sondergaard L, Ring P, Henriksen O. Myocardial perfusion modeling using MRI. Magn Reson Med. 1996;35:716–26.
39. Kitkungvan D, Lai D, Zhu H et al. Optimal adenosine stress for maximum stress perfusion, coronary flow reserve, and pixel distribution of coronary flow capacity by Kolmogorov-Smirnov analysis. Circ Cardiovasc Imaging 2017;10:e005650.
40. Slomka PJ, Alexanderson E, Jacome R, et al. Comparison of clinical tools for measurements of regional stress and rest myocardial blood flow assessed with 13N-ammonia PET/CT. J Nucl Med. 2012;53:171–81.
41. Christian TF, Aletras AH, Arai AE. Estimation of absolute myocardial blood flow during first-pass MR perfusion imaging using a dual-bolus injection technique: comparison to single-bolus injection method. J Magn Reson Imaging. 2008;27:1271–7.

14

CMR fluoroscopy right heart catheterization for cardiac output and pulmonary vascular resistance: results in 102 patients

Toby Rogers[1], Kanishka Ratnayaka[1,2], Jaffar M. Khan[1], Annette Stine[1], William H. Schenke[1], Laurie P. Grant[1], Jonathan R. Mazal[1], Elena K. Grant[1,3], Adrienne Campbell-Washburn[1], Michael S. Hansen[1], Rajiv Ramasawmy[1], Daniel A. Herzka[1], Hui Xue[1], Peter Kellman[1], Anthony Z. Faranesh[1] and Robert J. Lederman[1,4*]

Abstract

Background: Quantification of cardiac output and pulmonary vascular resistance (PVR) are critical components of invasive hemodynamic assessment, and can be measured concurrently with pressures using phase contrast CMR flow during real-time CMR guided cardiac catheterization.

Methods: One hundred two consecutive patients underwent CMR fluoroscopy guided right heart catheterization (RHC) with simultaneous measurement of pressure, cardiac output and pulmonary vascular resistance using CMR flow and the Fick principle for comparison. Procedural success, catheterization time and adverse events were prospectively collected.

Results: RHC was successfully completed in 97/102 (95.1%) patients without complication. Catheterization time was 20 ± 11 min. In patients with and without pulmonary hypertension, baseline mean pulmonary artery pressure was 39 ± 12 mmHg vs. 18 ± 4 mmHg ($p < 0.001$), right ventricular (RV) end diastolic volume was 104 ± 64 vs. 74 ± 24 ($p = 0.02$), and RV end-systolic volume was 49 ± 30 vs. 31 ± 13 ($p = 0.004$) respectively. 103 paired cardiac output and 99 paired PVR calculations across multiple conditions were analyzed. At baseline, the bias between cardiac output by CMR and Fick was 5.9% with limits of agreement −38.3% and 50.2% with $r = 0.81$ ($p < 0.001$). The bias between PVR by CMR and Fick was −0.02 WU.m^2 with limits of agreement −2.6 and 2.5 WU.m^2 with $r = 0.98$ ($p < 0.001$). Correlation coefficients were lower and limits of agreement wider during physiological provocation with inhaled 100% oxygen and 40 ppm nitric oxide.

Conclusions: CMR fluoroscopy guided cardiac catheterization is safe, with acceptable procedure times and high procedural success rate. Cardiac output and PVR measurements using CMR flow correlated well with the Fick at baseline and are likely more accurate during physiological provocation with supplemental high-concentration inhaled oxygen.

Keywords: Interventional MRI catheterization, Right heart catheterization, Invasive hemodynamics, Phase contrast MRI flow, Real-time MRI, CMR, Cardiac MRI

* Correspondence: lederman@nih.gov
Dr. Dana C. Peters served as a JCMR guest editor for this manuscript
[1]Cardiovascular and Pulmonary Branch, Division of Intramural Research, National Heart Lung and Blood Institute, National Institutes of Health, Bethesda, MD, USA
[4]Division of Intramural Research, National Heart Lung and Blood Institute, National Institutes of Health, Building 10, Room 2c713, Bethesda, MD 20892-1538, USA
Full list of author information is available at the end of the article

Background

Quantification of cardiac output in the cardiac catheterization laboratory is a central component of hemodynamic assessment. The most commonly used methods, thermodilution and the Fick principle, are subject to substantial error from intrinsic inaccuracy or imprecise assumptions. Thermodilution is particularly unreliable in the setting of intracardiac shunts or tricuspid regurgitation [1]. Calculations using the Fick principle require knowledge of oxygen consumption (VO_2) that is rarely measured directly, and instead is usually assumed from age, sex and heart rate [2–4]. Both methods commonly are inaccurate by over 25%.

In contrast, velocity encoded phase contrast cardiovascular magnetic resonance (CMR) is a well-validated technique to directly measure stroke volume through a major vessel [5], for example the pulmonary artery or aorta, from which cardiac output can be derived. CMR flow measurements have been shown to be superior to Fick for calculation of hemodynamic parameters such as cardiac output and pulmonary vascular resistance that establish diagnosis, guide treatment and inform prognosis [6].

Pressures and cardiac output should preferably be measured simultaneously. Right heart catheterization (RHC) can be safely performed in the CMR scanner using CMR fluoroscopy (also known as real-time CMR) to guide catheter navigation through the vasculature and cardiac chambers [7, 8], avoiding ionizing radiation, and affording full anatomic and functional evaluation with CMR together with invasive hemodynamic assessment [9].

We report our experience of CMR fluoroscopy guided RHC in 102 patients, and compare cardiac output and pulmonary vascular resistance measurements using CMR flow versus Fick, under resting conditions and under physiological provocation with inhaled oxygen and nitric oxide.

Methods

Consecutive patients referred for cardiac catheterization between February 2011 and March 2016 were invited to undergo CMR guided RHC. The research protocol was approved by the Institutional Review Board (NCT01287026). All patients gave written informed consent. Patients were excluded for cardiovascular instability (including ST-elevation myocardial infarction, refractory angina, or refractory congestive heart failure), pregnancy or nursing, an estimated glomerular filtration rate < 30 mL/min/1.73m^2, or ineligibility for CMR. Baseline demographic and clinical characteristics, invasive hemodynamic and CMR findings, technical details, and procedural complications were prospectively recorded.

Real-time CMR guided cardiac catheterization

CMR guided RHC procedures were performed under moderate sedation. Moderate sedation is a drug-induced depression of consciousness during which patients respond purposefully to verbal commands, either alone or accompanied by light tactile stimulation, with no interventions required to maintain a patent airway or spontaneous ventilation. All procedures were performed in the catheterization laboratory at the NIH Clinical Center in Bethesda, Maryland (Fig. 1). The laboratory comprises a 1.5 Tesla CMR scanner adjacent to a conventional X-ray fluoroscopy catheterization laboratory, with the ability to easily transfer patients between the two modalities. More details of the physical setup of an CMR catheterization laboratory and technique for CMR fluoroscopy guided RHC have been published previously [8, 10]. At our institution, in addition to the interventional cardiologist operator, a cardiovascular technologist, CMR technologist, cath lab nurse and moderate sedation nurse are present for every procedure. Vascular access was obtained in the adjoining X-ray room using ultrasound guidance. If indicated, left heart catheterization and selective coronary angiography was performed under X-ray guidance. Patients were then transferred to the CMR room, by docking the X-ray and CMR tables (Fig. 1). Seamless hemodynamic monitoring with 12-lead ECG, O_2 saturation, end-tidal CO_2 and invasive pressure waveforms was maintained throughout the transfer. Baseline CMR scanning was performed followed by CMR guided RHC using an intrinsically CMR-safe balloon wedge end-hole catheter (Fig. 2), with the balloon filled with dilute gadolinium contrast. The catheter was navigated through the heart under real-time CMR guidance (Fig. 3). Catheterization time was defined as the total time required to navigate catheters through the heart and vasculature, perform pressure measurements, acquire CMR data and sample blood for oxygen saturation (Fig. 4).

Patients underwent vasoreactivity testing if there was a clinical indication, specifically elevated pulmonary artery pressures, using a combination of inhaled nitric oxide (40 ppm) and 100% oxygen. If procedural workflow time permitted, additional patients with normal pulmonary artery pressures also underwent vasoreactivity testing to serve as controls. Pulmonary vascular resistance (PVR) was calculated using the formula PVR = (mean pulmonary artery pressure – mean pulmonary artery wedge pressure)/cardiac output. Cardiac output was obtained with phase contrast CMR and the Fick principle, resulting in two PVR measurements. Indexed PVR (PVRi) was calculated using the formula PVRi = PVR / body surface area. Estimated oxygen consumption (VO_2) using the LaFarge-Miettinen formula was used for cardiac output calculations with the Fick principle [2]. CMR flow analyses for cardiac output were performed using syngo Argus (Siemens, Erlangen, Germany) or QMass (Medis Medical Imaging Systems, Leiden, Netherlands).

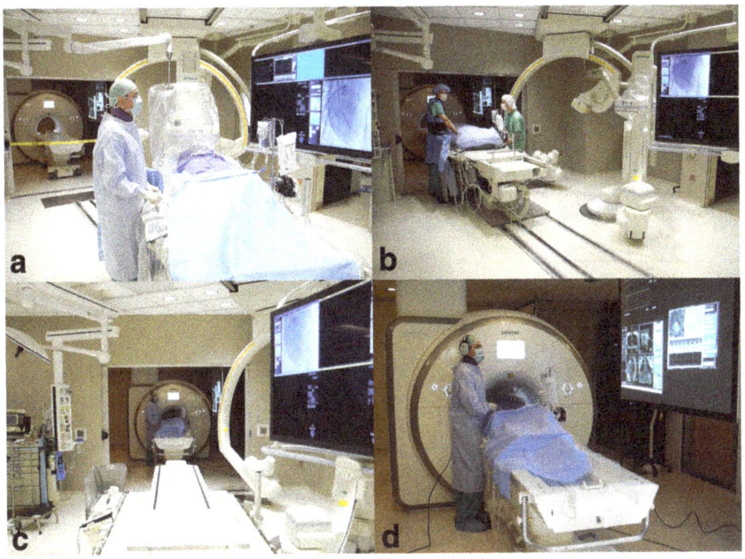

Fig. 1 Interventional CMR (iCMR) cardiac catheterization laboratory. **a** Vascular access is obtained in the X-ray room. **b** The patient is transferred from X-ray to CMR using a transfer table that docks with the CMR table. Hemodynamic monitoring is seamless between the two modalities. **c** View of the CMR room from the X-ray side of the iCMR laboratory. **d** Transfemoral cardiac catheterization under CMR guidance. Real-time images are projected in the CMR room for the operator to view. Noise-cancelling headsets permit open communication with the iCMR control room

CMR sequences

Cardiac volumes and function were obtained from real-time balanced steady state free precession (bSFP) cine imaging with repetition time (TR)/echo time (TE) 3.01/1.29 ms; flip angle 62°; bandwidth 558 Hz/pixel; field of view (FOV) 350mmx262mm; matrix 160x92pixels; slice thickness 8 mm; 30 cardiac phases; 11–13 short-axis slices. Images were acquired free-breathing and reconstructed with retrospective gating and respiratory motion correction. Reconstruction was implemented in a distributed cloud computing environment to limit reconstruction latency [11, 12]. To measure cardiac output, phase contrast flow imaging was used with TR/TE 5.0 ms/2.77; flip angle 20°; bandwidth 454 Hz/pixel; FOV 350mmx350mm; matrix 256x256pixels; slice thickness

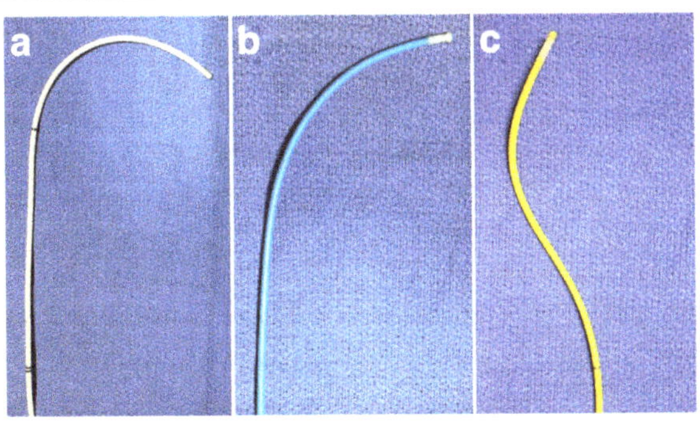

Fig. 2 Example CMR-safe catheters for right heart catheterization. A selection of different shape and stiffness CMR-safe balloon catheters is useful to navigate different right heart anatomies. **a** Vascor Balloon Wedge Pressure Catheter, Model #172-110P; (**b**) Medtronic Pulmonary Wedge Pressure Catheter, Model #150075; (**c**) Edwards True Size Monitoring 'S' Tip Catheter, Model #S111F7

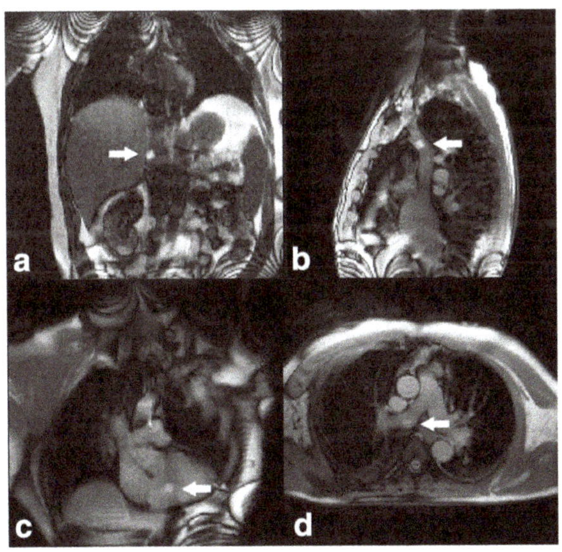

Fig. 3 CMR fluoroscopy guided right heart catheterization. **a** Coronal view with the gadolinium filled balloon at the tip of the catheter in the inferior vena cava (arrow), (**b**) sagittal view of the superior vena cava, (**c**) coronal view of the right ventricle, and (**d**) axial view of the main pulmonary artery bifurcation with the balloon in the right pulmonary artery

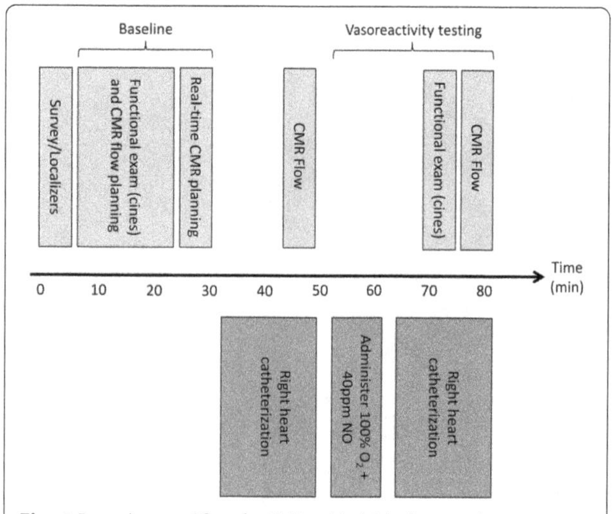

Fig. 4 Procedure workflow for CMR guided right heart catheterization

6 mm; 3 averages; velocity encoding (VENC) set appropriately for individual patient. Surface ECG or invasive arterial blood pressure waveform was used for cardiac gating. RHC was performed with an interactive real-time bSFP sequence with up to 3 interleaved slice planes and with TR/TE 2.6 ms/1.3 ms; flip angle 45°; bandwidth 1008 Hz/pixel; FOV 400mx400mm; matrix 160x120pixels; slice thickness 8 mm. A flow sensitive dark-blood saturation pulse was used for passive visualization of contrast filled balloon. The generalized autocalibrating partially parallel acquisition (GRAPPA) acceleration factor was adjusted interactively by the user between 1 and 4 to balance spatial and temporal resolution as needed for each procedure step.

Statistical analysis

Data were analyzed with SPSS v19.0. (International Business Machines, Chicago, IL) Categorical variables are presented as percentages and continuous variables as mean ± standard deviation. All tests were two-tailed, and a p value of <0.05 was considered significant.

Results

One hundred ten consecutive patients were invited to participate. Eight patients consented but did not ultimately undergo CMR guided RHC, including 2 patients with claustrophobia, 4 with coronary artery disease and acute chest pain and/or shortness of breath prior to starting the procedure, 1 patient who exceeded the CMR table weight limit and 1 patient with occluded external iliac veins. Therefore, 102 patients underwent CMR guided RHC, including the first 16 patients reported previously [8]. Table 1 summarizes baseline demographic and clinical details of these 102 patients. Ages ranged from 26 to 88 years. Body surface area ranged from 1.2 to 2.4m^2. RHC was clinically indicated in 75% of patients. The remaining 25% of patients were referred for other procedures such as selective coronary angiography, and consented to undergo additional CMR guided RHC for research purposes only. Of those patients with a clinical indication for RHC, 51% were under investigation for unexplained dyspnea, 25% required investigation of pulmonary hypertension suggested by echocardiography, 21% had a non-invasive diagnosis of congenital heart abnormality (most commonly unrepaired atrial septal defect), and the remaining 3% were referred for other reasons.

Table 1 Baseline demographics and clinical details

	All patients (n = 102)
Age (years)	53 ± 14
Women	47%
Body surface area (m^2)	1.8 ± 0.2
Hypertension (%)	53%
Diabetes mellitus (%)	20%
Hyperlipidemia (%)	25%
Tobacco prior or current (%)	30%
Coronary artery disease (%)	37%
Congenital heart disease (%)	16%
Prior cardiac surgery (%)	9%
Valvular heart disease (%)	14%
DVT or PE	14%
Congestive heart failure (%)	16%
Pulmonary arterial hypertension (%)	18%
Pulmonary parenchymal disease (%)	4%
Connective tissue disease (%)	6%
Sickle cell disease (%)	6%

Categorical variables are presented as percentages and continuous variables as mean ± standard deviation. *DVT* deep vein thrombosis; *PE* pulmonary embolism

Procedural success and timings

Procedural success, defined as successful completion of a full RHC, was met in 95% of patients. In 5 patients, the pulmonary artery could not be reached with a catheter alone. These patients were transferred back to the X-ray room. RHC was successfully completed in all 5 patients under X-ray guidance with the aid of a guidewire. Overall, procedure time was 83 ± 22 min including a combination determined by clinical necessity of left heart catheterization, selective coronary angiography, CMR imaging, baseline RHC and RHC under physiological provocation with inhaled 100% O_2 and 40 ppm NO. Time to complete a baseline RHC was 20 ± 11 min, and time to complete a second RHC under physiological provocation with inhaled 100% O_2 and 40 ppm NO was 22 ± 10 min.

Safety

With moderate sedation, all 102 patients tolerated CMR scanning. No complications related to CMR guided

RHC occurred in any patient, and no patient required evacuation from the CMR scanner for hemodynamic instability or resuscitation. Nonetheless, we perform regular emergency evacuation drills and can evacuate a patient from the CMR room to a safe location for defibrillation (the X-ray room in our institution) within less than 1 min. Post-procedure, 7 patients reported access site bruising, of which 2 had palpable hematoma. All were managed conservatively. 1 patient reported generalized urticaria, presumed due to allergy to iodinated contrast administered for selective coronary angiography in X-ray before CMR guided RHC.

CMR guided RHC hemodynamic findings

Thirty-eight patients (37%) had baseline pulmonary hypertension (mean PA pressure greater than or equal to 25 mmHg). Baseline mean PA pressure was 39 ± 12 mmHg vs. 18 ± 4 mmHg ($p < 0.001$) in patients with and without pulmonary hypertension respectively. Baseline RV end diastolic volume was 104 ± 64 mL vs. 74 ± 24 mL ($p = 0.02$), RV end-systolic volume was 49 ± 30 mL vs. 31 ± 13 mL ($p = 0.004$), RV stroke volume was 55 ± 36% vs. 43 ± 16 mL ($p = 0.09$), and RV ejection fraction was 50 ± 14 vs. 54 ± 17% ($p = 0.22$) in patients with and without pulmonary hypertension respectively.

Baseline cardiac index was 2.8 ± 1.0 L/min/m^2 vs. 2.9 ± 1.1 L/min/m^2 ($p = 0.12$) by CMR flow vs. Fick. With inhaled 100% O2 and 40 ppm NO, cardiac index was 2.6 ± 0.7 L/min/m^2 vs. 2.9 ± 1.0 L/min/m^2 ($p = 0.01$) by CMR flow vs. Fick. For patients with and without pulmonary hypertension respectively, baseline cardiac index using CMR flow was 3.1 ± 1.3 L/min/m^2 vs. 2.6 ± 0.8 L/min/m^2 ($p = 0.07$). This discrepancy was largely the result of higher baseline heart rate (76 ± 16 bpm vs. 65 ± 11 bpm, $p < 0.001$) rather than a difference in stroke volume (42 ± 12 mL vs. 40 ± 42 mL, $p = 0.79$).

Table 2 summarizes cardiac catheterization findings in all patients at baseline and in the fifty eight patients (57%) tested for pulmonary arterial vasoreactivity with inhaled 100% O_2 and 40 ppm NO. Only 5 patients met current guideline criteria for positive vasoreactivity, defined as a reduction in mean pulmonary artery pressure of at least 10 mmHg and to below 40 mmHg [13]. Median baseline pulmonary artery pressure in these 5 patients was 48 mmHg (41–50 mmHg). Using the earlier definition of ≥20% reduction in pulmonary vascular resistance index, 29% of vasoreactivity studies were positive.

A total of 103 paired cardiac index calculations were available for both CMR flow and Fick principle (56 at baseline on room air, and 47 on inhaled 100% O_2 and 40 ppm NO). At baseline, the mean difference (or bias) between methods was 5.9% with limits of agreement −38.3% and 50.2%. The correlation coefficient between

Table 2 Cardiac catheterization findings

	Baseline (n = 102)	100% O_2 and 40 ppm NO (n = 58)
Heart rate (bpm)	70 ± 14	67 ± 13
RA mean (mmHg)	7 ± 4	7 ± 4
RV pressure systolic/diastolic (mmHg)	45 ± 22/8 ± 5	43 ± 24/7 ± 4
PA pressure systolic/diastolic (mmHg)	43 ± 21/18 ± 9	40 ± 20/17 ± 9
PA mean (mmHg)	26 ± 13	25 ± 10
PA pulse pressure (mmHg)	25 ± 13	23 ± 13
PAWP (mmHg)	13 ± 6.3	13 ± 6
Transpulmonary gradient (mmHg)	13 ± 10	11 ± 10
Cardiac index (L/min/m^2) by CMR flow	2.9 ± 1.0	2.8 ± 0.9
PVRi (WU.m^2) by CMR flow	4.5 ± 3.5	4.0 ± 4.7
BP systolic/diastolic (mmHg)	136 ± 22/67 ± 12	140 ± 23/70 ± 11
LVEDP (mmHg)	15 ± 7	n/a
SVC sat (%)	69 ± 8	82 ± 5
IVC sat (%)	70 ± 8	83 ± 4
Mixed venous sat (%)	69 ± 7	83 ± 4
RA sat (%)	71 ± 7	84 ± 9
RV sat (%)	71 ± 7	85 ± 7
PA sat (%)	71 ± 7	84 ± 6
Aorta sat (%)	94 ± 4	98 ± 1

Categorical variables are presented as percentages and continuous variables as mean ± standard deviation. *BP* blood pressure, *IVC* inferior vena cava, *LVEDP* left ventricular end-diastolic pressure, *PA* pulmonary artery, *PAWP* pulmonary artery wedge pressure, *PVRi* pulmonary vascular resistance index, *RA* right atrium, *RV* right ventricle, *SVC* superior vena cava

the two methods was 0.81 ($p < 0.001$) (Fig. 5). Under physiological provocation with inhaled 100% O_2 and 40 ppm NO, the bias was 14.2% with limits of agreement −57.4% and 85.8%. The correlation coefficient between the two methods was 0.67 ($p < 0.001$) (Fig. 6).

A total of 99 paired PVRi calculations (invasive pressure and cardiac output with CMR flow or Fick principle) were obtained. Baseline PVRi was 4.5 ± 3.5 WU.m^2 vs. 4.8 ± 3.9 WU.m^2 ($p = 0.01$) by CMR flow vs. Fick. With inhaled 100% O2 and 40 ppm NO, PVRi was 3.9 ± 4.7 WU.m^2 vs 3.5 ± 3.9 WU.m^2 ($p = 0.15$) by CMR flow vs. Fick. Across both conditions, the bias between indexed PVR by CMR and Fick was −0.02 WU.m^2 with limits of agreement −2.6 and 2.5 WU.m^2. At baseline, mean PVRi was 4.5 ± 3.5WU.m^2 by CMR flow and 4.8 ± 4.5 WU.m^2 by Fick principle. The correlation coefficient between the two methods was 0.98 ($p < 0.001$) (Fig. 7). Bland-Altman analysis revealed a bias of −6.8% with limits of agreement −41.2% and 27.6%. Under physiological provocation with inhaled 100% O_2 and

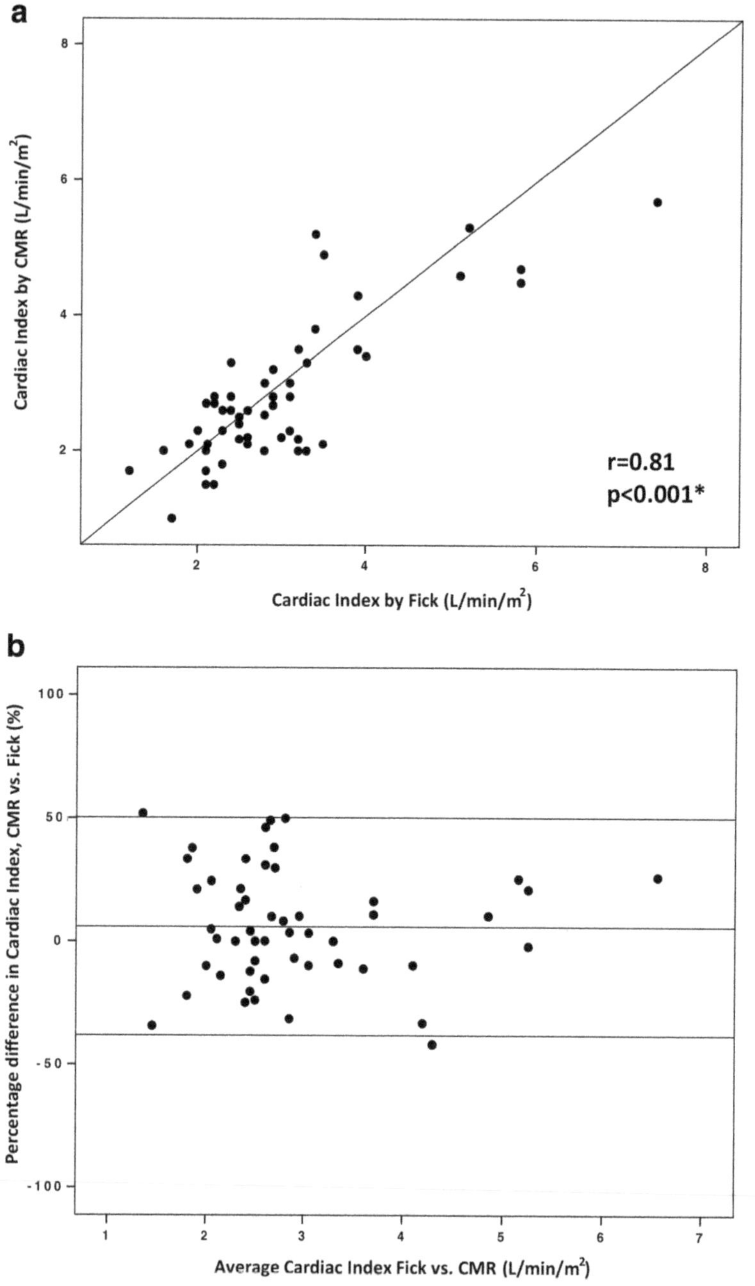

Fig. 5 Comparison of cardiac index calculated with the Fick principle and with CMR flow at baseline on room air. **a** Correlation between cardiac index calculated with the Fick principle and with CMR flow at baseline on room air (n = 56 paired calculations). **b** Bland-Altman plot of the difference in cardiac index calculated with the two methods, and mean cardiac index with the two methods

40 ppm NO, mean PVRi was 4.0 ± 4.7 WU.m^2 by CMR flow and 3.9 ± 4.1 WU.m^2 by Fick principle. The correlation coefficient between the two methods was 0.95 (p < 0.001) (Figure 8). Bland-Altman analysis revealed a bias of 4.8% with limits of agreement −44.5% and 54.1%.

Table 3 summarizes hemodynamic and CMR findings in response to inhaled 100% O_2 and 40 ppm NO in patients with or without pulmonary hypertension defined by baseline mean pulmonary artery pressure. Table 4 summarizes hemodynamic and CMR findings in response to inhaled 100% O_2 and 40 ppm NO according to whether patients were vasoactive or not (defined as ≥20% reduction in PVRi). Analysis per current guideline definition of vasoreactivity (defined as reduction in mean pulmonary artery pressure of at least 10 mmHg and to below 40 mmHg) was not

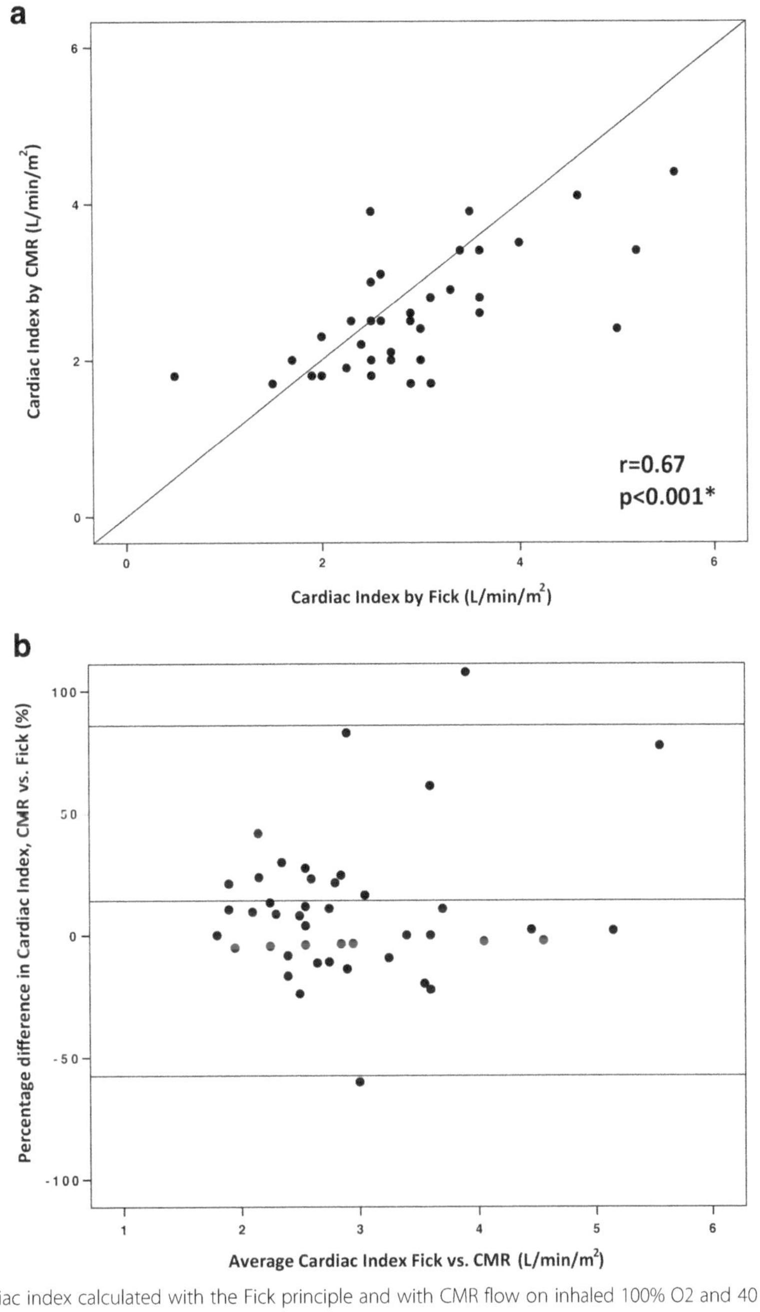

Fig. 6 Comparison of cardiac index calculated with the Fick principle and with CMR flow on inhaled 100% O2 and 40 ppm NO. **a** Correlation between cardiac index calculated with the Fick principle and with CMR flow on inhaled 100% O_2 and 40 ppm NO (n = 47 paired calculations). **b** Bland-Altman plot of the difference in cardiac index calculated with the two methods, and mean cardiac index with the two methods

possible due to the low number of patients with positive response (n = 5).

Discussion

CMR fluoroscopy (also known as real-time CMR) allowed catheter navigation for complete RHC in 97/102 patients with a range of cardiovascular diagnoses. The procedure was safe, had a high success rate, and had acceptable catheterization times. This is the largest published series of paired comparisons of cardiac output and PVRi measured by both CMR flow and Fick techniques. We demonstrated excellent agreement between the two methods at baseline and reasonable agreement during physiological provocation with inhaled 100% oxygen and 40 ppm NO, which is a circumstance when Fick is less accurate because of reduced signal-to-noise due to narrow arteriovenous oxygen difference.

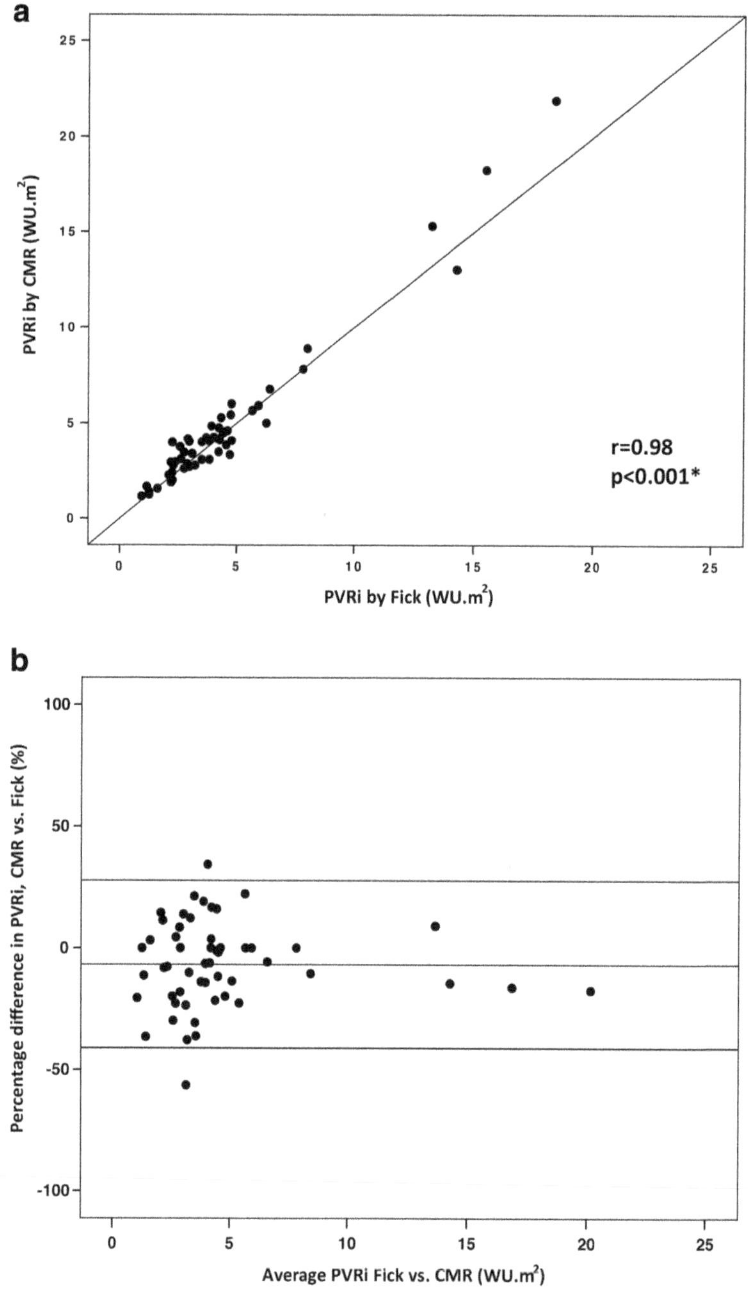

Fig. 7 Comparison of PVRi calculated with the Fick principle and with CMR flow at baseline on room air. **a** Correlation between PVRi calculated with the Fick principle and with CMR flow at baseline on room air (n = 54 paired calculations). **b** Bland-Altman plot of the difference in PVRi calculated with the two methods, and mean PVRi with the two methods. PVRi: pulmonary vascular resistance index

We previously tested feasibility of CMR guided RHC, comparing timings of specific procedural steps with X-ray guided RHC [8]. In that experiment, total RHC times ('sheath to sheath') were equivalent irrespective of image guidance modality (X-ray 19.4 + 11.5 min, CMR with air-filled balloon 21.4 + 6.0 min, CMR with gadolinium-filled balloon 21.0 + 8.8 min, p = 0.347). We also compared relative conspicuity of air-filled versus gadolinium-filled catheter balloons, with a clear operator preference for gadolinium. Integration of dedicated pulse sequences that darken blood while preserving background tissue signal further facilitates catheter visualization. Only the balloon at the tip of the catheter can be visualized, not the catheter shaft, and so the operator must learn to interpret catheter configuration based on balloon tip movement. This is not difficult for an experienced interventional cardiologist to learn. CMR guided RHC has been designated a standard clinical procedure at NIH. All patients are now

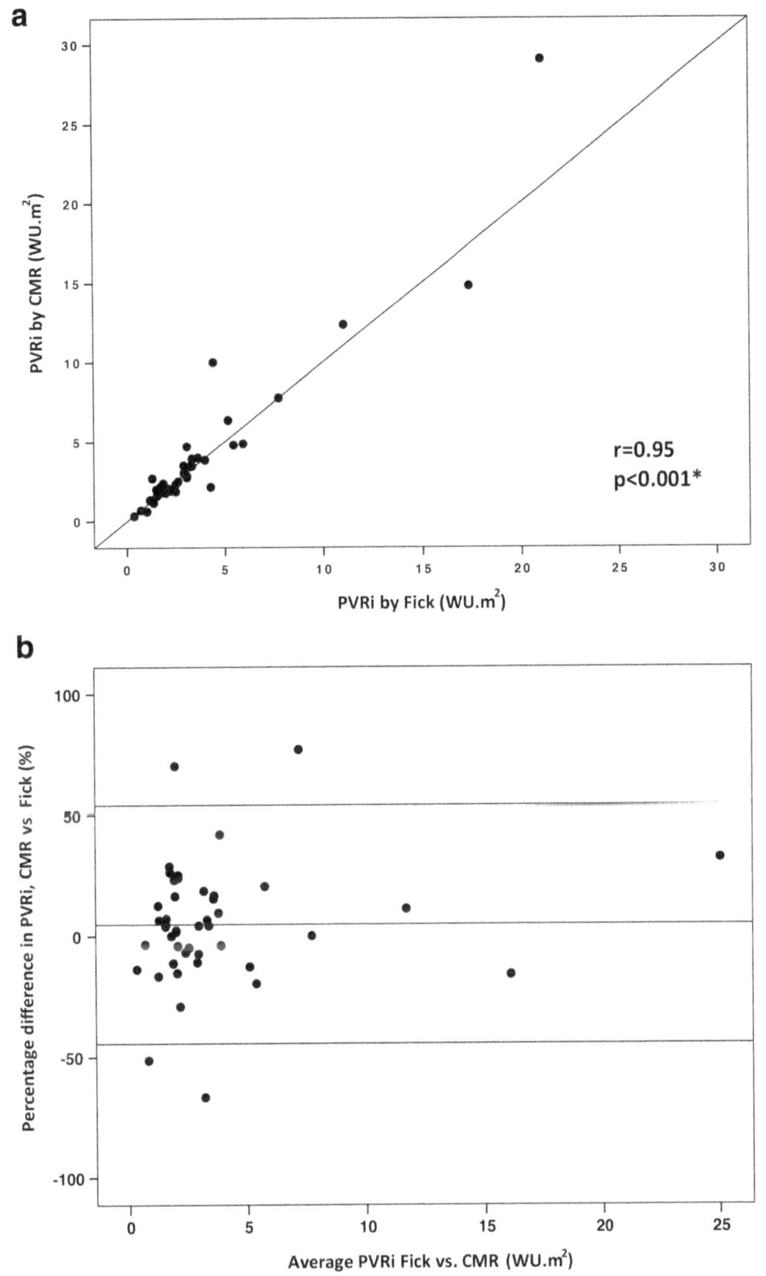

Fig. 8 Comparison of PVRi calculated with the Fick principle and with CMR flow on inhaled 100% O2 and 40 ppm NO. **a** Correlation between PVRi calculated with the Fick principle and with CMR flow on inhaled 100% O_2 and 40 ppm NO (*n* = 45 paired calculations). **b** Bland-Altman plot of the difference in PVRi calculated with the two methods, and mean PVRi with the two methods. PVRi: pulmonary vascular resistance index

offered CMR guided catheterization, even if they are not participating in research.

Vascular access was obtained in the adjoining X-ray room using ultrasound guidance, as there are currently no commercially available CMR-conditional guidewires to enable access to be obtained close to the CMR scanner. Fluoroscopy is certainly not required and therefore any adjoining room could be used for vascular access. An adjoining X-ray room does allow selective coronary angiography to be performed in the same sitting as CMR guided RHC. If needed, a patient can also be transferred from CMR to X-ray for a planned or bailout intervention. If general anesthesia is used, as is common in pediatrics, both CMR and cardiac catheterization can be performed during a single general anesthesia, sparing the child the need for a second.

We have learned that in the absence of available CMR-conditional guidewires, it is prudent to have

Table 3 Hemodynamic and CMR findings in response to inhaled 100% O2 and 40 ppm NO in patients with and without pulmonary hypertension

	Baseline	100% O_2 + 40 ppm NO	*p* value
Normal pulmonary pressures (n = 30)			
Mean PA pressure (mmHg)	18 ± 4	16 ± 5	0.01*
Mean PAWP (mmHg)	9 ± 3	10 ± 3	0.008*
Cardiac index (L/min/m^2) by CMR flow	2.6 ± 0.1	2.5 ± 0.1	0.65
RV end diastolic volume (mL)	74 ± 24	73 ± 24	0.41
RV end systolic volume (mL)	27 ± 12	25 ± 13	0.22
RV stroke volume (mL)	47 ± 15	47 ± 15	0.61
RV ejection fraction (%)	64 ± 9	66 ± 11	0.03*
LV end diastolic volume (mL)	75 ± 20	76 ± 20	0.11
LV end systolic volume (mL)	32 ± 18	33 ± 18	0.10
LV stroke volume (mL)	43 ± 9	43 ± 9	0.93
LV ejection fraction (%)	60 ± 11	59 ± 11	0.18
Pulmonary hypertension (n = 28)			
Mean PA pressure (mmHg)	39 ± 12	34 ± 12	<0.001*
Mean PAWP (mmHg)	16 ± 6	16 ± 8	0.75
Cardiac index (L/min/m^2) by CMR flow	3.1 ± 0.3	3.0 ± 0.2	0.44
RV end diastolic volume (mL)	120 ± 73	112 ± 74	0.01*
RV end systolic volume (mL)	57 ± 35	52 ± 40	0.06
RV stroke volume (mL)	64 ± 41	61 ± 37	0.22
RV ejection fraction (%)	54 ± 12	56 ± 11	0.17
LV end diastolic volume (mL)	89 ± 33	92 ± 34	0.045*
LV end systolic volume (mL)	39 ± 21	42 ± 25	0.07
LV stroke volume (mL)	50 ± 14	50 ± 10	0.94
LV ejection fraction (%)	59 ± 10	58 ± 9	0.22

Categorical variables are presented as percentages and continuous variables as mean ± standard deviation. Cardiac index was derived from CMR flow. *denotes statistical significance. *PA* pulmonary artery, *PAWP* pulmonary artery wedge pressure; *PVRi* pulmonary vascular resistance index, *RV* right ventricle

several differently shaped balloon catheters to maximize procedural success (Fig. 2). Depending on operator choice of central venous approach and patient anatomy, straight or angled catheters are more appropriate to reach target chambers or vessels. We failed to reach the pulmonary artery in 5 patients with severely dilated right heart chambers caused by pulmonary hypertension. In all 5 patients, pulmonary artery catheterization under X-ray guidance was also unsuccessful without the aid of a guidewire. CMR-conditional guidewires are in development, which should improve the procedural success rate [14, 15]. CMR-conditional guidewires will also permit more complex interventions to be performed under CMR guidance.

Mean PVRi at baseline was 5.1 ± 6.3WU.m^2 in the original report by Muthurangu et al. in which PVRi comparisons using the Fick principle and CMR flow were made in 15 patients [6]. The correlation coefficient at baseline on room air was excellent in their study (r = 0.91, p < 0.05). The bias between the two methods was 2.3% with limits of agreement −45.5% and 50.2%. On inhaled 100% O_2 and 20 ppm NO, the correlation coefficient was poor (r = 0.59, p = 0.02). Bias between the two methods was 54.2% with limits of agreement −66.0% and 174.4%. Our results, with substantially larger number of paired calculations, also showed a strong correlation between the two methods at baseline on room air. We observed a stronger correlation on inhaled 100% O_2 and 40 ppm than that reported by Muthurangu et al., although the limits of agreement were still much wider than at baseline. This may be due to a number of factors, including higher number of paired calculations in our study, use of estimated rather than measured VO_2, and lower mean PVRi at baseline.

We tested the hypothesis that current criteria for positive vasoreactivity to inhaled 100% O_2 and 40 ppm NO, defined as ≥10 mmHg reduction in mean pulmonary artery pressure and to below 40 mmHg, may miss subtle RV changes to pulmonary vasodilation. Using the older and less stringent criterion for positive vasoreactivity of

Table 4 Hemodynamic and CMR findings in response to inhaled 100% O2 and 40 ppm NO in patients with and without a 20% reduction in PVRi

	Baseline	100% O_2 + 40 ppm NO	*p* value
Positive vasodilatory response (n = 29)			
Mean PA pressure (mmHg)	26 ± 12	22 ± 10	<0.001*
Mean PAWP (mmHg)	13 ± 6	14 ± 7	0.11
Cardiac index (L/min/m²) by CMR flow	3.0 ± 0.2	2.9 ± 0.2	0.06
PVRi (WU.m²) by CMR flow	4.2 ± 3.2	2.6 ± 2.2	<0.001*
RV end diastolic volume (mL)	96 ± 63	91 ± 63	0.014*
RV end systolic volume (mL)	39 ± 32	36 ± 35	0.12
RV stroke volume (mL)	57 ± 34	55 ± 32	0.14
RV ejection fraction (%)	62 ± 11	63 ± 12	0.19
Negative vasodilatory response (n = 15)			
Mean PA pressure (mmHg)	25 ± 12	24 ± 11	0.08
Mean PAWP (mmHg)	11 ± 5	11 ± 4	0.65
Cardiac index (L/min/m²) by CMR flow	2.7 ± 0.8	2.7 ± 0.8	0.98
PVRi (WU.m²) by CMR flow	4.9 ± 3.8	4.9 ± 3.4	0.97
RV end diastolic volume (mL)	79 ± 23	81 ± 26	0.44
RV end systolic volume (mL)	35 ± 15	33 ± 17	0.33
RV stroke volume (mL)	45 ± 14	48 ± 12	0.014*
RV ejection fraction (%)	58 ± 11	62 ± 13	0.008*

Categorical variables are presented as percentages and continuous variables as mean ± standard deviation. Cardiac index and PVRi were derived from CMR flow. *PA* pulmonary artery, *PAWP* pulmonary artery wedge pressure, *PVRi* pulmonary vascular resistance index, *RV* right ventricle

≥20% reduction in PVRi, we did observe small differences in RV volumes and ejection fraction between groups (Table 4). Although some of these differences met statistical significance, they were not clinically meaningful. More information is needed to address whether evaluating RV response to pulmonary arterial vasodilators has prognostic or therapeutic merit. Even without vasodilator testing, patients in this study with pulmonary hypertension had increased RV end-diastolic and end-systolic volumes, and a trend towards lower stroke volumes and ejection fraction at baseline. For these patients, this incremental anatomic and functional information proved useful to guide treatment and inform prognosis because RV function is one of the strongest prognostic factors in patients with pulmonary hypertension.

Future directions

We believe that exercise CMR catheterization is a very promising clinical tool to unmask latent pathology, particularly in patients with unexplained dyspnea and normal non-invasive and invasive testing at rest. Most cardiac symptoms are not apparent at rest, and only manifest with stress. Exercise is unquestionably the most physiological form of stress. Barber et al. elegantly demonstrated the feasibility and value of cardiopulmonary exercise testing in a CMR scanner [16]. Quantification of RV dimensions and function during exercise is feasible using real-time CMR sequences [17]. We previously validated free-breathing motion-corrected cine imaging for cardiac chamber volume and function analysis [18]. Other groups have shown that exercise during CMR catheterization is feasible [19, 20] and CMR ergometers that permit carefully titrated workload are already commercially available.

Limitations

Due to protocol-specified procedure time limitations, we did not perform repeated measurements of cardiac output using CMR flow and Fick principle. Therefore, it is not possible to comment on repeatability of either technique. Neither did we perform an analysis of intra- or inter-observer variability.

CMR guided cardiac catheterization requires additional infrastructure. Most important, noise-suppressing headsets for communication, screens to visualize real-time images for the operator in the CMR room, and hemodynamic recording system. Many of these elements are now commercially available. It is possible to equip existing diagnostic CMR rooms to perform CMR guided invasive cardiac catheterization. The major limitation to performing more complex CMR guided interventions remains lack of CMR-conditional devices, catheters and guidewires. However, key components are now commercially available or under development, including electrophysiology ablation and mapping system [21], CMR endomyocardial bioptome [22], and CMR-conditional guidewires.

Conclusion

In conclusion, real-time CMR fluoroscopy guided RHC is feasible with high procedural success rate, acceptable procedure times and excellent safety. Cardiac output and pulmonary vascular resistance quantification with CMR flow correlated well with Fick principle at baseline, and under physiological provocation with inhaled 100% oxygen and NO. Using this approach, it is possible to perform high quality invasive hemodynamic studies together with anatomic and functional assessment in patients with cardiopulmonary disease using solely CMR guidance.

Abbreviations

CMR: Cardiovascular magnetic resonance; GRAPPA: Generalized autocalibrating partially parallel acquisition; LV: Left ventricle; PVR: Pulmonary vascular resistance; RHC: Right heart catheterization; RV: Right ventricle

Acknowledgements

Not applicable.

Funding

This work was supported by the Division of Intramural Research, National Heart, Lung, and Blood Institute, National Institutes of Health, USA (Z01-HL005062 and Z01-HL006061).

Authors' contributions

TR Designed, executed, analyzed experiments including CMR interpretation and drafted the manuscript. KR Designed and executed experiments and revised the manuscript. JMK Executed and analyzed experiments including CMR interpretation and revised the manuscript. AMS, WHS, JRM Designed and executed experiments and revised the manuscript. LPG, EKG Executed experiments and revised the manuscript. ACW, RR, DAH, MSH, HX, PK, AZF, RJL Designed, executed, analyzed experiments and revised the manuscript. All authors read and approved the final manuscript.

Authors' information

Not applicable.

Consent for publication

The protocol and NHLBI IRB approval include permission to use de-identified subject images in scientific communications.

Competing interests

NIH and Siemens Medical Systems have a collaborative research and development agreement for interventional CMR.

Author details

[1]Cardiovascular and Pulmonary Branch, Division of Intramural Research, National Heart Lung and Blood Institute, National Institutes of Health, Bethesda, MD, USA. [2]Department of Cardiology, Rady Children's Hospital, San Diego, CA, USA. [3]Department of Cardiology, Children's National Medical Center, Washington, DC, USA. [4]Division of Intramural Research, National Heart Lung and Blood Institute, National Institutes of Health, Building 10, Room 2c713, Bethesda, MD 20892-1538, USA.

References

1. Winniford MD, Kern MJ, Lambert CR. Blood flow measurement and quantification of vascular stenoses. In: Pepine CJ, Hill JA, Lambert CR, editors. Diagnostic and therapeutic cardiac catheterization 3/e. Baltimore: Williams & Wilkins; 1998. p. 399–441.
2. LaFarge CG, Miettinen OS. The estimation of oxygen consumption. Cardiovasc Res. 1970;4:23–30.
3. Dehmer GJ, Firth BG, Hillis LD. Oxygen consumption in adult patients during cardiac catheterization. Clin Cardiol. 1982;5:436–40.
4. Narang N, Thibodeau JT, Levine BD, Gore MO, Ayers CR, Lange RA, et al. Inaccuracy of estimated resting oxygen uptake in the clinical setting. Circulation. 2014;129:203–10.
5. Nayak KS, Nielsen JF, Bernstein MA, Markl M, Gatehouse PD, Botnar RM, et al. Cardiovascular magnetic resonance phase contrast imaging. J Cardiovasc Magn Reson. 2015;17:71.
6. Muthurangu V, Taylor A, Andriantsimiavona R, Hegde S, Miquel ME, Tulloh R, et al. Novel method of quantifying pulmonary vascular resistance by use of simultaneous invasive pressure monitoring and phase-contrast magnetic resonance flow. Circulation. 2004;110:826–34.
7. Razavi R, Hill DL, Keevil SF, Miquel ME, Muthurangu V, Hegde S, et al. Cardiac catheterisation guided by MRI in children and adults with congenital heart disease. Lancet. 2003;362:1877–82.
8. Ratnayaka K, Faranesh AZ, Hansen MS, Stine AM, Halabi M, Barbash IM, et al. Real-time MRI-guided right heart catheterization in adults using passive catheters. Eur Heart J. 2013;34:380–9.
9. Rogers T, Ratnayaka K, Lederman RJ. MRI catheterization in cardiopulmonary disease. Chest. 2014;145:30–6.
10. Rogers T, Lederman RJ. Interventional CMR: Clinical applications and future directions. Curr Cardiol Rep. 2015;17:31.
11. Xue H, Kellman P, Larocca G, Arai AE, Hansen MS. High spatial and temporal resolution retrospective cine cardiovascular magnetic resonance from shortened free breathing real-time acquisitions. J Cardiovasc Magn Reson. 2013;15:102.
12. Xue H, Kellman P, Larocca G, Arai AE, Hansen MS. Distributed MRI reconstruction using Gadgetron-based cloud computing. Magn Reson Med. 2015;73:1015–25.
13. Galie N, Humbert M, Vachiery JL, Gibbs S, Lang I, Torbicki A, et al. 2015 ESC/ERS Guidelines for the diagnosis and treatment of pulmonary hypertension: The Joint Task Force for the Diagnosis and Treatment of Pulmonary Hypertension of the European Society of Cardiology (ESC) and the European Respiratory Society (ERS): Endorsed by: Association for European Paediatric and Congenital Cardiology (AEPC), International Society for Heart and Lung Transplantation (ISHLT). Eur Heart J. 2016;37:67–119.
14. Sonmez M, Saikus CE, Bell JA, Franson DN, Halabi M, Faranesh AZ, et al. MRI active guidewire with an embedded temperature probe and providing a distinct tip signal to enhance clinical safety. J Cardiovasc Magn Reson. 2012; 14:38.
15. Basar B, Rogers T, Ratnayaka K, Campbell-Washburn AE, Mazal JR, Schenke WH, et al. Segmented nitinol guidewires with stiffness-matched connectors for cardiovascular magnetic resonance catheterization: preserved mechanical performance and freedom from heating. J Cardiovasc Magn Reson. 2015;17:105.
16. Barber NJ, Ako EO, Kowalik GT, Cheang MH, Pandya B, Steeden JA, et al. Magnetic resonance-augmented cardiopulmonary exercise testing: comprehensively assessing exercise intolerance in children with cardiovascular disease. Circ Cardiovasc Imaging. 2016;9
17. La Gerche A, Claessen G, Van de Bruaene A, Pattyn N, Van Cleemput J, Gewillig M, et al. Cardiac MRI: a new gold standard for ventricular volume quantification during high-intensity exercise. Circ Cardiovasc Imaging. 2013; 6:329–38.
18. Cross R, Olivieri L, O'Brien K, Kellman P, Xue H, Hansen M. Improved workflow for quantification of left ventricular volumes and mass using free-breathing motion corrected cine imaging. J Cardiovasc Magn Reson. 2016; 18:10.
19. Claessen G, La Gerche A, Wielandts JY, Bogaert J, Van Cleemput J, Wuyts W, et al. Exercise pathophysiology and sildenafil effects in chronic thromboembolic pulmonary hypertension. Heart. 2015;101:637–44.
20. Claessen G, La Gerche A, Voigt JU, Dymarkowski S, Schnell F, Petit T, et al. Accuracy of Echocardiography to Evaluate Pulmonary Vascular and RV Function During Exercise. JACC Cardiovasc Imaging. 2016;9:532–43.

Quantitative cardiovascular magnetic resonance perfusion imaging identifies reduced flow reserve in microvascular coronary artery disease

Benjamin Zorach[1†], Peter W. Shaw[2†], Jamieson Bourque[1,3], Sujith Kuruvilla[4], Pelbreton C. Balfour Jr[1], Yang Yang[1,5], Roshin Mathew[1], Jonathan Pan[1], Jorge A. Gonzalez[6], Angela M. Taylor[1], Craig H. Meyer[3,5], Frederick H. Epstein[3,5], Christopher M. Kramer[1,3*] and Michael Salerno[1,3,5*]

Abstract

Background: Preliminary semi-quantitative cardiovascular magnetic resonance (CMR) perfusion studies have demonstrated reduced myocardial perfusion reserve (MPR) in patients with angina and risk factors for microvascular disease (MVD), however fully quantitative CMR has not been studied. The purpose of this study is to evaluate whether fully quantitative CMR identifies reduced MPR in this population, and to investigate the relationship between epicardial atherosclerosis, left ventricular hypertrophy (LVH), extracellular volume (ECV), and perfusion.

Methods: Forty-six patients with typical angina and risk factors for MVD (females, or males with diabetes or metabolic syndrome) who had no obstructive coronary artery disease by coronary angiography and 20 healthy control subjects underwent regadenoson stress CMR perfusion imaging using a dual-sequence quantitative spiral pulse sequence to quantify MPR. Subjects also underwent T1 mapping to quantify ECV, and computed tomographic (CT) coronary calcium scoring to assess atherosclerosis burden.

Results: In patients with risk factors for MVD, both MPR (2.21 [1.95,2.69] vs. 2.93 [2.763.19], $p < 0.001$) and stress myocardial perfusion (2.65 ± 0.62 ml/min/g, vs. 3.17 ± 0.49 ml/min/g $p < 0.002$) were reduced as compared to controls. These differences remained after adjusting for age, left ventricular (LV) mass, body mass index (BMI), and gender. There were no differences in native T1 or ECV between subjects and controls.

Conclusions: Stress myocardial perfusion and MPR as measured by fully quantitative CMR perfusion imaging are reduced in subjects with risk factors for MVD with no obstructive CAD as compared to healthy controls. Neither myocardial hypertrophy nor fibrosis accounts for these differences.

Keywords: Cardiovascular magnetic resonance, Microvascular disease, Myocardial perfusion reserve, Non-obstructive coronary artery disease, Angina, Women, Diabetes, Metabolic syndrome

* Correspondence: ckramer@virginia.edu; ms5pc@virginia.edu
†Equal contributors
[1]Department of Medicine, Cardiology Division, University of Virginia Health System, Charlottesville, VA, USA
Full list of author information is available at the end of the article

Background

Coronary artery disease (CAD) is a major cause of morbidity in the United States. It is estimated that 15.5 million Americans have heart disease and 8.2 million suffer from angina pectoris [1]. In a retrospective analysis of the NCDR Cath Registry, among patients with suspected CAD undergoing elective coronary angiography without known CAD, only 37.6% of patients demonstrated obstructive epicardial CAD [2]. It is now widely recognized that obstructive epicardial CAD is not the sole cause of myocardial ischemia [3].

Indeed, microvascular disease (MVD), or coronary microvascular dysfunction (CMD), is increasingly seen as an important contributor in the pathophysiology of ischemic heart disease and chest pain syndromes [4, 5]. In the WISE study, abnormal coronary microvascular reactivity to adenosine was highly prevalent and a significant predictor of adverse cardiovascular outcomes in women even in the absence of obstructive CAD [6]. In a population of men and women undergoing coronary angiography, women had more cardiovascular events despite less significant obstructive CAD, attributable in part to reduced coronary flow reserve (CFR) [7].

The cause of MVD is thought to be multifactorial likely due impaired vasodilatation of the microcirculation supplying the myocardium, as well as from an increased response to factors that promote vasoconstriction [5]. The risk factors associated with MVD include – but are not limited to – female gender, diabetes, and the metabolic syndrome [8–10]. The cumulative number of risk factors was previously shown to be inversely related to coronary flow reserve [11]. A recent review by a working group in the study of myocardial ischemia and no obstructive coronary artery disease (MINOCA) comprehensively highlights the data behind the current understanding of MVD and proposes future directions of research including detection with noninvasive imaging [12].

The diagnosis of MVD has traditionally been ascertained by means of invasive cardiac catheterization using vasomotor testing with acetylcholine during coronary angiography and/or by CFR during adenosine infusion using invasive coronary Doppler flow measurements [12]. More recently, there has been growing interest in assessing abnormal myocardial perfusion reserve (MPR) in MVD non-invasively using techniques such as positron emission tomography (PET) and cardiovascular magnetic resonance (CMR).

A number of CMR methods have been applied to the measurement of myocardial perfusion for the detection of obstructive CAD, including semi-quantitative and fully quantitative techniques [13, 14]. To date, the efficacy of using fully quantitative CMR to assess MVD has yet to be examined. The aim of the present study is to demonstrate that quantitative CMR identifies reduced MPR in patients with angina and risk factors for MVD who have *no* evidence of obstructive CAD by coronary angiography. A secondary aim of the study was to investigate any relationship between myocardial hypertrophy, inflammation, fibrosis, and epicardial atherosclerosis with myocardial perfusion in this patient population.

Methods

Subjects

Patients with risk factors for MVD (women, or men with diabetes mellitus or metabolic syndrome) were prospectively recruited from the University of Virginia Health System. All patients had undergone coronary angiography for evaluation of typical exertional angina and were found to have no obstructive CAD (defined as stenosis > 50% by quantitative coronary angiography in at least one coronary artery or fractional flow reserve < 0.80 in at least one artery and no prior revascularization). Twenty healthy controls without angina and without risk factors for MVD were also recruited as a comparison group. The University of Virginia Health System institutional review board approved this study (Protocol #16056) and all subjects gave written informed consent. An electrocardiogram (ECG) was obtained before the CMR study and resting heart rate and blood pressure were recorded.

Image acquisition

CMR

Cine imaging CMR was performed on a 1.5 T scanner (Avanto or Aera, Siemens Healthineers, Erlangen, Germany) using the standard spine and body phased-array coils. Anatomic and functional assessment of the left ventricle (LV) was performed using a balanced steady-state free precession (bSSFP) cine sequence. The parameters included repetition time (TR) 2.7 ms, echo time (TE) 1.3 ms, flip angle (FA) 73^0, field of view (FOV) 300-350 mm, and resolution $1.8 \times 1.4 \times 8.0$ mm. A stack of 8 mm thick short axis images with 2 mm gap covered the LV from apex to base. Three long-axis images were obtained (2, 3, and 4-chamber views).

Perfusion imaging For assessment of MPR, quantitative first-pass myocardial perfusion imaging was performed first at rest and then during regadenoson stress following a 15 min contrast washout period. Resting perfusion assessment was performed before regadenoson stress to avoid confounding effects from regadenoson infusion, as it has been previously demonstrated that resting perfusion obtained 20 min after regadenoson with aminophylline reversal was higher than rest perfusion performed before regadenoson [15, 16].

For each perfusion assessment 3 short axis slice locations were imaged per heart beat over a 50 heart beat acquisition during an IV bolus of 0.075 mmol/kg of gadolinium contrast (Magnevist, Bayer Healthcare, Whippany, New Jersey, USA) injected via power injector (Medrad Continuum, Warrendale, Pennsylvania, USA) at 4 cm^3/s. Images were acquired using an accelerated saturation recovery (SR) variable-density spiral perfusion pulse sequence with integrated proton density (PD) and arterial input function (AIF) acquisitions for perfusion quantification [17–19]. Pulse sequence parameters included: SR time of 80 ms (time to first radiofrequency pulse of the readout), TE 1 ms, TR 9 ms, slice thickness 8 mm, FA 30 degrees, FOV 320 mm, 8 spiral interleaves, 6.1 ms readout duration per spiral and nominal spatial resolution of 1.5 mm^2. Arterial input function (AIF) images were acquired with a single-shot spiral acquisition with the following parameters: flip angle (FA) 45°, in-plane resolution 6.95mm^2, SR time 20 ms. The PD images were collected in the first 2 heart beats without a saturation pulse using FA 10° and were used for both quantification and calibration of the SPIRiT kernel for image reconstruction.

Native T1 maps were obtained at base and mid short-axis slice locations prior to the vasodilator stress protocol. T1 maps were obtained at 10 min following the first contrast injection, and at 10 and 15 min following the second contrast injection. A Modified Look-Locker Inversion Recovery (MOLLI) sequence with a 5 (4) 3 acquisition strategy was used with parameters as follows: TE 1.1 ms, TR 2.5 ms FA 35°, FOV 340 × 260 mm, resolution 1.8 mm × 1.8 mm × 8 mm.

Late gadolinium enhancement (LGE) was performed at least 5 min following the second gadolinium bolus injection for stress perfusion imaging, using a phase sensitive inversion recovery sequence (TR 650 ms, TE 4.2 ms, FA 25°, FOV 300-340 mm, resolution 1.8 × 1.3 × 8 mm).

Cardiac computed tomography (CT)

Calcium scoring Additionally, subjects with risk factors for MVD underwent coronary artery calcium scoring (CAC) to measure coronary atherosclerotic plaque burden. CAC scoring was performed on a Siemens FLASH CT Scanner (Siemens Healthineers, Munich, Germany) using high-pitch spiral mode. Non-contrast CT acquisition parameters included 120 kV, 80 mAs ref. mAs, and reconstructed slice thickness of 3 mm.

Image analysis

Functional assessment and LGE analysis

CMR images were analyzed by an experienced investigator using QMASS (Medis Medical Imaging Systems, Leiden, the Netherlands) on a Leonardo workstation. Cine images were semi-automatically contoured for each short-axis slice, with total LV mass, end-diastolic volume, end-systolic volume, stroke volume and ejection fraction measured [20]. LGE images were visually assessed for the presence of myocardial infarction or scar by an experienced cardiologist.

Perfusion quantification

Perfusion images were reconstructed using non-Cartesian SPIRiT [21], and then aligned with non-rigid registration using the ANTs toolbox [22]. Perfusion images were normalized by the PD images and Bloch simulation was used to convert normalized signal intensity to gadolinium concentration prior to Fermi-function deconvolution [23]. Quantification of first-pass perfusion was performed on a pixel-wise basis using the constrained Fermi function deconvolution method implemented in MATLAB (Mathworks, Natick, Massachusetts, USA) [14]. Global stress and rest perfusion were determined for each subject. MPR was calculated as a ratio of the stress perfusion divided by rest perfusion for each subject.

T1 analysis

T1 quantification was performed by manual segmentation of the myocardium with care to avoid partial volume effects with the LV cavity. The partition coefficient of gadolinium, λ, was determined from the slope of the linear fit of the plot of 1/T1 myocardium versus 1/T1 blood. The extracellular volume fraction (ECV) was calculated as λ *(1-Hematocrit). Hematocrit was measured on the day of the CMR study.

CT calcium scoring

The CAC studies were analyzed by determining the Agatston score on a per-patient basis using a package on a Carestream PACs system (Carestream Health, Rochester, New York, USA).

Statistical analysis

Analysis was conducted using SAS, version 9.4 (SAS Institute, Inc., Cary, North Carolina, USA). Continuous normally distributed data are presented as mean ± SD, and were compared using two-sided t-tests. Normality of continuous variables was assessed using the Shapiro-Wilk Test. Non-normally distributed data are presented as median and interquartile range (quartile 1 and quartile3 in brackets) and were compared using the Exact Wilcoxon-Mann-Whitney test. Categorical data are presented as N and percentages and compared using the Fisher Exact Test. For all statistics a $p < 0.05$ was considered statistically significant.

The effects of LV mass, body mass index (BMI), age, and gender on the differences in MPR, and rest and stress myocardial perfusion between the subjects and controls were assessed using PROC GLM to perform linear modelling. The goal of this linear modelling was to determine if the mean perfusion parameters were different between subjects and controls when other covariates were included in the model. The LSMEANS statement was used to determine the adjusted group means for the subjects and controls, and to determine whether they remained statistically different after appropriately adjusting for the other covariates in the model. When appropriate multiple comparisons were adjusted for using the Tukey method.

Results

Patient characteristics

A total of 46 subjects with risk factors for MVD and no obstructive CAD, and 20 healthy control subjects were included in the study. The subjects' and controls' baseline characteristics are summarized in Table 1. The subjects and controls had similar ages (57.5 ± 11.2 years vs 53.4 ± 11.9 $p = 0.20$). The percentage of female subjects were similar between the groups ($p = 0.38$). The subjects had a higher BMI as compared to the controls (31.3 ± 6.0 vs 24.3 ± 3.6, $p < 0.001$). The study group had a higher incidence of diabetes, hypertension, hyperlipidemia, and smoking than the control subjects. The median calcium score in the study population was 0.6.

CMR data analysis

Subjects and controls had a normal mean LV ejection fraction (LVEF) (61.2 ± 6.7% versus 59.7 ± 4.3%, respectively, $p = 0.26$). Native T1 values (988 ± 42 ms subjects vs. 987 ± 35 ms controls, $p = 0.87$), and extracellular volume fraction (ECV) (26.6 ± 2.9subjects vs. 27.1 ± 2.2controls, $p = 0.44$) were similar between groups. LV mass was similar in subjects and controls, 76.3 g [63.6, 94.8] g as compared to 67.8 g [56.9, 88.8] ($p = 0.1806$). These findings are listed in Table 2. No LGE was visualized in any subjects or controls.

Quantitative perfusion analysis

Figure 1 shows pixel-wise quantitative stress perfusion maps and regional absolute stress myocardial blood flow (MBF) per AHA 17 segment model mid-ventricular slice

Table 1 Patient Characteristics

Characteristic	Subjects (*n* = 46)	Healthy Controls (*n* = 20)	*P* value
Age	57.5 ± 11.2	53.4 ± 11.9	0.195
BMI	31.3 ± 6.0	24.3 ± 3.6	< 0.001
Female	34 (74)	12 (60)	0.382
Diabetes	37 (80)	0 (0)	0.048
History of smoking	25 (54)	1 (5)	< 0.001
Hypertension	37 (80)	1 (5)	< 0.001
Hyperlipidemia	40 (87)	1 (5)	< 0.001

Values listed are mean ± SD or n (%). BMI = body mass index

Table 2 MRI Parameters

Parameter	Subjects (*n* = 46)	Controls (*n* = 20)	*P*-value
Rest Perfusion (ml/g/min)	1.11 [0.99,1.37]	1.11 [0.92,1.23]	0.25
Stress Perfusion (ml/g/min)	2.65 ± 0.62	3.17 ± 0.49	0.002
MPR	2.21 [1.95,2.69]	2.93 [2.763.19]	< 0.001
LVEF (%)	61.2 ± 6.7	59.7 ± 4.3	0.26
LV mass (g)	76.3 [63.6,94.8]	67.8 [56.9,88.8]	0.18
ECV (%)	26.6 ± 2.9	27.1 ± 2.2	0.44
Native T1 (ms)	988 ± 42	987 ± 35	0.87

ECV extracellular volume fraction, *LV* left ventricular, *LVEF* left ventricular ejection fraction, *MPR* myocardial perfusion reserve

in (a) a subject with risk factors for MVD and (b) a control subject. Median resting MBF was similar in subjects and controls, with values of 1.11 [0.99, 1.37] ml/min/g in subjects versus 1.11 [0.92, 1.23]ml/min/g in controls ($p = 0.25$). Across both groups, female subjects had higher mean resting flow then male subjects, 1.26 ± 0.25 ml/min/g versus 0.93 ± 0.14 ml/min/g, respectively ($p < 0.001$). In linear modelling, age ($p = 0.27$) and BMI ($p = 0.55$), and LV mass ($p = 0.57$) were not significant linear predictors of resting MBF (Additional file 1).

The findings regarding stress MBF and MPR are presented in Fig. 2. Stress MBF was significantly lower in the subjects 2.65 ± 0.62 ml/min/g, when compared to the mean stress flow in controls, 3.17 ± 0.49 ml/min/g ($p = 0.002$). In the adjusted linear model for stress MBF, the differences in stress MBF between subjects and controls remained significant ($p = 0.028$). The covariates of gender (p < 0.001), and BMI ($p = 0.002$) but not age ($p = 0.15$) were also significantly predictive of stress MBF (Additional file 1).

Median MPR was lower in study subjects versus controls (2.21 [0.73] vs. 2.93 [0.44], p < 0.001). In the adjusted linear model for MPR, the differences in MPR between subjects and controls (p < 0.001) and BMI ($p = 0.03$) were the only significant effects. Covariates of gender ($p = 0.58$) and age ($p = 0.78$) were not significant predictors of MPR (Additional file 1). There was no significant correlation of MPR and stress perfusion with ECV or native T1.

A total of 57% ($N = 26$) of the MVD group subjects had a CAC score < 1 Agatston units, and 13 subjects (28%) had a CAC score > 10 Agatston units. However, there was no difference in median resting MBF between subjects with or without CAC, (1.10 [1.03 1.38] ml/min/g vs 1.14 [0.90,1,36] $p = 0.50$). Similarly, there was no difference in mean stress MBF between subjects when stratified above and below the median CAC score of 0.6 Agatston units, 2.56 ± 0.74 ml/min/g versus 2.72 ± 0.53 ml/min/g ($p = 0.40$). Consequently, median MPR was not significantly different above and below the

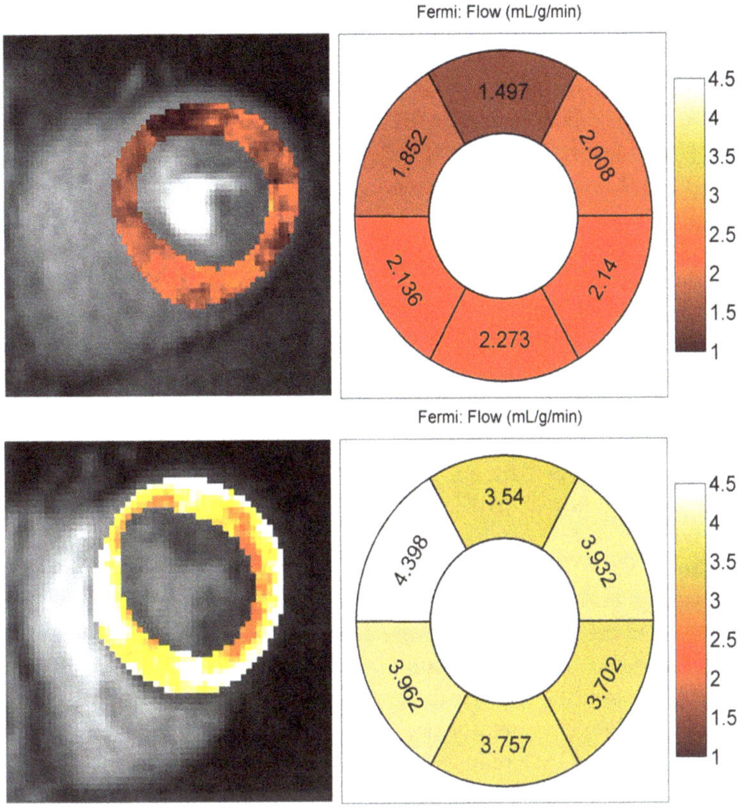

Fig. 1 Stress and Rest Absolute Perfusion Quantification. Comparison of absolute stress flow values of mid-ventricular short axis slice. Left column: Pixel based flow map. Top Row: Patient with microvascular disease (MVD). Bottom Row: Control subject

median CAC score, (2.22 [1.81,2.82] as compared to 2.29 [2.02,2.58] $p = 0.61$).

Per the inclusion criteria, none of the patients had a stenosis greater than 50%. There were 9 subjects (20%) with non-flow limiting stenosis in the 25%-45%. There was no significant difference resting perfusion, stress perfusion, or MPR between those with non-obstructive CAD > 25% as compared to those without a 25% luminal narrowing ($p = 0.17, p = 0.25, p = 0.23$ respectively).

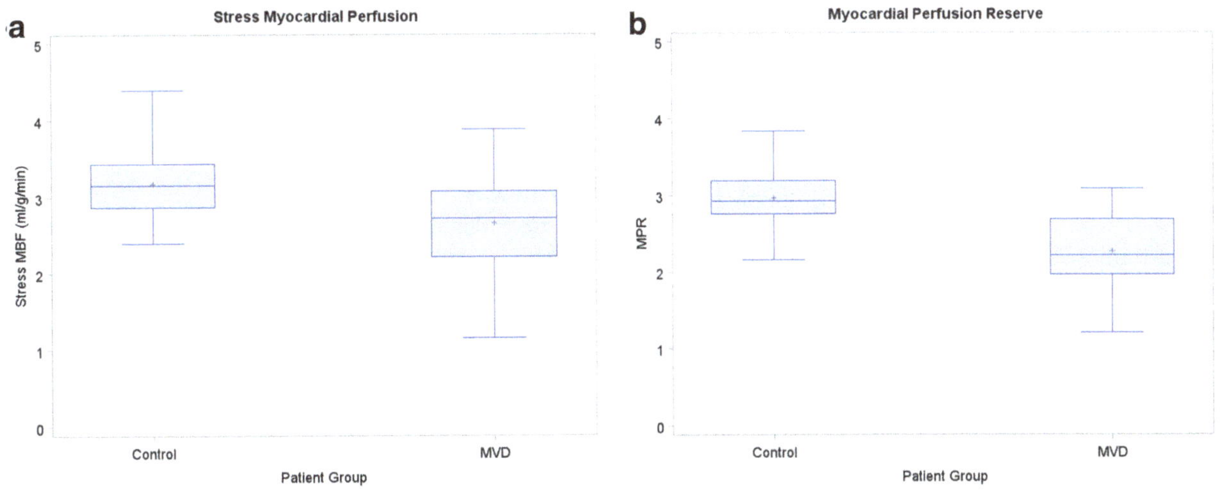

Fig. 2 Comparison of Stress myocardial blood flow (MBF) and myocardial perfusion reserve (MPR). Box and whisker plots representing stress MBF (**a**) and MPR (**b**), between study patients and controls. Stress MBF and MPR were lower in study patients by statistically significant values, $p < 0.002$ and $p < 0.001$, respectively. The + sign indicates the mean of each patient group

Discussion

Using quantitative CMR first pass perfusion imaging, the present study demonstrates that patients who are at high risk for MVD with angina or angina equivalent symptoms with no obstructive CAD have reduced stress MBF and reduced MPR compared with normal controls. This suggests that these patients likely have CMD as a cause for their symptoms. The subjects had an increased LV mass index and BMI, but neither accounted for the reduced MPR. Coronary arteriolar vasomotor dysfunction in response to adenosine is likely a contributing factor, as our group has demonstrated abnormal vasodilatory response of arterioles to graded doses of adenosine in a murine model of MVD [24].

CMR first-pass perfusion imaging has been used primarily in the assessment of perfusion in patients with obstructive CAD, with multiple studies showing high diagnostic accuracy when compared to invasive techniques [13, 25, 26]. In one study, MPR assessed by CMR and PET demonstrated a strong correlation; however, due to differential biases between the techniques absolute MBF was more weakly correlated [27]. When using quantitative coronary angiography as the gold standard, quantitative stress perfusion CMR demonstrates superior performance for detecting obstructive CAD than visual and semi-quantitative methods [26]. Additionally, our group has previously demonstrated that quantitative CMR perfusion imaging detected a larger burden of ischemia in multi-vessel disease as compared to visual analysis [13]. Thus, given the relative efficacy of quantitative assessment of MPR using stress perfusion CMR in obstructive disease, quantitative stress perfusion CMR is important to study in the evaluation of MVD.

This study's findings extend beyond previous assessments of MPR in those with MVD by qualitative and semi-quantitative perfusion CMR techniques. In a small cohort of patients with normal coronary arteries, Wohrle et al. demonstrated a correlation between CMD and MPR index measured by semi-quantitative analysis [28]. Thomson et al., as part of the WISE study group, examined 118 subjects and demonstrated that women with CMD proven by coronary reactivity testing can be identified with semi-quantitative perfusion CMR [29], which expanded on earlier work with similar results [30]. However, absolute assessment of MPR by CMR has advantages over semi-quantitative methods. Semi-quantitative assessment, as calculated by the ratio of the contrast upslope in the myocardium during stress and rest normalized by the blood pool upslope, is simple to perform but can be biased by signal-saturation in the blood pool due to the high concentrations of gadolinium. Quantitative analysis of myocardial perfusion avoids this bias by curve fitting to the end of the first-pass; however, calculated blood flow values can differ significantly by the specifics of the pulse sequence, limiting direct comparison between studies or across modalities. Calculating MPR indices obviates this latter limitation.

Our data demonstrates that patients at risk for MVD have similar native T1 and ECV to control subjects suggesting that these subjects may not have significant myocardial fibrosis, or sufficient inflammation/edema to cause abnormalities in native T1 or ECV. Furthermore, we saw no correlation between ECV and Native T1 with stress perfusion or MPR. Similar findings were seen in the recent paper from the iPOWER group, which demonstrated no correlation between MVD and fibrosis, as measured by CMR [31].

Notably, while rest and stress flows were higher in females than males, there was no gender difference in MPR. This has also been demonstrated previously in the PET literature [32]. In our study age was not a significant predictor of perfusion parameters. While we saw no significant relationship between CAC score and perfusion reserve, the majority of patients had very low CAC scores, and none of the patients had obstructive CAD.

There are some limitations to the present study. This study investigated patients who were high risk for MVD and had no obstructive CAD by coronary angiography. Due to study enrollment after coronary angiography, invasive CFR and coronary reactivity testing were not acquired at the time of angiography to validate the diagnosis of MVD and to compare with the quantitative CMR findings. The control group had a lower mean BMI than the study group. While the sample sizes of the two groups are different, with the current sample sizes there was > 90% power to detect a difference in stress flow between the groups. Finally, while the sample size of the current study does not allow for detailed subgroup analysis, the findings persisted when corrected for age, gender, BMI, and LV mass. A larger study will be needed to clarify any relationships between subgroups of patients within the MVD group and myocardial perfusion.

Conclusion

We have demonstrated by quantitative CMR perfusion imaging that in patients at high risk for MVD with angina and no obstructive CAD, there is a reduction in absolute stress myocardial blood flow, and an overall reduction in MPR when compared with normal controls, suggesting that MVD may be a possible cause of symptoms. Further studies with larger sample sizes, comparison to invasive assessment of MVD, and outcome measures are warranted. Future studies of MVD utilizing quantitative CMR perfusion may provide novel insights into MVD pathophysiology and may be helpful in the development of novel therapies.

Abbreviations

AIF: Arterial input function; BMI: Body mass index; bSSFP: Balanced steady state free precession; CAC: Coronary artery calcium; CAD: Coronary artery disease; CFR: Coronary flow reserve; CMD: Coronary microvascular dysfunction; CMR: Cardiovascular magnetic resonance; CT: Computed tomography; ECV: Extracellular volume; FOV: Field of view; LV: Left ventricle/left ventricular; LVEF: Left ventricular ejection fraction; LVH: Left ventricular hypertrophy; MBF: Myocardial blood flow; MOLLI: Modified Look-Locker Inversion Recovery; MPR: Myocardial perfusion reserve; MVD: Microvascular disease; PD: Proton density; PET: Positron emission tomography; RPP: Rate-pressure product; SR: Saturation recovery; TE: Echo time; TR: Repetition time

Acknowledgements

The authors would like to acknowledge the help of our study coordinators and nurses Jayne Missel RN, Jennifer Kay RN, and Caroline Flournoy PhD, and our research CMR technologists Jamie Castle-Shifflett, MS,RT(R)MR and Joseph Hylton, RT(R)MR and Jose Reyes RT(R)MR.

Funding

The work was funded by UVA Health System Clinical Research Grant, NIH K23 HL112910, NIH K23 HL119620, R01 HL131919, 5T32EB003841, R01 EB001763, and Siemens Medical Solutions.

Authors' contributions

JB, AT, CM, CK and MS contributed to the study conception and design. PS, JB, SK, PB, YY, JG, CK and MS were involved in data collection. BZ, PS, JB, SK, PB, RM, JP, YY, CK and MS were involved in data analysis and interpretation. BZ, PS, JB, CK, MS were involved in drafting the article. BZ, PS, JB, PB, AT, RM, JP, CM, FE, CK and MS were involved in critical revision of the article. All authors contributed to and approved the final manuscript.

Competing interests

MS receives grant support from Astra Zeneca and is a consultant to IBM. CK is a consultant for Bayer and IBM, and has research support from Novartis, and JB receives grant support from Astellas. The authors declare that they have no competing interests.

Author details

[1]Department of Medicine, Cardiology Division, University of Virginia Health System, Charlottesville, VA, USA. [2]Berkshire Medical Center, Pittsfield, MA, USA. [3]Department of Radiology, Cardiovascular Imaging Center, University of Virginia Health System, Charlottesville, VA, USA. [4]Department of Medicine, Philadelphia VA Medical Center, University of Pennsylvania, Perelman School of Medicine, Philadelphia, PA, USA. [5]Department of Biomedical Engineering, University of Virginia Health System, Charlottesville, VA, USA. [6]Division of Cardiovascular Disease, Scripps Clinic, Division of Cardiology, Cardiovascular Imaging, Division of Radiology, La Jolla, San Diego, CA, USA.

References

1. Mozaffarian D, Benjamin EJ, Go AS, Arnett DK, Blaha MJ, Cushman M, et al. Executive summary: heart disease and stroke statistics–2016 update: a report from the American Heart Association. Circulation. 2016;133:447–54.
2. Patel MR, Peterson ED, Dai D, Brennan JM, Redberg RF, Anderson HV, et al. Low diagnostic yield of elective coronary angiography. N Engl J Med. 2010; 362:886–95.
3. Marzilli M, Merz CN, Boden WE, Bonow RO, Capozza PG, Chilian WM, et al. Obstructive coronary atherosclerosis and ischemic heart disease: an elusive link! J Am Coll Cardiol. 2012;60:951–6.
4. Lanza GA, Crea F. Primary coronary microvascular dysfunction: clinical presentation, pathophysiology, and management. Circulation. 2010;121: 2317–25.
5. Crea F, Camici PG, Bairey Merz CN. Coronary microvascular dysfunction: an update. Eur Heart J. 2014;35:1101–11.
6. Pepine CJ, Anderson RD, Sharaf BL, Reis SE, Smith KM, Handberg EM, et al. Coronary microvascular reactivity to adenosine predicts adverse outcome in women evaluated for suspected ischemia results from the National Heart, lung and blood institute WISE (Women's ischemia syndrome evaluation) study. J Am Coll Cardiol. 2010;55:2825–32.
7. Taqueti VR, Shaw LJ, Cook NR, Murthy VL, Shah NR, Foster CR, et al. Excess cardiovascular risk in women relative to men referred for coronary angiography is associated with severely impaired coronary flow reserve, Not Obstructive Disease. Circulation. 2017;135:566–77.
8. Reis SE, Holubkov R, Conrad Smith AJ, Kelsey SF, Sharaf BL, Reichek N, et al. Coronary microvascular dysfunction is highly prevalent in women with chest pain in the absence of coronary artery disease: results from the NHLBI WISE study. Am Heart J. 2001;141:735–41.
9. Murthy VL, Naya M, Foster CR, Hainer J, Gaber M, Di Carli G, et al. Association between coronary vascular dysfunction and cardiac mortality in patients with and without diabetes mellitus. Circulation. 2012;126:1858–68.
10. Di Carli MF, Charytan D, McMahon GT, Ganz P, Dorbala S, Schelbert HR. Coronary circulatory function in patients with the metabolic syndrome. J Nucl Med. 2011;52:1369–77.
11. Graf S, Khorsand A, Gwechenberger M, Novotny C, Kletter K, Sochor H, et al. Typical chest pain and normal coronary angiogram: cardiac risk factor analysis versus PET for detection of microvascular disease. J Nucl Med. 2007; 48:175–81.
12. Bairey Merz CN, Pepine CJ, Walsh MN, Fleg JL. Ischemia and no obstructive coronary artery disease (INOCA): developing evidence-based therapies and research agenda for the next decade. Circulation. 2017;135:1075–92.
13. Patel AR, Antkowiak PF, Nandalur KR, West AM, Salerno M, Arora V, et al. Assessment of advanced coronary artery disease: advantages of quantitative cardiac magnetic resonance perfusion analysis. J Am Coll Cardiol. 2010;56: 561–9.
14. Jerosch-Herold M. Quantification of myocardial perfusion by cardiovascular magnetic resonance. J Cardiovasc Magn Reson. 2010;12:57.
15. Vasu S, Bandettini WP, Hsu L, Kellman P, Wilson J, Leung S, et al. Optimal timing of rest perfusion with regadenoson stress testing – normal volunteer study of quantitative MRI perfusion. J Cardiovasc Magn Reson. 2011; 13(Suppl 1):P128.
16. Bhave NM, Freed BH, Chattanong Y, Kolanczyk D, Dill K, Lang RM, et al. Considerations when measuring myocardial perfusion reserve by cardiovascular magnetic resonance using regadenoson. J of Cardiovasc Magn Reson. 2012;14:89.
17. Yang Y, Kuruvilla S, Meyer CH, Kramer CM, Salerno M. Quantification of myocardial perfusion with spiral pulse sequences. J of Cardiovasc Magn Reson. 2013;15(Suppl 1):E12.
18. Yang Y, Kuruvilla S, Meyer CH, Epstein FH, Taylor AM, Kramer CM, et al. High-resolution quantitative spiral perfusion for microvascular coronary dysfunction detection. J of Cardiovasc Magn Reson. 2014;16(Suppl 1):P227.
19. Salerno M, Taylor A, Yang Y, Kuruvilla S, Ragosta M, Meyer CH, et al. Adenosine stress cardiovascular magnetic resonance with variable-density spiral pulse sequences accurately detects coronary artery disease: initial clinical evaluation. Circ Cardiovasc Imaging. 2014;7:639–46.
20. Schulz-Menger J, Bluemke DA, Bremerich J, Flamm SD, Fogel MA, Friedrich MG, et al. Standardized image interpretation and post processing in cardiovascular magnetic resonance: Society for Cardiovascular Magnetic Resonance (SCMR) board of trustees task force on standardized post processing. J Cardiovasc Magn Reson. 2013;15:35.
21. Lustig M, Pauly JM. SPIRiT: iterative self-consistent parallel imaging reconstruction from arbitrary k-space. Magn Reson Med. 2010;64:457–71.
22. Avants BB, Tustison NJ, Song G, Cook PA, Klein A, Gee JC. A reproducible evaluation of ANTs similarity metric performance in brain image registration. NeuroImage. 2011;54:2033–44.
23. Axel L. Tissue mean transit time from dynamic computed tomography by a simple deconvolution technique. Investig Radiol. 1983;18:94–9.
24. Naresh NK, Butcher JT, Lye RJ, Chen X, Isakson BE, Gan LM, et al. Cardiovascular magnetic resonance detects the progression of impaired myocardial perfusion reserve and increased left-ventricular mass in mice fed a high-fat diet. J Cardiovasc Magn Reson. 2016;18:53.
25. Costa MA, Shoemaker S, Futamatsu H, Klassen C, Angiolillo DJ, Nguyen M, et al. Quantitative magnetic resonance perfusion imaging detects anatomic

and physiologic coronary artery disease as measured by coronary angiography and fractional flow reserve. J Am Coll Cardiol. 2007;50:514–22.
26. Mordini FE, Haddad T, Hsu LY, Kellman P, Lowrey TB, Aletras AH, et al. Diagnostic accuracy of stress perfusion CMR in comparison with quantitative coronary angiography: fully quantitative, semiquantitative, and qualitative assessment. JACC Cardiovasc Imaging. 2014;7:14–22.
27. Morton G, Chiribiri A, Ishida M, Hussain ST, Schuster A, Indermuehle A, et al. Quantification of absolute myocardial perfusion in patients with coronary artery disease: comparison between cardiovascular magnetic resonance and positron emission tomography. J Am Coll Cardiol. 2012;60:1546–55.
28. Wohrle J, Nusser T, Merkle N, Kestler HA, Grebe OC, Marx N, et al. Myocardial perfusion reserve in cardiovascular magnetic resonance: correlation to coronary microvascular dysfunction. J Cardiovasc Magn Reson. 2006;8:781–7.
29. Thomson LE, Wei J, Agarwal M, Haft-Baradaran A, Shufelt C, Mehta PK, et al. Cardiac magnetic resonance myocardial perfusion reserve index is reduced in women with coronary microvascular dysfunction. A National Heart, Lung, and Blood Institute-sponsored study from the Women's ischemia syndrome evaluation. Circ Cardiovasc Imaging. 2015;8 https://doi.org/10.1161/CIRCIMAGING.114.002481.
30. Shufelt CL, Thomson LE, Goykhman P, Agarwal M, Mehta PK, Sedlak T, et al. Cardiac magnetic resonance imaging myocardial perfusion reserve index assessment in women with microvascular coronary dysfunction and reference controls. Cardiovasc Diagn Ther. 2013;3:153–60.
31. Mygind ND, Michelsen MM, Pena A, Qayyum AA, Frestad D, Christensen TE, et al. Coronary microvascular function and myocardial fibrosis in women with angina pectoris and no obstructive coronary artery disease: the iPOWER study. J Cardiovasc Magn Reson. 2016;18:76.
32. Manabe O, Yoshinaga K, Katoh C, Naya M, deKemp RA, Tamaki N. Repeatability of rest and hyperemic myocardial blood flow measurements with 82Rb dynamic PET. J Nucl Med. 2009;50:68–71.

16

Adenosine stress CMR T1-mapping detects early microvascular dysfunction in patients with type 2 diabetes mellitus without obstructive coronary artery disease

Eylem Levelt[1,2], Stefan K. Piechnik[1], Alexander Liu[1], Rohan S. Wijesurendra[1], Masliza Mahmod[1], Rina Ariga[1], Jane M. Francis[1], Andreas Greiser[3], Kieran Clarke[4], Stefan Neubauer[1], Vanessa M. Ferreira[1†] and Theodoros D. Karamitsos[1,5*†]

Abstract

Background: Type 2 diabetes mellitus (T2DM) is associated with coronary microvascular dysfunction in the absence of obstructive coronary artery disease (CAD). Cardiovascular magnetic resonance (CMR) T1-mapping at rest and during adenosine stress can assess coronary vascular reactivity. We hypothesised that the non-contrast T1 response to vasodilator stress will be altered in patients with T2DM without CAD compared to controls due to coronary microvascular dysfunction.

Methods: Thirty-one patients with T2DM and sixteen matched healthy controls underwent CMR (3 T) for cine, rest and adenosine stress non-contrast T1-mapping (ShMOLLI), first-pass perfusion and late gadolinium enhancement (LGE) imaging. Significant CAD (>50% coronary luminal stenosis) was excluded in all patients by coronary computed tomographic angiography.

Results: All subjects had normal left ventricular (LV) ejection and LV mass index, with no LGE. Myocardial perfusion reserve index (MPRI) was lower in T2DM than in controls (1.60 ± 0.44 vs 2.01 ± 0.42; $p = 0.008$). There was no difference in rest native T1 values ($p = 0.59$). During adenosine stress, T1 values increased significantly in both T2DM patients (from 1196 ± 32 ms to 1244 ± 44 ms, $p < 0.001$) and controls (from 1194 ± 26 ms to 1273 ± 44 ms, p < 0.001). T2DM patients showed blunted relative stress non-contrast T1 response (T2DM: ΔT1 = 4.1 ± 2.9% vs. controls: ΔT1 = 6.6 ± 2.6%, $p = 0.007$) due to a blunted maximal T1 during adenosine stress (T2DM 1244 ± 44 ms vs. controls 1273 ± 44 ms, $p = 0.045$).

(Continued on next page)

* Correspondence: tkaramitsos@auth.gr
[†]Equal contributors
[1]University of Oxford Centre for Clinical Magnetic Resonance Research, Division of Cardiovascular Medicine, Radcliffe Department of Medicine, University of Oxford, Oxford, UK
[5]1st Department of Cardiology, Aristotle University of Thessaloniki, AHEPA Hospital St. Kyriakidi 1, 54636 Thessaloniki, Greece
Full list of author information is available at the end of the article

(Continued from previous page)

Conclusions: Patients with well controlled T2DM, even in the absence of arterial hypertension and significant CAD, exhibit blunted maximal non-contrast T1 response during adenosine vasodilatory stress, likely reflecting coronary microvascular dysfunction. Adenosine stress and rest T1 mapping can detect subclinical abnormalities of the coronary microvasculature, without the need for gadolinium contrast agents. CMR may identify early features of the diabetic heart phenotype and subclinical cardiac risk markers in patients with T2DM, providing an opportunity for early therapeutic intervention.

Keywords: Cardiovascular magnetic resonance, Diabetes mellitus, Myocardial perfusion, ShMOLLI T1-mapping, Microvascular obstruction

Background

Type 2 diabetes mellitus (T2DM), independent of coronary artery disease (CAD) or hypertension, directly affects the structure and function of the myocardium [1], leading to adverse cardiovascular outcomes [2–4]. There is a robust association between T2DM and heart failure, and heart failure is the leading cause of mortality in patients with T2DM [5–8]. Coronary microvascular dysfunction in diabetes is a complex pathophysiological process, which involves structural, functional and metabolic alterations, and has emerged among the potential mechanisms leading to increased incidence of heart failure [9] and risk of cardiovascular mortality [4, 10] in patients with diabetes. Using cardiovascular magnetic resonance (CMR), myocardial perfusion during vasodilator stress has been shown to be impaired in patients with diabetes mellitus (DM) [11–13] and in the absence of epicardial coronary artery stenoses, this finding is indicative of coronary microvascular dysfunction.

CMR non-contrast T1-mapping may be used to assess myocardial ischaemia and coronary vasodilatory function. In CMR, T1 (or proton spin-lattice) relaxation time is a magnetic property of tissue. Each tissue type has a normal range of T1 values, deviation from each may indicate disease or a change in physiology. T1 is prolonged by increased free water content [14], which may have an intracellular or extracellular origin, including the interstitial and intravascular compartments. Healthy controls demonstrate normal myocardial T1 values at rest; during adenosine stress, coronary vasodilation leads to an increase in myocardial blood volume in the myocardium, which is detectable using myocardial T1-mapping, through the partial volume of blood T1 [14–16]. We have previously demonstrated the use of adenosine stress and rest non-contrast T1-mapping for detecting ischaemia in patients with CAD, and for assessing coronary vasodilatory reserve in patients without CAD [17, 18]. In the absence of obstructive CAD, the percentage change in non-contrast T1 values from rest to vasodilator stress (ΔT1) likely represents coronary vascular reactivity and has potential to assess the health and function of the micro coronary circulation.

We hypothesize that patients with T2DM but without obstructive CAD will have microvascular dysfunction detectable using adenosine stress and rest T1-mapping. In this study, we compared native myocardial T1 values at rest and during adenosine stress, as well as myocardial perfusion reserve index (MPRI) in patients with T2DM without obstructive CAD and in matching healthy controls using CMR at 3 Tesla.

Methods

The study was granted a favourable opinion by the National Research Ethics Committee (REC Ref 13/SW/0257), and written informed consent was obtained from each participant. The main project was set out to investigate the intricate interplay of perfusion, oxygenation and metabolic changes during stress in the diabetic heart. The wider aims and methods of the main project has been published elsewhere [13].

Study population

T2DM was diagnosed according to the World Health Organization criteria [19]. Patients with T2DM were excluded if they had a history of cardiovascular disease, chest pain, tobacco smoking, uncontrolled hypertension (resting systolic blood pressure (BP) >140 mmHg and diastolic BP >90 mmHg), contraindications to CMR imaging, ischemic changes on 12-lead electrocardiogram (ECG), or significant renal impairment (estimated glomerular filtration rate below 30 mL/min), and if they were taking insulin. Importantly, patients with T2DM were initially screened for obstructive epicardial CAD (>50% of luminal stenosis) with coronary computed tomographic angiography (CCTA). Only subjects with no evidence of significant epicardial CAD on CCTA underwent the study investigations.

Healthy subjects were age-, gender- and weight-matched to patients and served as controls. Healthy controls had no history of heart disease, DM, hypertension, or high cholesterol and were taking no medications. They had normal physical examinations and ECG.

Other study procedures

BP was recorded as an average of 3 supine measurements taken over 10 min (DINAMAP-1846-SX, Critikon Corporation, Tampa, Florida, USA). Fasting venous blood was drawn for glucose, triglyceride, haemoglobin A1c and renal function tests as previously described [20].

Coronary computed tomographic angiography

CCTA scans were performed on a 64-slice CT scanner (Discovery CT 690, GE Healthcare, Waukesha, Wisconsin, USA) in accordance with performance guidelines from the Society of Cardiovascular Computed Tomography [21]. In the absence of contraindications, patients received beta-blockade (intravenous metoprolol) and sublingual nitroglycerine prior to the scan to achieve a heart rate of <65 beats per minute and coronary dilation, respectively. A preliminary unenhanced scan was performed to assess coronary artery calcium score. During the CCTA acquisition, 80 ml of iodinated contrast (Visipaque, GE Healthcare, Princeton, New Jersey, USA) was injected followed by a 50 ml saline flush. Significant CAD was defined as >50% luminal stenosis. CCTA was carried out 1 week prior to CMR study for each participant withT2DM.

Cardiovascular magnetic resonance protocol

CMR was performed on a 3-Tesla system (Magnetom Trio Tim; Siemens Healthcare, Erlangen, Germany). All participants were instructed to refrain from caffeine ingestion in the 24 h preceding the study. All subjects were scanned after fasting overnight. Cine imaging was performed in long- and short-axis covering the left ventricle (LV) using standard balanced-steady state free precession (bSSFP) methods [22].

At rest, mid LV native T1 map was acquired using the shortened modified Look-Locker inversion recovery (ShMOLLI) prototype sequence as previously described [14], matched to the first-pass stress and rest perfusion mid-LV slices. Adenosine stress perfusion imaging was performed as previously described [23, 24] with acquisition of 3 matched short axis stress and rest perfusion images. Briefly, adenosine (140 μg/kg/min to 210 μg/kg/min to achieve adequate hemodynamic stress response) was infused intravenously for at least 3 min. Heart rate and blood pressure were recorded at baseline and at 1-min intervals during stress. This was followed by acquisition of a single mid-ventricular short-axis T1-map (matched to the mid-ventricular T1-map at rest). Subsequently (4–5 min after commencing the adenosine infusion), a 0.03-mmol/kg bolus of gadolinium-based contrast Gadoterate meglumine (Dotarem, Guerbet LLC, Villepinte, France) was injected, followed by 15 mL of normal saline at a rate of 6 mL/s for first-pass perfusion imaging. Adenosine was then discontinued, and after at least 20 min (to allow contrast washout adenosine), another 0.03-mmol/kg bolus of gadolinium was given for rest perfusion imaging.

For late gadolinium enhancement (LGE) CMR, a top-up bolus of 0.09 mmol/kg of contrast (Gadoteric acid, Guerbet, France) followed by a 15-mL saline flush was administered immediately after the rest perfusion image acquisition (total dose of gadolinium 0.15 mmol/kg). The LGE images were acquired using a T1-weighted phase-sensitive inversion recovery sequence 8–12 min after the last intravenous administration of contrast agent in the same long- and short-axis images as cine imaging, using imaging parameters as previously described [25]. A single mid-ventricular short-axis slice matching the pre-contrast T1-map was acquired 15 min after the administration of gadolinium contrast for extracellular volume fraction (ECV) quantification.

CMR data analysis

For each patient, LV volumes, ejection fraction, and mass were calculated using cmr42© software (Circle Cardiovascular Imaging Inc., Calgary, Canada) by manually tracing the endocardial and epicardial contours in end-diastolic and end-systolic images, as previously described [22].

For the analysis of ShMOLLI T1-maps, the LV myocardium of the mid ventricular short axis slice acquired at baseline was contoured by two operators (EL, SKP), using dedicated software, as previously described [26], providing a single average myocardial T1 value from the whole slice of T1 map per each individual with consensus of two operators. T1-maps were assessed for quality in three ways: examination of the T1-map, the raw T1 images and R^2 maps; ~11% of segments were excluded due to any combination of: off-resonance artifacts, partial-volume effects, poor T1 fit on the R^2 maps, patient movement or low signal to noise, similar to previous publications using T1-mapping from our center [27]. The myocardial T1 value from the stress mid-ventricular ShMOLLI non-contrast T1-map was obtained and compared to the non-contrast T1 at baseline (Fig.1).

T1 reactivity to adenosine stress was expressed in absolute terms: $\Delta T1(ms) = T1stress - T1rest$ and as percentages: $(\Delta T1)(\%) = \Delta T1 \div T1rest \times 100$. T1rest and T1stress represent mean T1 values at rest and during adenosine stress, respectively. Inter-observer variability of mid-ventricular ShMOLLI T1-map stress reactivity was assessed by further analysis performed by another independent operator in a blinded fashion (RSW). Inter-study variability of mid-ventricular ShMOLLI T1-map stress reactivity was assessed in 5 healthy subjects of another study performed at our research centre (REC reference: 13/SC/0376). These scans were anonymized and analyzed in random order in a blinded fashion (AL).

For analysis of myocardial perfusion, signal intensity over time curves were generated by tracing endocardial and epicardial contours (cmr42© software, Circle

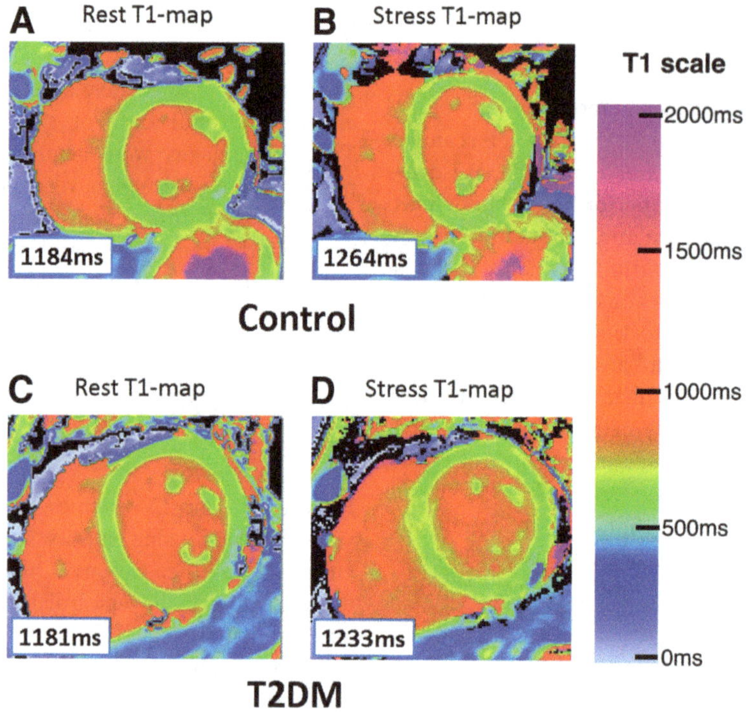

Fig. 1 Representative examples of rest and stress T1 maps. Normal control with **a** resting native T1-map, 1174 ms; **b** corresponding stress T1-map, 1271 ms. T2DM patient with **c** resting native T1-map, 1177 ms; **d** corresponding stress T1-map, 1195 ms. Values in graphic indicate the average mid-left-ventricular myocardial T1 values

Cardiovascular Imaging Inc.) after manual correction for displacement during breathing, by two operators (AL, EL). A region of interest was drawn in the LV blood pool, avoiding any papillary muscles, to permit the derivation of an arterial input function. The myocardium was divided into equiangular segments on the basis of the American Heart Association 16-segmentation model. Rest and stress myocardial perfusion up-slopes were calculated using a 5-point linear-fit model of SI versus time and normalized to the LV blood pool upslope. Myocardial perfusion reserve index (MPRI) was defined as the ratio of stress to rest relative upslope, as previously described [28].

For LGE analysis, areas of contrast enhancement were visually scored as absent or present by 2 operators with at least 3 years of CMR experience (EL, MM). LGE was considered present only if myocardial enhancement was confirmed on both short-axis and perpendicular long-axis locations. Consistent with established methods of estimating myocardial ECV using a delayed postcontrast bolus protocol [29, 30], we measured precontrast and postcontrast myocardial and blood T1 values. These assessments were carried out by two operators together by consensus (EL, SKP), using previously described methods [30].

Statistical analysis

All data are expressed as mean ± standard deviations and checked for normality using the Kolmogorov–Smirnov test. Categorical data are presented as numbers and percentages. Comparisons between the 2 groups were performed by Student's t-test. The chi-square test or Fisher's exact test was used to compare discrete data as appropriate. Bivariate correlations were performed using Pearson's or Spearman's method as appropriate. A p-value <0.05 was considered significant. All statistical analyses were performed with SPSS Statistics (version 20; International Business Machines, Inc., Armonk, New York, USA).

Results

Participant characteristics

Demographic, clinical, and biochemical data of patients with T2DM and controls matched for age, gender and body mass index (BMI) are shown in Table 1. 31 patients with T2DM (median duration of diabetes 7 years [IQR: 1–8] and mean glycated haemoglobin level 7.7 ± 1.4%) and 16 controls were studied. Although resting heart rates were statistically higher in patients, these remained within the normal range (T2DM resting heart rate: 69 ± 8 vs. controls: 58 ± 10 beats per minute, Table 1). Diastolic BP and resting heart rate were statistically higher in the diabetic cohort, although remained within the normal range. A significant proportion of patients (77%) were on statin therapy, hence total cholesterol and low-density

Table 1 Baseline characteristics of the study cohort

Variable	Healthy Controls $N = 16$	T2DM $N = 31$	P value
Age, y	51 ± 9	55 ± 9	0.162
BMI, kg/m^2	25.8 ± 4.2	28.7 ± 5.6	0.083
Male, %	53	58	0.739
Diabetes duration, y	...	7[IQR:1–8]	
Systolic blood pressure, mmHg	121 ± 13	125 ± 11	0.366
Diastolic blood pressure, mmHg	71 ± 9	77 ± 8	0.048
Resting heart rate, bpm	58 ± 10	69 ± 8	<0.001
Plasma fasting glucose	4.8 ± 0.5	9.1 ± 3.2	<0.001
Plasma triglycerides, mmol/L	1.25 ± 0.68	1.47 ± 0.71	0.391
Total cholesterol, mmol/L	3.58 ± 0.93	1.99 ± 0.63	<0.001
HDL, mmol/L	1.32 ± 0.37	1.22 ± 0.36	0.442
LDL, mmol/L	2.86 ± 0.56	1.99 ± 0.63	<0.001
Hematocrit, %	41 ± 4	42 ± 3	0.501
Medications, n (%)			
Metformin	–	30 (97)	
Sulphonylurea	–	21 (68)	
Aspirin	–	11 (35)	
Statin	–	24 (77)	
ACE-I	–	21 (68)	

Values are mean ± standard deviations or percentages. T2DM indicates type 2 diabetes mellitus; BMI, body mass index; y, years; bpm, beats per minute; HDL, high density lipoprotein; LDL, low density lipoprotein; ACE-I angiotensin-converting enzyme inhibitors

lipoprotein cholesterol levels were lower in diabetics compared to controls.

Myocardial structure and systolic function

CMR results for LV volumes and function are summarized in Table 2. There was no significant difference in LV ejection fraction between patients with T2DM and healthy controls. There was also no difference in LV mass and LV mass index between patients and healthy controls, though patients with T2DM exhibited concentric LV remodelling (LV mass to volume ratio T2DM: 0.96 ± 0.18 g/ml vs. healthy controls: 0.75 ± 0.23 g/ml; $p = 0.001$).

Myocardial fibrosis on late gadolinium enhancement imaging

On visual assessment of LGE images, there were no areas of myocardial enhancement indicative of myocardial infarction or focal replacement fibrosis in either patients or healthy controls.

Changes in myocardial perfusion reserve during adenosine stress

Rest and stress rate pressure product values are summarised in Table 3. Patients and healthy controls demonstrated a similar increase in rate pressure product during adenosine stress ($p = 0.206$). Despite the absence of significant obstructive epicardial CAD on CCTA and adequate response to adenosine vasodilatory stress, MPRI was significantly reduced in T2DM patients compared to controls (T2DM MPRI, 1.60 ± 0.44 vs healthy controls, 2.01 ± 0.42; $p = 0.008$). A sub-group analysis of lean T2DM patients (BMI < 25) vs lean controls for the MPRI was performed and our results showed in the absence of obesity or even overweight status T2D is associated with reduced MPRI (1.50 ± 0.27 vs lean controls 2.24 ± 0.36, $p = 0.005$).

Inter-study reproducibility, inter-observer and intra-observer variability of stress native T1 mapping

The inter-study reproducibility, inter-observer and intra-observer variability of mid-ventricular ShMOLLI T1-map stress reactivity were assessed.

Table 2 Cardiovascular magnetic resonance results in patients vs. controls

Variable	Healhty Controls $N = 16$	T2DM $N = 31$	P value
LV end-diastolic volume, ml	159 ± 33	128 ± 33	0.004
Indexed LV end-diastolic volume, ml/m^2	78 ± 19	64 ± 21	0.012
LV end-systolic volume, ml	49 ± 12	40 ± 17	0.087
Indexed LV end-systolic volume, ml/m^2	23 ± 13	20 ± 16	0.168
LV stroke volume, ml	110 ± 22	87 ± 23	0.002
Indexed LV stroke volume, ml/m^2	55 ± 25	45 ± 20	0.008
LV ejection fraction, %	69 ± 4	69 ± 8	0.786
LV mass index, g/m^2	53 ± 15	60 ± 13	0.075
LV mass, g	115 ± 29	120 ± 31	0.534
LV mass/end-diastolic volume g/ml	0.75 ± 0.23	0.96 ± 0.18	0.001

Values are mean ± standard deviations or percentages. T2DM indicates type 2 diabetes mellitus; CMR, cardiovascular magnetic resonance; LV, left-ventricular

Table 3 Haemodynamic measurements and myocardial perfusion reserve index

Adenosine Stress CMR

	Healthy Controls $N = 16$	T2DM $N = 31$	P value
Rest RPP, bpm*mmHg	7673 ± 1334	8862 ± 1745	0.025
Stress RPP, bpm*mmHg	11,181 ± 2750	11,827 ± 1736	0.365
Increase in RPP, %	49 ± 18	38 ± 29	0.206
MPRI, ratio	2.01 ± 0.42	1.60 ± 0.44	0.008

Values are mean ± standard deviations or percentages. T2DM indicates type 2 diabetes mellitus; CMR, cardiovascularmagnetic resonance; bpm, beats per minute; MPRI, myocardial perfusion reserve index; RPP, rate pressure product

5 healthy subjects (2 males, 3 females; age 41 ± 23 years; all 1.5 T, mid-ventricular slice stress/rest). All 10 scans anonymized and analyzed in random order. The interval between scans for these participants undergoing test-retest inter-study reproducibility was 3 ± 2 years apart. There was a good agreement between the first and second scans (0.33 ± 1.13%). Mean ΔT1 for the first scan (6.2 ± 1.0%) was not significantly different compared to the second scan (6.5 ± 1.0%), paired t-test $p = 0.55$.

There was a good agreement for inter-observer (−0.3 ± 1.7%) and intra-observer assessments (−0.2 ± 1.4%) by Bland-Altman plotting. Coefficient of determination showed strong relationship for inter-observer ($r^2 = 0.759$) and intra-observer ($r^2 = 0.837$) assessments.

Changes in rest and adenosine stress T1 mapping

There were no significant differences in native myocardial non-contrast T1 values between T2DM patients and healthy controls at rest. During adenosine stress, T1 values increased significantly in both T2DM patients (from 1196 ± 32 ms to 1244 ± 44 ms, $P < 0.001$) and healthy controls (from 1194 ± 26 ms to 1273 ± 44 ms, $p < 0.001$) (Fig.2). However, stress T1 response was significantly blunted in T2DM patients compared to healthy controls (T2DM ΔT1 = 4.1 ± 2.9% vs. healthy controls ΔT1 = 6.6 ± 2.6%, $p = 0.007$) (Fig.3), as was the maximal T1 during adenosine stress (T2DM: 1244 ± 44 ms vs. healthy controls: 1273 ± 44 ms, $p = 0.045$). A sub-group analysis of lean T2DM patients (BMI < 25) vs lean controls for the ΔT1 was performed and our results showed in the absence of obesity or even overweight status T2D is associated with T1 (3.51 ± 2.18 vs lean controls 6.21 ± 1.72, $p = 0.013$).

There was no significant correlation between the percent change of T1 and MPRI. However, there was a significant correlation between the adenosine stress T1 and MPRI ($r = 0.35$, $p = 0.031$), when there was no significant correlation between rest T1 and MPRI ($r = -0.19$, $p = 0.31$).

Maximal T1 during adenosine stress and T1 reactivity (ΔT1) correlated negatively with LV mass index

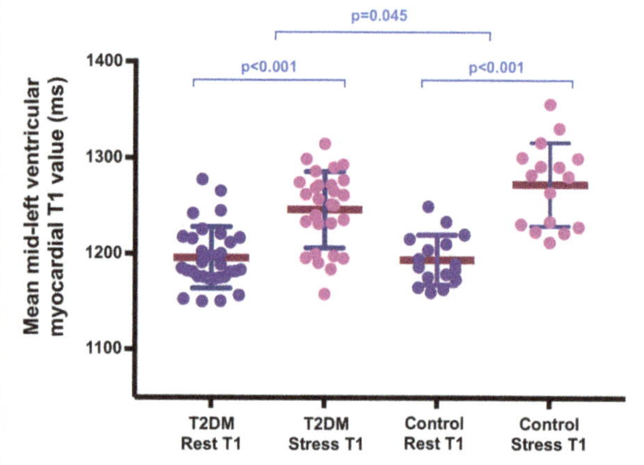

Fig. 2 Differences in rest and adenosine stress LV myocardial T1 values between healthy controls and patients with T2DM. Scatter columns show mean LV myocardial T1 relaxation times and error bars indicate standard deviations. The lower *p*-values represent the differences in rest and adenosine stress LV myocardial T1, the upper *p*-value represent the represent the statistical difference in relative T1 reactivity between controls and patients with T2DM

($r = -0.50$, $p = 0.001$; $r = -0.40$, $p = 0.018$) and LV concentricity (LV mass to LV EDV ratio)($r = -0.33$, $p = 0.027$; $r = -0.41$, $p = 0.005$) in the study group as a whole, but no significant correlation in separate groups.

Extra-cellular volume (ECV) quantification

There was no significant difference in ECV between T2DM patients and controls (T2DM 30 ± 3%, vs healthy controls 30 ± 2%, $p = 0.91$).

Discussion

In this study using CMR stress and rest T1-mapping, we demonstrate that T2DM is associated with blunted native T1 response under adenosine stress even in highly selected T2DM patients with stable disease and no other

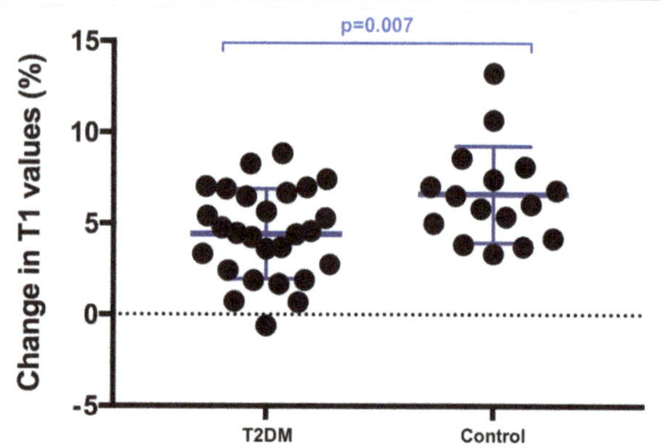

Fig. 3 LV myocardial T1 reactivity to adenosine stress in patients with T2DM and healthy controls. Scatter columns show mean percentage change in T1 with adenosine stress and error bars indicate standard deviations

comorbidities. The blunted maximal stress T1 response in T2DM, as well as the impaired myocardial perfusion reserve index, are consistent with attenuated vascular reactivity and coronary microvascular dysfunction. Additionally, we show a negative correlation between stress T1 and concentric LV remodelling, suggesting a link between the subclinical abnormalities in coronary vasodilatory function and adverse cardiac remodeling in diabetes. However, the causality of this relationship needs to be investigated in future studies.

Coronary microvascular dysfunction in diabetes is likely to be a multifactorial phenomenon, related to changes in perivascular and interstitial fibrosis [31], myocardial hypertrophy [32], reduced capillary density, and autonomic neuropathy [33]. Importantly, coronary microvascular dysfunction is an early precursor of cardiovascular events and was shown to be associated with a 2.5% annual major adverse event rate that includes cardiovascular mortality, nonfatal myocardial infarction, nonfatal stroke, and heart failure even among patients without epicardial coronary artery stenosis [34]. Consequently, early identification of coronary microvascular disease may be beneficial in prognosis evaluation and patient stratification for optimal medical therapy [35].

Myocardial perfusion is influenced by multiple factors including metabolic demand, diastolic time, and driving blood pressure [36]. The functional responsiveness of the microcirculation can be influenced by increased heart rate, reduced diastolic time, decreased driving BP. An increase in systolic intramyocardial and ventricular pressures, as it would be expected to occur in LV concentric remodelling, can also adversely affect myocardial perfusion. In this study, although it remained within the normal limits, the resting heart rates were higher in patients with T2DM compared to healthy controls. Furthermore, patients with T2DM also demonstrated LV concentric remodeling. The higher rate pressure product at rest in our patients with T2DM would be expected to cause a higher resting perfusion, as a result may lead to lower MPRI; on the other hand the LV concentric remodeling would be expected to reduce the resting perfusion. The influence of these important factors on the coronary physiology is intricate, and should be considered while interpreting the myocardial perfusion abnormalities in patients with diabetes.

CMR T1-mapping for the assessment of coronary vasodilatory function

Heart failure is the leading cause of mortality in patients with T2DM [5] and importantly coronary microvascular dysfunction is considered among the pathophysiological alterations in diabetes responsible for cardiac dysfunction [1]. In the context of the global epidemic of diabetes, coronary vascular reactivity, as assessed by rest and adenosine stress T1-mapping, may serve as an additional biomarker for disease severity and therapeutic response without the need for gadolinium-based contrast agents. Furthermore, this gadolinium-free technique is easily applicable, independent of heart rate and robust to tachyarrhythmias [14, 37], making it highly suitable for CMR scanning during vasodilator stress. This study shows that the technique is sensitive to detecting subtle changes in vascular reactivity in this patient group, in agreement with traditional first pass perfusion, paving the way to future mechanistic studies of further alterations of $\Delta T1$ in overt diabetic cardiomyopathy, or for use in patients with diabetes and more significant comorbidities, including renal failure. CMR stress/rest T1 mapping may prove a convenient tool to assess potential beneficial effects of novel therapies designed for patients with T2DM on the myocardium and coronary vasculature, and to monitor drug response, without the need for repeated exposure to gadolinium-based contrast agents.

First-pass myocardial perfusion CMR during vasodilatory stress directly assesses reductions in microvascular blood flow with high diagnostic accuracy. CMR studies of the coronary circulation exploit the first-pass kinetics of T1-enhancing extracellular gadolinium-based contrast media. During the first pass, the contrast medium diffuses into the interstitial space from the microvasculature, resulting in an increase in signal intensity that is proportional to the perfusion and blood volume of the tissue, the extravascular compartment size, and capillary permeability.

It is conceivable that in the future adenosine rest/stress T1 mapping may become a valuable test in addition to conventional clinical information and perfusion assessment for patients with diabetes. Early identification of changes using these techniques may lead to improved clinical outcomes by preventive interventions. This method may provide surrogate markers of long-term prognostic effects without the need for gadolinium, making it also available for diabetic patients with end-stage kidney disease. However, reproducibility assessments, transferability between centers, and translatability between field strengths and vendors, are requirements which are not yet all fulfilled with adenosine stress and rest T1 mapping [38] and future studies are needed to address these lacunae, innovatively. As a result, first pass perfusion imaging persists as the robust and validated tool for assessment of myocardial perfusion, despite its limitations in patients without contraindications to use contrast agents.

Study limitations

This study was limited by a relatively small sample size, and larger-scale future studies with long follow-up are necessary to determine the prognostic value of stress T1 response. Furthermore, as an observational study, we cannot determine the mechanisms for the observed differences in MPRI and T1 stress response.

Whilst the demonstration of a robust inter-study reproducibility for any technique is important to support the technique's clinical and research application, due to ethical considerations regarding a second administration of adenosine with an additional hospital visit in this study was deemed too high a burden on study subjects as this could lead to higher risk of adverse event rates, and high drop-out rates. Consequently, in our study we have not assessed the inter-study reproducibility of the adenosine stress T1 mapping. Further studies are needed to demonstrate the inter-study reproducibility of adenosine stress T1 mapping.

Although resting heart rates were statistically higher in patients, we have previously demonstrated that T1 estimation using the ShMOLLI technique is independent of heart rate variations (40 to 100 beats/min) over the applicable range of T1 values in phantoms and simulations at 1.5- and 3.0-Tesla [39]. Therefore, any potential confounding effects due to technical heart rate dependencies on the findings in this study are negligible, and the observed T1 values most likely reflect true physiologic and pathophysiologic changes in healthy controls and patients, respectively.

Despite statistical differences in stress ΔT1 between T2DM patients (4.1 ± 2.9%) and healthy controls (6.6 ± 2.6%), there are numerical overlaps between these values. The effect size to detect significant differences between diabetic patients and healthy controls using stress ΔT1 is respectable (Cohen's d 1.2), which is comparable to the difference in myocardial perfusion reserve index between fractional flow reserve -negative (MPRI 1.8 ± 0.5) and fractional flow reserve-positive (MPRI 1.2 ± 0.3) epicardial coronary lesions using gadolinium-enhanced stress perfusion CMR (Cohen's d 1.4 [40]). Liu et al., previously showed that stress T1-mapping is independent of field-strength between 1.5 and 3 T [18]. Considering the abolished stress ΔT1 values for ischemic myocardium (0.2 ± 0.8%) at 1.5 T [41], the effect size for detecting a significant difference between diabetic patients (4.1 ± 2.9%) vs. ischemic myocardium (0.2 ± 0.8%) is higher (Cohen's d 1.8). This suggests that the detection of myocardial ischemia in diabetic patients using gadolinium-free stress T1-mapping is possible, without the need for gadolinium contrast agents, and deserves further investigation.

Adenosine is the most commonly used agent for CMR perfusion studies, and it increases blood flow mostly by non-endothelial-dependent mechanisms via receptors on microvascular smooth muscle cells that modulate intracellular calcium [42]. Thus, the lower MPRIs and T1 stress responses observed in T2DM patients in this study might be the result of decreased vasodilation via both endothelium-dependent and -independent pathways. However, a complete characterisation of coronary microvascular function also requires the assessment of response to vasoconstrictor stimuli (acethylcholine, ergonovine), which can be performed only during an invasive coronary angiogram. Subjecting our participants to invasive coronary angiography, with even a small risk of complications, was deemed unacceptable for asymptomatic patients. Adenosine is shown to assess mostly non-endothelial-dependent coronary flow changes, and therefore we cannot completely rule out that endothelial-dependent coronary flow abnormalities may have affected our findings. Similarly, because we haven't carried out invasive assessment of coronary physiology, the diameter changes in response to an exogenous donor of nitric oxide, isosorbide dinitrate, could not be assessed, and therefore impaired responsiveness of underlying vascular smooth muscle cells or structural changes of the vascular wall cannot be excluded with certainty.

Absolute quantification of myocardial perfusion would have been interesting for direct comparison with absolute T1 quantification under stress and rest conditions. However, quantitative perfusion analysis is relatively cumbersome, requiring specialized computational software with mathematical assumptions and some recognized limitations [43].

The incidence of T2DM is driven predominantly by the obesity epidemic, and there is no doubt that obesity is a strong contributor to diabetic cardiomyopathy [44]. There is a significant overlap between the obesity related and diabetes related heart disease phenotypes. Both conditions are associated with LV concentric remodeling [4, 45–47], coronary microvascular dysfunction, myocardial energetic impairment [44] and increased risk of heart failure [4]. In our study, a third of (11 out of 31) T2DM patients were obese (35 > BMI > 30), 10 out of 31 patients were normal weight (BMI < 25), and the remaining 10 patients were overweight (25 < BMI < 30). This study aimed to prove the concept that adenosine rest and stress non-contrast T1 mapping would detect significant differences in patients with T2DM free of obstructive epicardial CAD on CTCA, in-keeping with coronary microvascular dysfunction. In sub-group analysis we have detected significant differences in MPRI and T1reactivity, suggesting that in the absence of obesity or even overweight status T2D is associated with coronary microvascular dysfunction. Given the comorbidity of obesity in a third of our patients with T2DM in this study, impact of obesity on the cardiac abnormalities cannot be dismissed; however, this is in fact not within the scope of our study aims.

Finally, CCTA was not performed in the healthy cohort to prevent unnecessary ionizing radiation exposure. Significant CAD was deemed to be very unlikely in this cohort.

Conclusions

Patients with well controlled T2DM, even in the absence of arterial hypertension and significant epicardial CAD, exhibit blunted maximal T1 response during adenosine vasodilatory stress, likely reflecting coronary microvascular dysfunction, as well as early signs of LV concentric remodelling without overt LVH. Adenosine stress and rest T1 mapping can detect subclinical functional abnormalities of the coronary microvasculature, without the need for gadolinium contrast agents.

In the future, CMR and particularly T1 mapping at stress may be used to identify early features of diabetic heart disease and subclinical risk markers in patients with T2DM, providing an opportunity for early therapeutic intervention.

Abbreviations

BMI: Body mass index; BP: Blood pressure; bSSFP: Balanced steady state free precession; CAD: Coronary artery disease; CCTA: Coronary computed tomographic angiography; CMR: Cardiovascular magnetic resonance; ECG: Electrocardiogram; ECV: Extracellular volume fraction; LGE: Late gadolinium enhancement; LV: Left ventricle/left ventricular; MPRI: Myocardial perfusion reserve index; RPP: Rate pressure product; ShMOLLI: Shortened modified Look-Locker inversion recovery; T2DM: Type 2 diabetes mellitus; ΔT1: Change in myocardial T1 values from rest to vasodilator stress

Acknowledgements

Not applicable.

Funding

The study was supported by the Oxford Partnership Comprehensive Biomedical Research Centre with funding from the Department of Health's National Institute for Health Research Biomedical Research Centers funding plan. S.N. acknowledges support from the Oxford British Heart Foundation Center of Research Excellence. S.K.P and V.M.F. are supported in part by the National Institute for Health Research (NIHR) Oxford Biomedical Research Centre based at The Oxford University Hospitals Trust at the University of Oxford.

Authors' contributions

All authors made appropriate contributions according to the ICMJE guidance, and as such have read and approved the final manuscript. All authors take public responsibility for appropriate portions of the manuscript content; and agree to be accountable in ensuring that questions related to the accuracy or integrity of the work are appropriately investigated and resolved. In addition, author specific contributions to the study are listed below: EL contributed to study conception and design, subject recruitment, data acquisition, analysis and interpretation; drafting of manuscript and revisions AL contributed to subject recruitment, data acquisition, analysis, interpretation, and manuscript revisions. RSW contributed to data analysis, interpretation and manuscript revision. RA, MM contributed to subject recruitment, data acquisition and manuscript revisions. SN contributed to study conception and design, data interpretation, study supervision and manuscript revisions. KC contributed to study supervision and manuscript revisions. SKP contributed to study conception and design, data analysis, interpretation and manuscript revisions. AG contributed to giving technical advice on T1-mapping and manuscript revisions. JMF contributed to data acquisition and manuscript revisions. VMF contributed to study conception and design, data interpretation and manuscript revisions. TK contributed to study conception and design, data interpretation, study supervision and manuscript revisions.

Competing interests

SKP has patent authorship rights for U.S. patent 9,285,446 B2. Systems and methods for shortenedLlook Locker inversion recovery (Sh-MOLLI) cardiac gated mapping of T1. Granted March 15, 2016. All rights transferred to Siemens Medical.
All other authors have no relationships relevant to the contents of this paper to disclose.

Author details

[1]University of Oxford Centre for Clinical Magnetic Resonance Research, Division of Cardiovascular Medicine, Radcliffe Department of Medicine, University of Oxford, Oxford, UK. [2]Department of Cardiovascular Sciences, University of Leicester, Leicester, UK. [3]Siemens Healthcare GmbH, Erlangen, Germany. [4]Department of Physiology, Anatomy and Genetics, University of Oxford, Oxford, UK. [5]1st Department of Cardiology, Aristotle University of Thessaloniki, AHEPA Hospital St. Kyriakidi 1, 54636 Thessaloniki, Greece.

References

1. Boudina S, Abel ED. Diabetic cardiomyopathy, causes and effects. Rev Endocr Metab Disord. 2010;11:31–9.
2. Galderisi M, Anderson KM, Wilson PWF, Levy D. Echocardiographic evidence for the existence of a distinct diabetic cardiomyopathy (the Framingham heart study). Am J Cardiol. 1991;68:85–9.
3. Garcia MJ, PM MN, Gordon T, Kannel WB. Morbidity and mortality in diabetics in the Framingham population: sixteen year follow-up study. Diabetes. 1974;23(2):105–11.
4. Kannel WB, McGee DL. Diabetes and cardiovascular disease: the framingham study. JAMA. 1979;241:2035–8.
5. Morrish JN, Wang S-L, Stevens KL, Fuller HJ, Keen H. Mortality and causes of death in the WHO multinational study of vascular disease in diabetes. Diabetologia. 2001;44:S14–21.
6. Stratton IM, Adler AI, Neil HAW, et al. Association of glycaemia with macrovascular and microvascular complications of type 2 diabetes (UKPDS 35): prospective observational study. BMJ. 2000;321:405–12.
7. Iribarren C, Karter AJ, Go AS, et al. Glycemic control and heart failure among adult patients with diabetes. Circulation. 2001;103:2668–73.
8. Bell DSH. Heart failure. Diabetes Care. 2003;26:2433–41.
9. Sucato V, Novo G, Evola S, Novo S. Coronary microvascular dysfunction in patients with diabetes, hypertension and metabolic syndrome. Int J Cardiol. 2015;186:96–7.
10. Murthy VL, Naya M, Foster CR, et al. Association between coronary vascular dysfunction and cardiac mortality in patients with and without diabetes mellitus. Circulation. 2012;126:1858–68.
11. Larghat AM, Swoboda PP, Biglands JD, Kearney MT, Greenwood JP, Plein S. The microvascular effects of insulin resistance and diabetes on cardiac structure, function, and perfusion: a cardiovascular magnetic resonance study, 2014.
12. Bratis K, Child N, Terrovitis J, et al. Coronary microvascular dysfunction in overt diabetic cardiomyopathy. IJC Metabolic & Endocrine. 2014;5:19–23.
13. Levelt E, Rodgers CT, Clarke WT, et al. Cardiac energetics, oxygenation, and perfusion during increased workload in patients with type 2 diabetes mellitus. Eur Heart J. 2016;37(46):3461–69. doi:10.1093/eurheartj/ehv442.
14. Piechnik SK, Ferreira VM, Dall'Armellina E, et al. Shortened modified look-locker inversion recovery (ShMOLLI) for clinical myocardial T1-mapping at 1. 5 and 3 T within a 9 heartbeat breathhold. J Cardiovasc Magn Reson. 2010; 12:69.
15. Piechnik SK, Ferreira VM, Lewandowski AJ, et al. Normal variation of magnetic resonance T1 relaxation times in the human population at 1.5 T using ShMOLLI. J Cardiovasc magnetic. Resonance. 2013;15:13.
16. McCommis KS, Goldstein TA, Abendschein DR, et al. Roles of myocardial blood volume and flow in coronary artery disease: an experimental MRI study at rest and during hyperemia. Eur Radiol. 2010;20:2005–12.
17. Mahmod M, Piechnik SK, Levelt E, et al. Adenosine stress native T1 mapping in severe aortic stenosis: evidence for a role of the intravascular compartment on myocardial T1 values. J Cardiovasc Magn Reson. 2014;16:92.

18. Liu A, Wijesurendra RS, Francis JM, et al. Adenosine stress and rest T1 mapping can differentiate between ischemic, infarcted, remote, and normal myocardium without the need for gadolinium contrast agents. J Am Coll Cardiol Img. 2016;9:27–36.
19. Alberti KG, Zimmet P. Definition, diagnosis and classification of diabetes mellitus and its complications. Part 1: diagnosis and classification of diabetes mellitus provisional report of a WHO consultation. Diabet Med. 1998;15(7):539–53.
20. Rider OJ, Tayal U, Francis JM et al. The effect of obesity and weight loss on aortic pulse wave velocity as assessed by magnetic resonance imaging. Obesity (silver spring), MD;18:2311–6.
21. Abbara S, Arbab-Zadeh A, Callister TQ, et al. SCCT guidelines for performance of coronary computed tomographic angiography: a report of the Society of Cardiovascular Computed Tomography Guidelines Committee. Journal of Cardiovascular Computed Tomography. 2009;3:190–204.
22. Karamitsos T, Hudsmith L, Selvanayagam J, Neubauer S, Francis J. Operator induced variability in left ventricular measurements with cardiovascular magnetic resonance is improved after training. J Cardiovasc Magn Reson. 2007:777–83.
23. Selvanayagam JB, Jerosch-Herold M, Porto I, et al. Resting myocardial blood flow is impaired in hibernating myocardium: a magnetic resonance study of quantitative perfusion assessment. Circulation. 2005;112:3289–96.
24. Karamitsos TD, Dass S, Suttie J, et al. Blunted myocardial oxygenation response during vasodilator stress in patients with hypertrophic cardiomyopathy. J Am Coll Cardiol. 2013;61:1169–76.
25. Kellman P, Arai AE, McVeigh ER, Aletras AH. Phase-sensitive inversion recovery for detecting myocardial infarction using gadolinium-delayed Hyperenhancement. Magnetic resonance in medicine : official journal of the Society of Magnetic Resonance in medicine/society of. Magn Reson Med. 2002;47:372–83.
26. Ferreira VM, Piechnik SK, Dall'Armellina E, et al. Non-contrast T1-mapping detects acute myocardial edema with high diagnostic accuracy: a comparison to T2-weighted cardiovascular magnetic resonance. J Cardiovasc Magn Reson. 2012;14:42.
27. Ferreira VM, Piechnik SK, Dall'Armellina E, et al. T1 mapping for the diagnosis of acute myocarditis using CMR: comparison to T2-weighted and late gadolinium enhanced imaging. J Am Coll Cardiol Img. 2013;6:1048–58.
28. Nagel E, Klein C, Paetsch I, et al. Magnetic resonance perfusion measurements for the noninvasive detection of coronary artery disease. Circulation. 2003;108:432–7.
29. White SK, Sado DM, Fontana M, et al. T1 mapping for myocardial extracellular volume measurement by CMR: bolus only versus primed infusion technique. J Am Coll Cardiol Img. 2013;6:955–62.
30. Moon JC, Messroghli DR, Kellman P, et al. Myocardial T1 mapping and extracellular volume quantification: a Society for Cardiovascular Magnetic Resonance (SCMR) and CMR working Group of the European Society of cardiology consensus statement. J Cardiovasc Magn Reson. 2013;15:92.
31. Asbun J, Villarreal FJ. The pathogenesis of myocardial fibrosis in the setting of diabetic cardiomyopathy. J Am Coll Cardiol. 2006;47:693–700.
32. Eguchi K, Boden-Albala B, Jin Z, et al. Association between diabetes mellitus and left ventricular hypertrophy in a multiethnic population. Am J Cardiol. 2008;101:1787–91.
33. Taskiran M, Fritz-Hansen T, Rasmussen V, Larsson HBW, Hilsted J. Decreased myocardial perfusion Reserve in Diabetic Autonomic Neuropathy. Diabetes. 2002;51:3306–10.
34. Rubinshtein R, Yang EH, Rihal CS, et al. Coronary microcirculatory vasodilator function in relation to risk factors among patients without obstructive coronary disease and low to intermediate Framingham score. Eur Heart J. 2009;31:936–42.
35. Lanza GA, Crea F. Primary coronary microvascular dysfunction: clinical presentation, pathophysiology, and management. Circulation. 2010;121: 2317–25.
36. Camici PG, d'Amati G, Rimoldi O. Coronary microvascular dysfunction: mechanisms and functional assessment. Nat Rev Cardiol. 2015;12:48–62.
37. Wijesurendra RS, Liu A, Casadei B, Robson MD, Neubauer S, Ferreira VM. Systolic ShMOLLI myocardial T1-mapping for improved robustness to partial-volume effects and applications in tachyarrhythmias. J Cardiovasc Magn Reson. 2015;17:77. doi:10.1186/s12968-015-0182-5.
38. Nagel E, Puntmann VOI. Myocardial native T1 the one answer for all? J Am Coll Cardiol Img. 2016;9:37.
39. Piechnik SK, Ferreira VM, Dall'Armellina E, Cochlin LE, Greiser A, Neubauer S. Shortened modified look-locker inversion recovery (ShMOLLI) for clinical myocardial T1-mapping at 1.5 and 3 T within a 9 heartbeat breathhold. J Cardiovasc Magn Reson. 2010;12
40. Rieber J, Huber A, Erhard I, et al. Cardiac magnetic resonance perfusion imaging for the functional assessment of coronary artery disease: a comparison with coronary angiography and fractional flow reserve. Eur Heart J. 2006;27:1465–71.
41. Liu A, Wijesurendra RS, Francis JM, et al. Adenosine stress and rest T1 mapping can differentiate between ischemic, infarcted, remote, and normal myocardium without the need for gadolinium contrast agents. JACC Cardiovascular imaging. 2016;9:27–36.
42. Mustafa SJ, Morrison RR, Teng B, Pelleg A. Adenosine receptors and the heart: role in regulation of coronary blood flow and cardiac electrophysiology. Handb Exp Pharmacol. 2009;193:161–88.
43. Lee DC, Johnson NP. Quantification of absolute myocardial blood flow by magnetic resonance perfusion imaging. J Am Coll Cardiol Img. 2009;2:761–70.
44. Rider OJ, Francis JM, Tyler D, Byrne J, Clarke K, Neubauer S. Effects of weight loss on myocardial energetics and diastolic function in obesity. Int J Cardiovasc Imaging. 2013;29:1043–50.
45. Jiang J, Ahn J, Huang W-Y, Hayes RB. Association of obesity with cardiovascular disease mortality in the PLCO trial. Prev Med. 2013;57:60–4.
46. Rider OJ, Lewis AJM, Neubauer S. Structural and metabolic effects of obesity on the myocardium and the aorta. Obesity Facts. 2014;7:329–38.
47. Turkbey EB, McClelland RL, Kronmal RA, et al. The impact of obesity on the left ventricle: the multi-ethnic study of atherosclerosis (MESA). JACC Cardiovascular imaging. 2010;3:266–74.

17

Site-specific association between distal aortic pulse wave velocity and peripheral arterial stenosis severity: a prospective cardiovascular magnetic resonance study

Harrie C M van den Bosch[1*], Jos J M Westenberg[2], Wikke Setz-Pels[1], John Wondergem[1], Ron Wolterbeek[3], Lucien E M Duijm[4], Joep A W Teijink[5] and Albert de Roos[2]

Abstract

Background: Vascular disease expression in one location may not be representative for disease severity in other vascular territories, however, strong correlation between disease expression and severity within the same vascular segment may be expected. Therefore, we hypothesized that aortic stiffening is more strongly associated with disease expression in a vascular territory directly linked to that aortic segment rather than in a more remote segment. We prospectively compared the association between aortic wall stiffness, expressed by pulse wave velocity (PWV), sampled in the distal aorta, with the severity of peripheral arterial occlusive disease (PAOD) as compared to atherosclerotic markers sampled in remote vascular territories such as PWV in the proximal aorta and the normalized wall index (NWI), representing the vessel wall thickness, of the left common carotid artery.

Methods: Forty-two patients (23 men; mean age 64±10 years) underwent velocity-encoded cardiovascular magnetic resonance (CMR) in the proximal and distal aorta, whole-body contrast-enhanced MR angiography (CE-MRA) and carotid vessel wall imaging with black-blood CMR in the work-up for PAOD. Strength of associations between aortic stiffness, carotid NWI and peripheral vascular stenosis grade were assessed and evaluated with multiple linear regression.

Results: Stenosis severity correlated well with PWV in the distal aorta (Pearson r_P=0.64, p<0.001, Spearman r_S=0.65, p<0.001) but to a lesser extent with PWV in the proximal aorta (r_P=0.48, p=0.002, r_S=0.22, p=0.18). Carotid NWI was not associated with peripheral stenosis severity (r_P=0.17, p=0.28, r_S=0.14, p=0.37) nor with PWV in the proximal aorta (r_P=0.22, p=0.17) nor in the distal aorta (r_P=0.21, p=0.18). Correlation between stenosis severity and distal aortic PWV remained statistically significant after correction for age and gender.

Conclusions: Distal aortic wall stiffness is more directly related to peripheral arterial stenosis severity than markers from more remote vascular territories such as proximal aortic wall stiffness or carotid arterial wall thickness. Site-specific evaluation of vascular disease may be required for full vascular risk estimation.

Keywords: Cardiovascular magnetic resonance, Atherosclerosis, Peripheral arterial occlusive disease, Pulse wave velocity, Carotid vessel wall

* Correspondence: harrie.vd.bosch@cze.nl
[1]Department of Radiology, Catharina Hospital, Michelangelolaan 2, 5623EJ, Eindhoven, The Netherlands
Full list of author information is available at the end of the article

Background

It is well known that the expression of vascular disease in one location may not be representative for the severity of disease in other vascular territories. From an observational cardiovascular magnetic resonance (CMR) study in 394 subjects, Barbier et al. reported that unrecognized myocardial infarction was not associated with manifestation of atherosclerosis depicted on whole-body MR angiography, nor with increased intima-media thickness (IMT) sampled in the carotid artery [1].

However, strong correlation has been reported between vascular disease expression and vascular wall changes within the same vascular segment. Increased wall thickness and wall stiffening in the carotid artery have been associated with the presence of atherosclerotic plaque in patients with hypertension and elderly patients [2]. Additionally, a stronger association between arterial vessel wall thickness and wall stiffness has been demonstrated when these markers were sampled regionally within the same vascular territory of either the aorta or the carotid artery, rather than across vascular territories [3]. Atherosclerosis involves both arterial wall thickening due to fatty degeneration (i.e., atherosis) and arterial wall stiffening due to media degeneration (i.e., sclerosis) [4,5]. Atherosclerosis is therefore not limited to luminal narrowing and structural changes in the arterial wall, but is also strongly associated with arterial wall stiffening [6]. The pulse wave velocity (PWV) has been acknowledged as an important indicator for increased aortic stiffness with prognostic value for cardiovascular events [7,8]. With velocity-encoded CMR, the PWV can be accurately assessed with high reproducibility, regionally in the aorta [9].

We hypothesized that aortic stiffening is more strongly associated with the expression of vascular disease in the vascular territory at risk directly linked to that aortic segment rather than in a more remote aortic segment or in other vascular territories. Accordingly, the purpose of this study was to prospectively compare the association between aortic wall stiffness, expressed by pulse wave velocity, sampled in the distal aorta with the severity of peripheral arterial occlusive disease as compared to atherosclerotic markers sampled in remote vascular territories such as PWV in the proximal aorta and normalized wall index [10] describing the vessel wall thickness of the left common carotid artery.

Methods

Patients

In our study, 42 consecutive patients (23 men; mean age 64±10 years) were included who were clinically referred for CE-MRA evaluation and were either suspected for PAOD due to clinical symptoms or already known to be suffering from PAOD and had to undergo follow-up evaluation. In all patients, a single comprehensive CMR examination was performed consisting of a moving-table CE-MRA of the run-off vessels, carotid vessel wall imaging and assessment of the aortic pulse wave velocity. In all patients, the glomerular filtration rate (GFR) was >60 mL/min/1.73 m^2. No adverse reactions or complications occurred during or after MRA. Institutional Review Board approval and written informed consent was obtained from all patients.

Of note, 16 patients of the present study have been described previously in a study comparing different MRA techniques of the run-off vessels [11].

CMR protocol

CMR was performed using a 3T CMR system (Achieva X-series, release 2.1; Philips Healthcare, Best, The Netherlands). Whole-body CE-MRA was performed and has been partially described before [11]. In short, first standardized 3-station single-injection CE-MRA was performed, including the abdominal aorta, iliac arteries and run-off vessels. The contrast protocol consisted of a biphasic contrast injection using an CMR-compatible injector (Spectris MR injector; Medrad, Indianola, PA). In total, 0.1 mmol/kg body weight gadoterate meglumine (Gd-DOTA, Guerbet, Paris, France) was administered. The first half of the contrast bolus was administered at 1.2 mL/s and the remaining half at 0.5 mL/s. Contrast injection was followed by 15 mL saline flush at 0.6 mL/s. Timing of the contrast arrival, required to start the acquisition of the CE-MRA, was determined by means of automatic bolus timing (BolusTrak; Philips Healthcare, Best, The Netherlands). For signal transmission and reception a quadrature body coil was used in all three stations. Imaging parameters of the 3D fast gradient-echo (FFE) CE-MRA were as follows: for the pelvic arteries repetition time (TR) 3.6 ms, echo time (TE) 1.25 ms, flip angle 20°, field-of-view (FOV) 410 mm, acquired voxel size 1.25×1.84×3.70 mm^3, reconstructed voxel size 0.73×0.73×1.85 mm^3; for the upper-leg arteries TR/TE 3.6/1.26, flip angle 20°, FOV 410 mm, acquired voxel size 1.30×1.75×3.00 mm^3, reconstructed voxel size 0.73×0.73×1.50 mm^3;for the lower-leg arteries TR/TE 4.7/1.60, flip angle 30°, FOV 410 mm, acquired voxel size 0.80×0.90×1.40 mm^3, reconstructed voxel size 0.71×0.71×0.70 mm^3. The first station was acquired with reversed linear k-space filling, the second and third station were acquired with centric k-space filling. Table speed was set at 180 mm/s between all imaged stations. The fourth station consisting of the thoracic aorta and its supra-aortic braches, including the carotid arteries, was acquired after a second contrast injection (0.1 mmol/kg body weight Gd-DOTA). Timing of contrast arrival was determined by means of automatic bolus timing. For signal transmission and reception a quadrature body coil was used. Imaging parameters were as follows:

TR/TE 5.5/1.80, flip angle 30°, FOV 410 mm, acquired voxel size 0.96×0.97×2.00 mm^3, reconstructed voxel size 0.64×0.64×1.00 mm^3. Data were acquired with centric k-space filling.

Preceding to the whole-body CE-MRA procedure, the vessel wall of the left common carotid artery was examined in all patients using multi-slice two-dimensional black blood imaging. On oblique sagittal and oblique coronal survey scans axial slices were planned perpendicular to the course of the common carotid artery (Figure 1A). Starting from the carotid flow divider, eight contiguous slices of 2 mm thick were acquired in caudal direction. To maximize contrast between the carotid vessel wall, the lumen blood pool and the surrounding tissue, a 2D dual-inversion-recovery (black-blood) gradient echo technique with spectral selective fat suppression was used. VCG-triggering was used for gated data acquisition at end-diastole. For signal reception, a 2-element Flex-M surface coil was positioned around the neck of the patient. Images were acquired at each RR interval with the following typical parameters: TR/TE 12/3.5, flip angle 45°, FOV 140 mm, two signal averages, acquired voxel size 0.46×0.46×2 mm^3.

The pulse wave velocity, defined as the wave propagation speed, was assessed regionally in the aorta, between the ascending and descending thoracic aorta (i.e., the proximal aorta), and between the thoracic descending and distal abdominal aorta (i.e., the distal aorta) (Figure 1B), using a 6-element cardiac coil. Two one-directional through-plane velocity-encoded CMR acquisitions were performed to assess the flow waveform propagation through the aorta. First, a double-oblique sagittal survey of the aorta was obtained (1C) and used for planning of the velocity-encoded acquisitions. The first velocity-encoded acquisition was planned perpendicular to the ascending aorta at the level of the pulmonary trunk, and transecting both the ascending and thoracic descending aorta. The second acquisition was planned at the most distal aortic location still present in the sagittal survey. Velocity-encoded CMR was performed using a retrospectively VCG-gated gradient-echo sequence with velocity-encoding in through-plane direction: TR/TE 4.9/3.0, flip angle 10°, FOV 320 mm, one signal average, acquired voxel size 2.50×2.50×8.00 mm^3. The maximum number of phases was reconstructed in order to obtain high temporal resolution (the true temporal resolution was 2×TR =9.8 ms). At the proximal level, a velocity sensitivity V_{enc} of 150 cm/s was used and at the distal level, V_{enc} =100 cm/s. Free breathing was allowed during the acquisition.

Image analysis

MR angiographic images were reviewed at random and in consensus by two MR radiologists (HvdB and JW; 15 and 17 years of experience with CE-MRA, respectively). CE-MRA images were analyzed on a remote workstation. The arterial tree from infrarenal aorta down to the peripheral arteries was divided into 27 segments (Figure 2): the infrarenal aorta, common iliac arteries, external iliac arteries, common femoral arteries, superficial femoral arteries, popliteal arteries in the thigh station, popliteal arteries in the calf station, tibiofibular trunk, and the proximal and distal halves of the anterior and posterior tibial arteries and peroneal arteries. The severity of each stenosis was visually graded according to a five point scale: class 1 (0%-

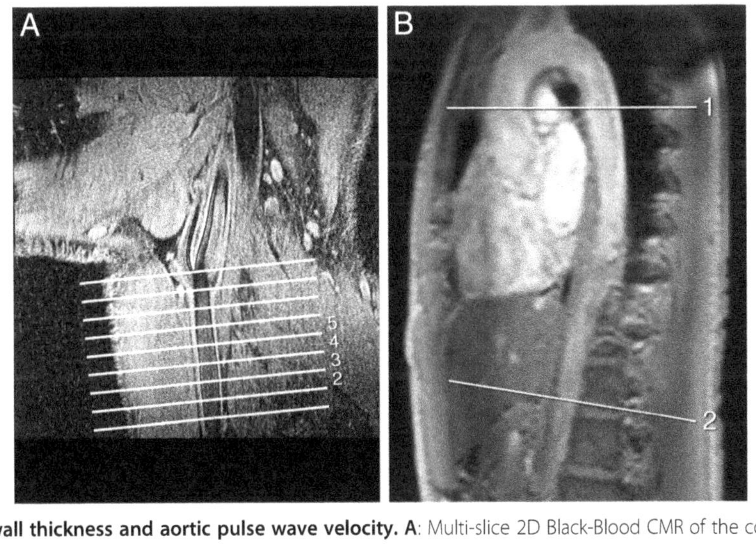

Figure 1 Carotid vessel wall thickness and aortic pulse wave velocity. A: Multi-slice 2D Black-Blood CMR of the common carotid artery for assessment of vessel wall thickness. Eight cross-sectional slices of the left common carotid artery were acquired, with the last slice adjacent to the bifurcation, however only slice 2 to 5 were included in the analysis. **B**: Proximal and distal aortic Pulse Wave Velocity (PWV) was assessed by two one-directional velocity-encoded CMR acquisitions in through-plane direction, planned perpendicular to the aorta at the level of the pulmonary trunk and at the abdominal aorta, respectively.

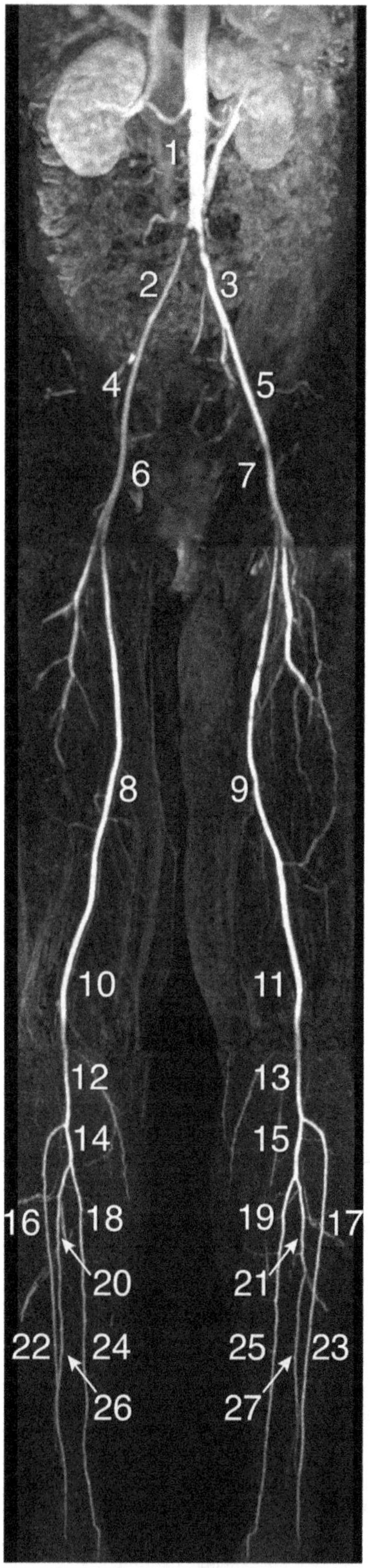

Figure 2 Segments of arterial tree from infrarenal aorta to peripheral arteries. Contrast-enhanced MRA of the infra-renal aorta down to the lower leg arteries in a patient with a subtotal stenosis in the right common iliac artery. For each patient, mean and maximal stenosis class were obtained by dividing the arterial tree into 27 segments: the infrarenal aorta (1), common iliac arteries (2 +3), external iliac arteries (4 +5), common femoral arteries (6 +7), superficial femoral arteries (8 +9), popliteal arteries in the thigh station (10 +11), popliteal arteries in the calf station (12 +13), tibiofibular trunk (14 +15), and the proximal (16-21) and distal (22-27) halves of the anterior and posterior tibial arteries and peroneal arteries.

stenosis), 2 (1-50%), 3 (51-75%), 4 (76-99%) and 5 (100%). The highest stenosis class per segment was determined, and next, the highest stenosis class over all available segments (maximal 27), presenting one value per patient (Max SC), was determined. Also, the mean stenosis class (Mean SC), averaged over all available segments was calculated. While both parameters relate to the severity of PAOD, Max SC relates to the stenosis severity and Mean SC relates to distribution of stenoses in peripheral arterial tree. Stenosis classification per patient was performed blinded from carotid vessel wall and aortic PWV analysis.

Cross-sectional carotid vessel wall area (VWA) and total vessel area were obtained using the previously validated in-house developed software package VesselMass software (Leiden University Medical Center, Leiden, the Netherlands [12]. Inner and outer lumen contours were manually defined. Analysis was performed in four slices out of eight. The mean cross-sectional carotid VWA and total vessel area were averaged over the four included slices, and subsequently the normalized wall index (NWI) [10] was calculated as follows: NWI=VWA/total vessel area.

The aortic PWV was obtained from systolic wave propagation analysis based on the transit-time method which has been validated before [9]. The aortic path length (Δx), describing the distance between sampling sites in the ascending and the thoracic descending aorta for proximal aortic PWV ($PWV_{proximal}$) and between the thoracic and abdominal descending aorta for distal aortic PWV (PWV_{distal}), respectively, was manually determined using MASS software (Leiden University Medical Center, Leiden, The Netherlands), by placing a poly-line along the centerline of the aorta in the sagittal survey images. Each aortic path length measurement was performed twice and averaged. Wave propagation was evaluated from maximal velocity-time curves that were obtained at each sampling site by using FLOW software (Leiden University Medical Center, Leiden, the Netherlands) with automated contour detection for image segmentation. The transit-time defining the wave propagation was assessed from the onset of each wave front, automatically calculated from the intersection of the horizontal line modeling the diastolic flow (averaged over the final 250 ms of the velocity-time curve) and the upslope of the systolic wave which was modeled by a straight line, using linear regression of all values between 20% and 80% of the range of velocity values that are part of the upslope.

Statistical analysis

Kolmogorov-Smirnov tests were performed to test normality of data distribution. Continuous variables are expressed as mean ± standard deviation (SD). Associations between atherosclerotic disease severity (Mean SC and Max SC) and atherosclerotic markers $PWV_{proximal}$, PWV_{distal} and carotid NWI were explored. Furthermore, association between NWI and PWV was examined. Correlation between Mean SC and Max SC and $PWV_{proximal}$, PWV_{distal} and carotid NWI was examined by calculating Pearson (for continuous variables) or Spearman (in case of association with an ordinal variable) correlation coefficients, where appropriate. Multiple linear regression analyses were performed with Mean SC as dependent variable and age, gender and respectively alternating proximal and distal aortic PWV and carotid NWI as predictors. Additionally, interaction between predictors was analyzed. A p-value of <0.05 is considered statistically significant. Statistical analysis was performed using IBM SPSS software version 20 (Armonk, NY, USA).

Results

Patient characteristics are presented in Table 1. Thirty-four patients (81%) presented with intermittent claudication (Fontaine classification 2), of which twenty-three patients (55%) with pain-free claudication walking ≥200 m and eleven patients (26%) with pain-free claudication walking <200 m. Five patient (12%) presented with rest pain (Fontaine classification 3) and three patients (7%) with necrosis (Fontaine classification 4). Mean ankle-brachial index (ABI) in rest was 0.75±0.21. CE-MRA was successful in all patients. No imaging artefacts or venous contamination affected the image analysis and image quality was sufficient for stenosis scoring in all segments. Mean SC per patient ranged between 1 (no stenosis) and 3.6, with a mean value ± standard deviation of 1.6 ±0.5. Max SC ranged between 1 and 5, with mean ± SD 4.4 ±1.0 (median 5, interquartile range from 4 to 5). Carotid NWI ranged from 0.20 to 0.59, with mean ± SD of 0.46 ±0.07. PWV ranged from 4.5 m/s to 45.3 m/s in the proximal aorta (mean ± SD 10.1±6.5 m/s) and from 4.4 m/s to 24.4 m/s in the distal aorta (mean ± SD 9.3 ±3.8 m/s). All continuous data were normally distributed according to Kolmogorov-Smirnov tests (all p>0.05). In Figure 3, scatter plots and box plots are presented to illustrate data distribution and associations between markers. From the distribution of the data in these figures it is obvious that one outlier for Mean SC (Figures 3A to 3C: data point with Mean SC =3.6) and one outlier for PWV in the proximal aorta (Figures 3A, 3D and 3G: data point with PWV =45.3 m/s) might contribute substantially to the correlations. For the patient with Mean SC of 3.6, $PWV_{proximal}$ was 8.8 m/s, PWV_{distal} 9.2 m/s and carotid NWI 0.48. For the patient with $PWV_{proximal}$ 45.3 m/s, the Mean SC was 1.6, PWV_{distal} 13.2 m/s and carotid NWI 0.57. Analysis was performed on the full dataset as well as on the dataset with these two outliers removed. For the data with outliers removed, mean values ± SD changed for Mean SC 1.5 ±0.4 and for $PWV_{proximal}$ 9.3 ±3.5 m/s.

In two patients, significant stenoses were found in the carotid arteries: in one patient, a class 3 stenosis was depicted in the right internal carotid artery and in the other patient, a full occlusion was present in the right internal carotid artery while the left internal carotid artery presented with a class 3 stenosis. All other patients were free from stenoses in the carotid arteries. In 28 patients, no stenosis was present in the distal aorta; 11 patients were graded with a class 2 stenosis in the abdominal aorta, 1 patient with class 3 stenosis, 1 patient with class 4 stenosis and one patient with an occlusion. Spearman correlation coefficients indicated no significant correlations between stenosis severity in the distal aorta and proximal aortic PWV (r_S=-0.09, p=0.59) and distal aortic PWV (r_S=-0.21, p=0.21), respectively. Low correlation was found between stenosis severity in the distal aorta and the carotid NWI (r_S=0.38, p=0.02).

In two patients, no stenoses were depicted on any of the CE-MRA images. Correlations between Mean SC in the complete run-off and proximal and distal aortic PWV and carotid VWA/BSA were evaluated by Pearson correlation coefficients, while correlations between Max SC, proximal and distal aortic PWV and carotid NWI were evaluated by Spearman correlation coefficients, respectively. The results are presented in Table 2, both for all data point as well as for the data with two outliers removed.

Table 1 Patient characteristics

Gender (male/female)	23/19
Age (years)	64 ± 10
Hypertension (yes/no)	28/14
Fontaine Class (stages I/IIa/IIb/III/IV)	0/23/11/5/3
ABI in rest	0.75 ± 0.21
Mean SC	1.6 ± 0.5
Max SC (median (interquartile range))	5 (4–5)
Carotid NWI	0.46 ± 0.07
$PWV_{proximal}$ (m/s)	10.1 ± 6.5
PWV_{distal} (m/s)	9.3 ± 3.8

ABI: ankle-brachial index; *SC*: stenosis class; *NWI*: normalized wall index; *PWV*: pulse wave velocity.

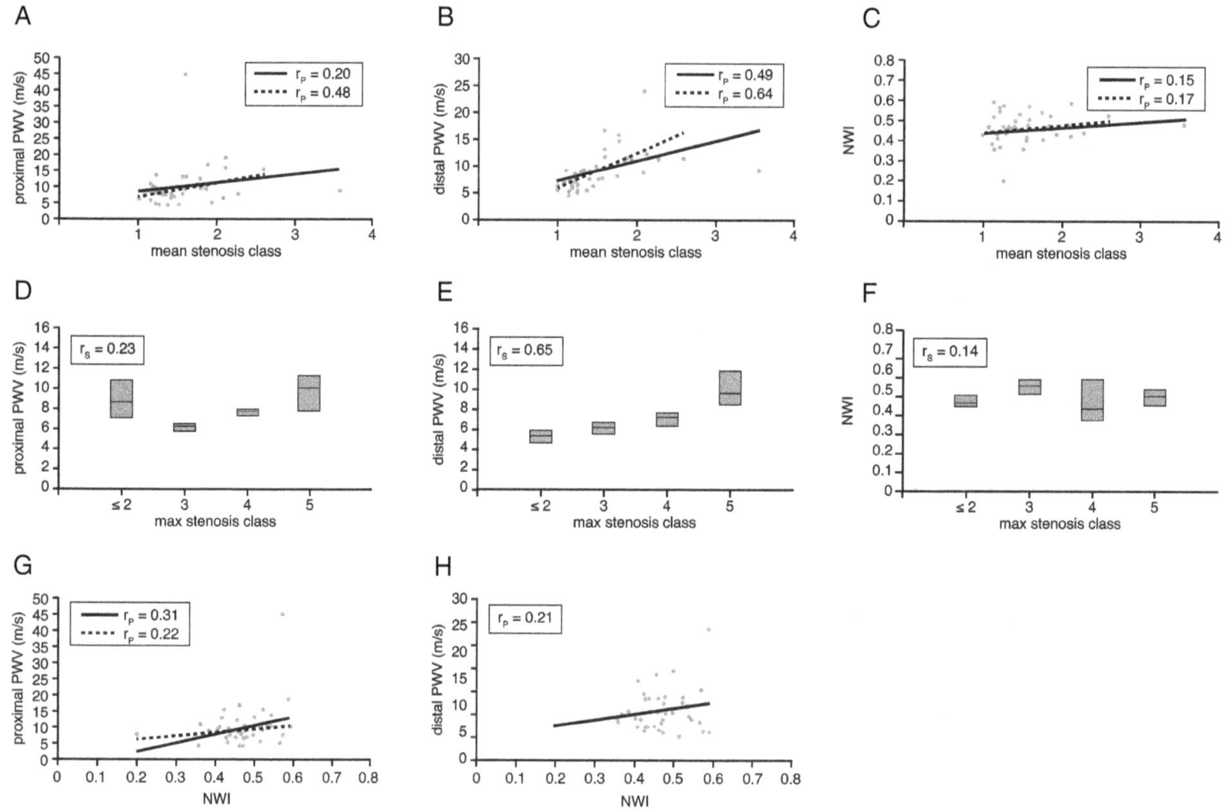

Figure 3 Association stenosis severity, PWV, and carotid wall thickness (A-H). Associations between stenosis severity (expressed in mean and max stenosis class), the proximal and distal aortic pulse wave velocity and normalized wall index sampled in the left common carotid artery. Solid line represents correlation between parameters for the full dataset, dashed line represents correlation for dataset with two outliers removed.

None to moderate association between PWV in the proximal aorta and stenosis class (r_P=0.46 for Mean SC and r_P=0.22 for Max SC) was found. Associations between distal aortic PWV and stenosis class are good. However, associations are absent between carotid NWI and stenosis class as well as between carotid NWI and proximal and distal aortic PWV.

In Table 3, the results of multiple linear regression between Mean SC and proximal and distal aortic PWV, carotid NWI, age and gender are presented. No significant interaction was found between these predictors (all p>0.05). These tests show that proximal and distal aortic PWV and carotid NWI are all statistically significantly associated with age, but none of these predictors is associated with gender. However, for these patients, only distal aortic PWV remained significantly associated with Mean SC (with β=0.46, p=0.003), when corrected for age (β=0.30, p=0.04) and gender (β=−0.06, p=0.61).

Discussion

This study prospectively evaluated the association between aortic wall stiffness, expressed by PWV, sampled in the distal aorta and the severity of PAOD as compared to atherosclerotic markers sampled in remote vascular territories such as the PWV in the proximal aorta and vessel wall thickness of the left common carotid artery. The main findings of our study are: 1) In patients with PAOD, the PWV in the distal aorta is well associated with

Table 2 Pearson and Spearman correlation coefficients between mean and maximal stenosis severity, proximal and distal aortic PWV and cross-sectional carotid NWI, both for the total dataset as well as for one outlier removed

	All patients included			Two outliers removed		
	Mean SC r_P	Max SC r_S	NWI r_P	Mean SC r_P	Max SC r_S	NWI r_P
$PWV_{proximal}$	0.20 (p=0.22, N=42)	0.23 (p=0.14, N=42)	0.31 (p=0.048, N=42)	0.48 (p=0.002, N=40)	0.22 (p=0.18, N=41)	0.22 (p=0.17, N=41)
PWV_{distal}	0.49 (p=0.001, N=42)	0.65 (p<0.001, N=42)	0.21 (p=0.18, N=42)	0.64 (p<0.001, N=41)	0.65 (p<0.001, N=42)	0.21 (p=0.18, N=42)
NWI	0.15 (p=0.34, N=42)	0.14 (p=0.37, N=42)		0.17 (p=0.28, N=41)	0.14 (p=0.37, N=42)	

PWV: pulse wave velocity, *NWI*: normalized wall index, *SC*: stenosis class, r_P: Pearson correlation coefficient, r_S: Spearman correlation coefficient, *N*: number of samples.

Table 3 Multiple linear regression analysis with mean stenosis class as dependent variable and age, gender and respectively alternating cross-sectional carotid normalized wall index, proximal and distal aortic pulse wave velocity as predictors

	NWI				$PWV_{proximal}$				PWV_{distal}		
	B (SE)	β	p		B (SE)	β	p		B (SE)	β	p
Constant	0.13 (0.39)		0.75	**Constant**	0.31 (0.33)		0.36	**Constant**	0.40 (0.29)		0.18
Age	0.02 (0.005)	0.50	0.001	**Age**	0.02 (0.01)	0.41	0.01	**Age**	0.01 (0.005)	0.30	0.04
Gender	−0.15 (0.11)	−0.21	0.17	**Gender**	−0.11 (0.10)	−0.15	0.28	**Gender**	−0.04 (0.09)	−0.06	0.61
NWI	0.59 (0.76)	0.12	0.44	**$PWV_{proximal}$**	0.03 (0.02)	0.27	0.08	**PWV_{distal}**	0.05 (0.01)	0.46	0.003

NWI: normalized wall index, *PWV*: pulse wave velocity, *SE*: standard error.

peripheral arterial stenosis severity. 2) Correlation between peripheral arterial stenosis severity with markers sampled in remote vascular territories such as PWV in the proximal aorta and carotid VWA NWI, are weak to absent, only moderate at best, indicating site-specific association between aortic wall stiffness and peripheral arterial disease severity. 3) Only the correlation between stenosis severity and distal aortic PWV remains statistically significant after correction for age and gender.

PAOD is an important clinical manifestation of atherosclerosis, for which 3T CE-MRA is a reliable diagnostic tool, widely used to detect and grade stenosis severity [11]. However, CE-MRA is not without risks, especially in patients with impaired renal function [13]. The initial test in clinical routine for diagnosing patients with clinical symptoms of PAOD is assessment of the ankle-brachial index (ABI) [14]. A low ABI is a strong indicator of the presence of PAOD [15] but a normal ABI, however, does not rule out risk due to the false negative rates [16]. Furthermore, Wikström et al. reported that ABI<0.9 may underestimate the prevalence of PAOD when assessed with CE-MRA [17]. Therefore, the evaluation of other markers associated with the severity of PAOD is warranted. Atherosclerosis is a systemic disease which affects the arterial wall both by thickening and stiffening. Structural changes in the wall usually occur over a larger part of the arterial tree rather than confined to a localized arterial segment (i.e., diffuse preintrusive wall thickening in contrast to focal intrusive thickening [2]). Maroules et al. recently demonstrated a strong association between wall thickness sampled in the abdominal aorta and the occurrence of cardiovascular events in a large population-based study [18]. Additionally, arterial wall stiffening has been described as an independent predictor of cardiovascular events in patients with hypertension, diabetes and end-stage renal disease [19,20] as well as in the aging population [21]. Moreover, increased carotid arterial wall thickness is associated with carotid wall stiffening and with the presence of atherosclerotic plaque in the carotid artery and the aorta in patients with hypertension and elderly patients [22].

However, it is well known that the expression of vascular disease in one location may not be representative for the severity of disease in other vascular territories and it is conceivable that disease severity is stronger associated with atherosclerotic markers sampled within the same vascular territory than when sampled in a more remote vascular territory. Barbier et al. demonstrated that unrecognized myocardial infarction is not necessarily associated with atherosclerotic disease severity, depicted from whole-body MR angiography nor with increased intima-media thickness (IMT) sampled in the carotid artery [1]. Furthermore, in a recent publication, Turkbey et al. found no independent association between imaging biomarkers of atherosclerosis such as carotid IMT and distensibility sampled in the ascending aorta [23]. This finding was confirmed by our results, as the association between carotid NWI and the PWV in the proximal aorta was not statistically significant. Furthermore, in a study by Brandts et al. it was shown both in healthy volunteers as well as in patients with hypertension that the aortic PWV correlated more strongly with the aortic VWA than when compared to the carotid VWA [24]. Kröner et al. [3] confirmed these findings in healthy volunteers and added stronger correlations between arterial vessel wall thickness and stiffness when sampled within the same vascular territory of either the aorta or the carotid artery, rather than across vascular territories. These reports underline the suggestion of a strong site-specific coupling between morphologic and functional degenerative changes of the arterial wall and the possible effect on future cardiovascular events.

In our study, 42 consecutive patients referred for CE-MRA for the evaluation of severity of PAOD were included. In these patients, the prevalence of significant stenoses in the distal aorta was low (i.e., 7%), and therefore, no association with PWV in this part of the aorta could be demonstrated. However, the stenosis severity detected with CE-MRA in the peripheral arteries correlated well with the PWV sampled in the distal aorta, but to a lesser extent with PWV in the proximal aorta, and no association was found with carotid NWI. Taniwaki et al. [25] showed that in patients with type 2 diabetes mellitus, the presence of PAOD symptoms was more closely associated with increased femoral arterial wall stiffness compared to increased femoral arterial wall thickness, suggesting that stiffening has a significant impact on clinical symptoms in patients with peripheral vascular disease. In our study, aortic wall stiffness is represented by the PWV, which is defined as the systolic wave front velocity propagating through the aorta. The assessment of PWV by CMR has shown good agreement with invasive pressure measurements, the gold standard for defining PWV [9,26]. Still, data on reproducibility of this assessment is scarce. Grotenhuis et al. [9] evaluated the reproducibility by repeating acquisitions on the same day and reported a coefficient of variation of 9% for PWV assessment in the total aorta by CMR. In a study by Suever et al. [27], reproducibility of CMR-assessed PWV was compared to applanation tonometry by performing repeated studies on volunteers on the same day. However, no data has been published for repeated acquisitions on separate days, therefore information on the physiological variation of this marker is missing, although CMR-assessed PWV is widely used in clinical research. To our knowledge, this is the first clinical study to evaluate the association between peripheral arterial stenosis severity and regional aortic wall stiffness and carotid vessel wall thickness, all assessed from one comprehensive CMR examination. The results from our study and from literature underline a potentially important role for the site-specific assessment of arterial wall stiffness by PWV regionally in the aorta as this may be required for full estimation of vascular risk in patients with atherosclerosis. The strong site-specific association between distal aortic wall stiffening and the degree of stenosis in the peripheral arteries suggests that sampling within the same vascular territory may be preferred over sampling across vascular territories.

We acknowledge certain limitations of our study. First, it involves a cross-sectional design in a relatively small prospectively included patient population in which the association between atherosclerotic markers and stenosis severity was evaluated. Association, however, does not prove causality. Population-based long-term follow-up studies are required to prove whether distal aortic stiffening indeed is a precursor to PAOD and to elucidate the predictive value of increased wall stiffness in the distal aorta with respect to further development of flow-limiting stenoses in the peripheral arteries. Carotid arterial vessel wall sampling was limited to the left common carotid artery. Prevalence of stenoses in the carotid circulation in this patient population was very low. Adding VWA sampling of the right carotid artery would be possible but this was not performed, however, as it requires additional scan time. Also, no comparison with ultrasound-assessed IMT was performed, additionally to VWA sampling with Black-Blood CMR, but from literature it is known that CMR shows good agreement with ultrasound when sampling IMT [28]. The higher spatial resolution on ultrasound potentially may improve the association between IMT and PAOD stenosis severity, however, CMR has the advantage of providing increased vessel coverage with information on the complete circumference over the length of a vessel, which permits assessment of localized abnormalities without assuming vessel uniformity.

Conclusions

Peripheral arterial stenosis severity is well correlated with aortic PWV sampled in the distal aorta but correlation with markers sampled in remote vascular territories such as PWV in the proximal aorta and carotid arterial wall thickness, is only moderate at best. The association between aortic wall stiffening and stenosis severity in a vascular territory directly linked to this aortic segment suggests that site-specific evaluation of vascular disease may be required for full vascular risk assessment and therefore, regional aortic PWV assessment by CMR may be considered in the clinical workup of PAOD.

Abbreviations

ABI: Ankle-brachial index; BSA: Body surface area; CE-MRA: Contrast-enhanced MR angiography; FFE: Fast gradient-echo; FOV: Field-of-view; GFR: Glomerular filtration rate; IMT: Intima-media thickness; Max Sc: Highest stenosis class per patient; Mean Sc: Mean stenosis class per patient; NWI: Normalized wall index; PAOD: Peripheral arterial occlusive disease; PWV: Pulse wave velocity; TE: Echo time; TR: Repetition time; VWA: Vessel wall area.

Competing interests

The authors declare that they have no competing interests. There are no non-financial competing interests (political, personal, religious, ideological, academic, intellectual, commercial or any other) to declare in relation to this manuscript.

Authors' contributions

All authors have made substantial contributions to conception and design, acquisition of data, and analysis and interpretation of data. All authors have been involved in drafting the manuscript or revising it critically for important intellectual content. All authors have given final approval of the version to be published; and agree to be accountable for all aspects of the work in ensuring that questions related to the accuracy or integrity of any part of the work are appropriately investigated and resolved.

Author details

[1]Department of Radiology, Catharina Hospital, Michelangelolaan 2, 5623EJ, Eindhoven, The Netherlands. [2]Department of Radiology, Leiden University Medical Center, Leiden, The Netherlands. [3]Department of Medical Statistics, Leiden University Medical Center, Leiden, The Netherlands. [4]Department of Radiology, Canisius-Wilhelmina Hospital, Nijmegen, The Netherlands. [5]Department of Vascular Surgery, Catharina Hospital, Eindhoven, The Netherlands.

References

1. Barbier CE, Nylander R, Themudo R, Ahlström H, Lind L, Larsson EM, Bjerner T, Johansson L. **Prevalence of unrecognized myocardial infarction detected with magnetic resonance imaging and its relationship to cerebral ischemic lesions in both sexes.** *J Am Coll Cardiol.* 2011; **58**:1372–77.

2. Simon A, Megnien J-L, Gariepy J, Levenson J. **Early atherosclerosis in human hypertension.** *Am J Hypertens.* 1998; **11:**882–83.
3. Kröner ES, Lamb HJ, Siebelink HM, Putter H, van der Geest RJ, van der Wall EE, de Roos A, Westenberg JJ. **Coupling of vessel wall morphology and function in the aorta and the carotid artery: an evaluation with MRI.** *Int J Cardiovasc Imaging.* 2014; **30:**91–8.
4. Selvin E, Najjar S, Cornish T, Halushka MK. **A comprehensive histopathological evaluation of vascular medial fibrosis: Insights into the pathophysiology of arterial stiffening.** *Atherosclerosis.* 2010; **208:**69–74.
5. Blankenhorn DH, Kramsch DM. **Reversal of atherosis and sclerosis. The two components of atherosclerosis.** *Circulation.* 1989; **79:**1–7.
6. Van Popele NM, Grobbee DE, Bots ML, Asmar R, Topouchian J, Reneman RS, Hoeks AP, van der Kuip DA, Hofman A, Witteman JC. **Association between arterial stiffness and atherosclerosis: the Rotterdam study.** *Stroke.* 2001; **32:**454–60.
7. Mitchell GF, Hwang SJ, Vasan RS, Larson MG, Pencina MJ, Hamburg NM, Vita JA, Levy D, Benjamin EJ. **Arterial stiffness and cardiovascular events: the Framingham Heart Study.** *Circulation.* 2010; **121:**505–11.
8. Karras A, Haymann JP, Bozec E, Metzger M, Jacquot C, Maruani G, Houillier P, Froissart M, Stengel B, Guardiola P, Laurent S, Boutouyrie P, Briet M. **Large artery stiffening and remodeling are independently associated with all-cause mortality and cardiovascular events in chronic kidney disease.** *Hypertension.* 2012; **60:**1451–57.
9. Grotenhuis HB, Westenberg JJ, Steendijk P, van der Geest RJ, Ottenkamp J, Bax JJ, Jukema JW, de Roos A. **Validation and reproducibility of aortic pulse wave velocity as assessed with velocity-encoded MRI.** *J Magn Reson Imaging.* 2009; **20:**521–26.
10. Saam T, Yuan C, Chu B, Takaya N, Underhill H, Cai J, Tran N, Polissar NL, Neradilek B, Jarvik GP, Isaac C, Garden GA, Maravilla KR, Hashimoto B, Hatsukami TS. **Predictors of carotid atherosclerotic plaque progression as measured by noninvasive magnetic resonance imaging.** *Atherosclerosis.* 2007; **194:**34–42.
11. Van den Bosch HCM, Westenberg JJM, Caris R, Duijm LE, Tielbeek AV, Cuypers PW, de Roos A. **Peripheral arterial occlusive disease: 3.0-T versus 1.5-T MR angiography compared with digital subtraction angiography.** *Radiology.* 2013; **266:**337–46.
12. Alizadeh DR, Doornbos J, Tamsma JT, Stuber M, Putter H, van der Geest RJ, Lamb HJ, de Roos A. **Assessment of the carotid artery by MRI at 3T: a study on reproducibility.** *J Magn Reson Imaging.* 2007; **25:**1035–43.
13. Prince MR, Zhang HL, Roditi GH, Leiner T, Kucharczyk W. **Risk factors for NSF: a literature review.** *J Magn Reson Imaging.* 2009; **30:**1298–308.
14. Langham MC, Englund EK, Mohler ER III, Li C, Rodgers ZB, Floyd TF, Wehrli FW. **Quantitative CMR markers of impaired vascular reactivity associated with age and peripheral artery disease.** *J Cardiovasc Magn Reson Imaging.* 2013; **15:**17.
15. Ouriel K, McDonnell AE, Metz CE, Zarins CK. **Critical evaluation of stress testing in the diagnosis of peripheral vascular disease.** *Surgery.* 1982; **91:**686–93.
16. Doobay AV, Anand SS. **Sensitivity and specificity of the ankle-brachial index to predict future cardiovascular outcomes: a systematic review.** *Arterioscler Thromb Vasc Biol.* 2005; **25:**1463–69.
17. Wikström J, Hansen T, Johansson L, Lind L, Ahlström H. **Ankle brachial index <0.9 underestimates the prevalence of peripheral artery occlusive disease assessed with whole-body magnetic resonance angiography in the elderly.** *Acta Radiol.* 2008; **49:**143–49.
18. Maroules CD, Rosero E, Ayers C, Peshock RM, Khera A. **Abdominal aortic atherosclerosis at MR imaging is associated with cardiovascular events: the Dallas heart study.** *Radiology.* 2013; **269:**84–91.
19. Laurent S, Katsahian S, Fassot C, Tropeano AI, Gautier I, Laloux B, Boutouyrie P. **Aortic stiffness is an independent predictor of fatal stroke in essential hypertension.** *Stroke.* 2003; **34:**1203–06.
20. Blacher J, Guerin A, Pannier P, Marchais SJ, Safar ME, London GM. **Impact of Aortic Stiffness on Survival in End-Stage Renal Disease.** *Circulation.* 1999; **99:**2434–39.
21. Sutton-Tyrrell K, Najjar S, Boudreau R, Venkitachalam L, Kupelian V, Simonsick EM, Havlik R, Lakatta EG, Spurgeon H, Kritchevsky S, Pahor M, Bauer D, Newman A. **Elevated Aortic Pulse Wave Velocity, a Marker of Arterial Stiffness, Predicts Cardiovascular Events in Well-Functioning Older Adults.** *Circulation.* 2005; **111:**3384–90.
22. Zureik M, Temmar M, Adamopoulos C, Bureau JM, Courbon D, Thomas F, Bean K, Touboul PJ, Ducimetière P, Benetos A. **Carotid plaques, but not common carotid-media thickness, are independently associated with aortic stiffness.** *Hypertension.* 2002; **20:**85–93.
23. Turkbey EB, Redheuil A, Backlund JY, Small AC, Cleary PA, Lachin JM, Lima JA, Bluemke DA. **Aortic Distensibility in Type 1 Diabetes.** *Diabetes Care.* 2013; **36:**2380–87.
24. Brandts A, Westenberg J, Van Elderen S, Kroft LJ, Roes SD, Tamsma JT, van der Geest RJ, Lamb HJ, Doornbos J, Putter H, Stuber M, de Roos A. **Site-specific coupling between vascular wall thickness and function.** *Invest Rad.* 2013; **48:**86–91.
25. Taniwaki H, Shoji T, Emoto M, Kawagishi T, Ishimura E, Inaba M, Okuno Y, Nishizawa Y. **Femoral artery wall thickness and stiffness in evaluation of peripheral vascular disease in type 2 diabetes mellitus.** *Atherosclerosis.* 2001; **158:**207–14.
26. Westenberg JJ, Van Poelgeest EP, Steendijk P, Grotenhuis HB, Jukema JW, de Roos A. **Bramwell-Hill modeling for local aortic pulse wave velocity estimation: a validation study with velocity-encoded cardiovascular magnetic resonance and invasive pressure assessment.** *J Cardiovasc Magn Reson Imaging.* 2012; **14:**2.
27. Suever JD, Oshinski J, Rojas-Campos E, Huneycutt D, Cardarelli F, Stillman AE, Raggi P. **Reproducibility of pulse wave velocity measurements with phase contrast magnetic resonance and applanation tonometry.** *Int J Cardiovasc Imaging.* 2012; **28:**1141-1146.
28. Crowe LA, Ariff B, Keegan J, Mohiaddin RH, Yang GZ, Hughes AD, McG Thom SA, Firmin DN. **Comparison between three-dimensional volume-selective turbo spin-echo imaging and two-dimensional ultrasound for assessing carotid artery structure and function.** *J Magn Reson Imaging.* 2005; **21:**282–89.

Use of a 1.0 Tesla open scanner for evaluation of pediatric and congenital heart disease

Jimmy C Lu[1,2*], James C Nielsen[3], Layne Morowitz[3], Muzammil Musani[4], Maryam Ghadimi Mahani[2], Prachi P. Agarwal[5], El-Sayed H. Ibrahim[5] and Adam L. Dorfman[1,2]

Abstract

Background: Open cardiovascular magnetic resonance (CMR) scanners offer the potential for imaging patients with claustrophobia or large body size, but at a lower 1.0 Tesla magnetic field. This study aimed to evaluate the efficacy of open CMR for evaluation of pediatric and congenital heart disease.

Methods: This retrospective, cross-sectional study included all patients ≤18 years old or with congenital heart disease who underwent CMR on an open 1.0 Tesla scanner at two centers from 2012–2014. Indications for CMR and clinical questions were extracted from the medical record. Studies were qualitatively graded for image quality and diagnostic utility. In a subset of 25 patients, signal-to-noise (SNR) and contrast-to-noise (CNR) ratios were compared to size- and diagnosis-matched patients with CMR on a 1.5 Tesla scanner.

Results: A total of 65 patients (median 17.3 years old, 60% male) were included. Congenital heart disease was present in 32 (50%), with tetralogy of Fallot and bicuspid aortic valve the most common diagnoses. Open CMR was used due to scheduling/equipment issues in 51 (80%), claustrophobia in 7 (11%), and patient size in 3 (5%); 4 patients with claustrophobia had failed CMR on a different scanner, but completed the study on open CMR without sedation. All patients had good or excellent image quality on black blood, phase contrast, magnetic resonance angiography, and late gadolinium enhancement imaging. There was below average image quality in 3/63 (5%) patients with cine images, and 4/15 (27%) patients with coronary artery imaging. SNR and CNR were decreased in cine and magnetic resonance angiography images compared to 1.5 Tesla. The clinical question was answered adequately in all but 2 patients; 1 patient with a Fontan had artifact from an embolization coil limiting RV volume analysis, and in 1 patient the right coronary artery origin was not well seen.

Conclusions: Open 1.0 Tesla scanners can effectively evaluate pediatric and congenital heart disease, including patients with claustrophobia and larger body size. Despite minor artifacts and differences in SNR and CNR, the majority of clinical questions can be answered adequately, with some limitations with coronary artery imaging. Further evaluation is necessary to optimize protocols and image quality.

Keywords: Open scanner, Congenital heart disease, 1.0 Tesla

* Correspondence: jimmyl@umich.edu
[1]Department of Pediatrics and Communicable Diseases, Division of Pediatric Cardiology, University of Michigan, Ann Arbor, MI, USA
[2]Department of Radiology, Section of Pediatric Radiology, University of Michigan, Ann Arbor, MI, USA
Full list of author information is available at the end of the article

Background

Cardiovascular magnetic resonance (CMR) is an indispensible tool for evaluation of cardiac anatomy and physiology in pediatric and congenital heart disease. CMR is particularly useful for adults with congenital heart disease, in whom acoustic windows often limit the utility of echocardiography [1, 2]. However, this population may be at increased risk for obesity [3, 4], which can limit use of CMR. Short bore 1.5 Tesla scanners, the primary tool in this population, or 3.0 Tesla scanners can be limited by patient size and difficulty with claustrophobia, as patients must lie still within a circumferential bore. "Open" scanners allow more room to the sides of the patient, and may be more tolerable for patients with claustrophobia or larger body size [5]. At a lower magnetic field of 1.0 Tesla, there are also theoretical advantages, e.g. lower specific absorption rate (SAR) and less B1 shading artifact. However, there is a paucity of data regarding application of 1.0 Tesla scanners in pediatric and congenital heart disease [6, 7], and it is unclear whether the lower magnetic field and signal to noise ratio is adequate to evaluate pediatric patients with smaller body size, or adult congenital heart disease patients, with more complicated cardiac anatomy. This retrospective study aimed to evaluate the efficacy of open scanners in this population.

Methods

Patient selection

This multicenter retrospective cohort study included all patients who underwent CMR for evaluation of pediatric or congenital heart disease on an open scanner at Stony Brook University or the University of Michigan C.S. Mott Children's Hospital, between 2/8/2012 and 7/24/2014. This study was approved by the Institutional Review Boards at both centers, and requirement for informed consent in this retrospective study was waived. Patients of any age with congenital heart disease were included; patients without congenital heart disease were included if they were 18 years or younger at the time of CMR. Patients were excluded if digital images were not available for review. Medical records were reviewed for patient demographics, indication for the study, and reason for performing the study on the open scanner.

For quantitative comparison of signal-to-noise ratio (SNR) and contrast-to-noise ratio (CNR), a subset of 25 CMR studies were matched 1:1 by patient body surface area and diagnosis with CMR studies performed on a 1.5 Tesla scanner at the same institution. It should be noted that SNR and CNR depend on a number of imaging parameters, including voxel size, acceleration factor, readout bandwidth, and number of averages. Therefore, imaging parameters on both scanners are summarized in Table 1.

CMR imaging

CMR was performed with a Panorama High Field Open 1.0 Tesla scanner (Philips, Best, The Netherlands), using a solenoid body coil (medium, large or extra large as appropriate for patient size). Gradient amplitude is 28 mT/m; maximum slew rate is 120 mT/m/ms. Sensitivity encoding (SENSE) was not used for image acquisition, i.e. SENSE acceleration factor = 1, to maintain adequate signal-to-noise ratio (SNR). Typical imaging parameters are presented in Table 1, with some minor differences by center. Cine imaging was performed with a breathhold, electrocardiographic gated, segmented k-space balanced steady-state with free precession (SSFP) sequence. Black blood imaging was performed with a breathhold, electrocardiographic gated, double inversion recovery turbo spin echo sequence. Imaging parameters varied by weighting of the sequence. Phase contrast imaging was performed free-breathing. Magnetic resonance angiogram (MRA) was performed with a T1-weighted fast field echo sequence, after injection of 0.2 mmol/kg of gadoteridol (ProHance, Bracco, Monroe Township, New Jersey) for studies performed at the University of Michigan, or gadopentetate dimeglumine (Magnevist, Bayer, Leverkusen, Germany) for studies performed at Stony Brook University. Two post-contrast dynamics were performed to highlight the anatomy of interest (e.g. pulmonary arteries or aorta) as well as the venous phase. Coronary artery imaging was performed with a respiratory navigator gated, electrocardiographic gated, three-dimensional SSFP sequence. Late gadolinium enhancement (LGE) was performed 12–15 minutes after contrast injection, using a breathhold, electrocardiographic gated, phase-sensitive inversion recovery sequence. In 12 patients at the University of Michigan, LGE imaging was performed with a three-dimensional, respiratory navigator gated, electrocardiographic gated, phase-sensitive inversion recovery sequence, to improve in-plane spatial resolution while maintaining adequate SNR.

CMR at 1.5 Tesla was performed on a commercially available scanner (Ingenia, Philips, Best, The Netherlands), using a phased-array body surface coil. Gradient amplitude is 33 mT/m; maximum slew rate is 200 mT/m/ms. Typical imaging parameters are presented in Table 1. It should be noted that TR was longer on the 1.0 Tesla scanner than the 1.5 Tesla scanner due to the lower gradient performance characteristics (maximum gradient strength and slew rate) of the 1.0 Tesla scanner. Phase contrast imaging was performed free-breathing. MRA was performed with two post-contrast dynamics, which was sufficient to highlight the anatomy of interest, e.g. pulmonary arteries or aorta, as well as the venous phase of the contrast uptake. LGE was performed using a breathhold, electrocardiographic gated, phase-sensitive inversion recovery sequence.

Table 1 Typical imaging parameters at 1.0 Tesla and 1.5 Tesla

	1.0 Tesla	1.5 Tesla
Cine SSFP		
TR (ms)/TE (ms)	4.1-4.4/2.0-2.2	3.1-3.3/1.6
Flip angle (°)	55-60	60
Receive bandwidth (Hz/pixel)	578 or 1014	954
In-plane spatial resolution (mm)	1.9-2.0	1.7-1.9
Slice thickness (mm)	8	8
Phases per cardiac cycle	24-30	30
SENSE	1	2
SAR*	<74-92%	<95%
Black blood		
In-plane spatial resolution (mm)	1.6-1.7	1.2-1.5
Slice thickness (mm)	5-7	4-5
Number of signals averaged	1-2	1
SENSE	1	2
SAR (for proton density)	<34%	<15%
Phase contrast		
TR (ms)/TE (ms)	6.5-6.9/4.1-4.7	3.1-3.3/1.6
Flip angle (°)	12-25	12
Receive bandwidth (Hz/pixel)	318-364	717
In-plane spatial resolution (mm)	2.0-2.2	1.6-1.8
Slice thickness (mm)	6	6
Phases per cardiac cycle	20-40	40
Number of signals averaged	2-3	3
SENSE	1	2
SAR	<2%	<2%
Magnetic resonance angiogram		
TR (ms)/TE (ms)	4.0/1.5	4.8/1.5
Flip angle (°)	40	40
Receive bandwidth (Hz/pixel)	482 or 789	249
In-plane spatial resolution (mm)	1.8-2.2	1.7-1.8
Slice thickness (mm)	3.0-3.4	2.6-2.8
SENSE	1	1.5 AP, 1.5 LR
SAR	<82-92%	<51%
3-dimensional SSFP		
TR (ms)/TE (ms)	5.1-5.5/2.6-2.8	4.3/2.2
Flip angle (°)	90	90
Receive bandwidth (Hz/pixel)	578	618
Isotropic voxel size (mm)	1.9-2.6	1.6
SENSE	1	1.5 AP, 1.5 LR
SAR	<62%	<36%

Table 1 Typical imaging parameters at 1.0 Tesla and 1.5 Tesla *(Continued)*

LGE		
TR (ms)	6.0	6.1
TE (ms)	3.0	3.0
Flip angle (°)	25	25
Receive bandwidth (Hz/pixel)	299 or 495	232
In-plane spatial resolution (mm)	2.0-2.2	1.7-1.8
Slice thickness (mm)	8	8
SENSE	1	1
SAR	<10%	<8%
3-dimensional LGE		
TR (ms)/TE (ms)	5.3/2.6	Not performed
Flip angle (°)	25	
Receive bandwidth (Hz/pixel)	299	
In-plane spatial resolution (mm)	1.9	
Slice thickness (mm)	5	
SAR	<17%	

SSFP, balanced steady-state free precession; TR, repetition time; TE echo time; SENSE, sensitivity encoding; SAR, systemic absorption rate; LGE, late gadolinium enhancement

*SAR measurements are based on level 0 (normal operating mode) with whole body SAR < 2 W/kg

Scan time for both scanners was measured from the start of the first imaging sequence through the final imaging sequence. Thus, this included patient rest time between breath-holds, and potential need to pause during imaging if there was any patient discomfort.

Image analysis

All images were evaluated by a single experienced observer. For each sequence type, image quality was scored qualitatively, taking into consideration resolution, blurring effects, low SNR, delineation of structures, and artifacts, according to a 4-point scale (4 – excellent with no artifacts; 3 – good with minor artifacts; 2 – below average, with significant artifacts affecting interpretation; 1 – poor, nondiagnostic) [8]. Imaging examples are presented in Fig. 1.

Clinical questions were extracted from the medical record, and were categorized as: ventricular size/function, pulmonary artery anatomy, regurgitant fraction, LGE, aortic root dimensions, coronary artery anatomy, aortic arch anatomy, ratio of pulmonary to systemic blood flow (Qp:Qs ratio), and pulmonary venous anatomy. A given study could have multiple clinical questions. Studies were scored for diagnostic utility on a 4-point scale, based on the interpreter's confidence in their ability to answer the specific clinical questions (4 – high confidence of diagnosis; 3 – answers question adequately; 2 – low confidence; 1 – could not answer the clinical question). Ventricular

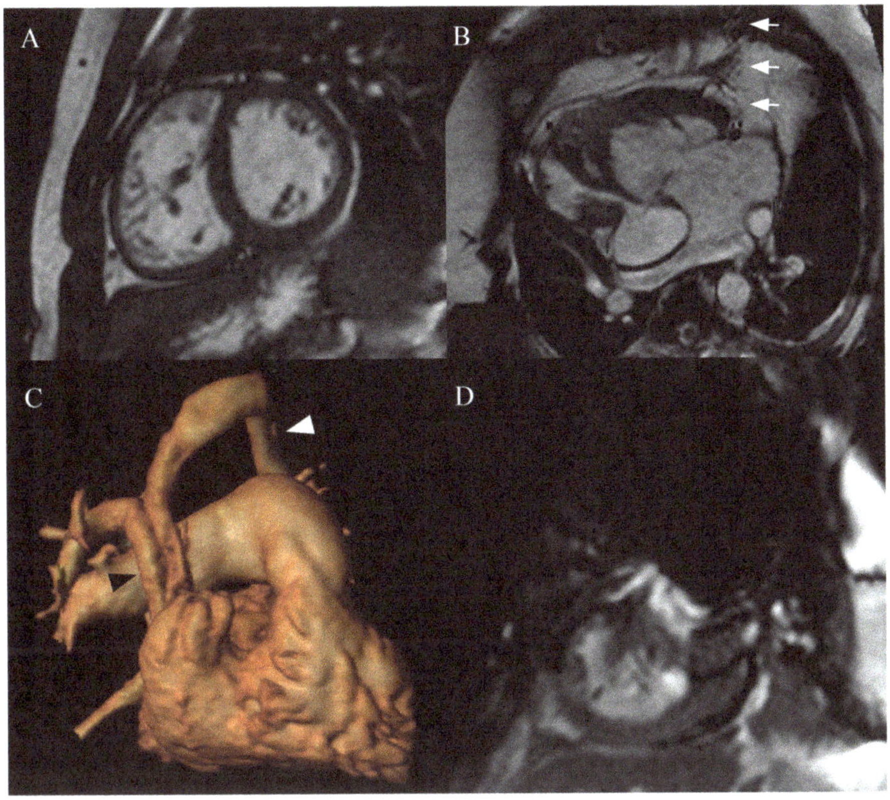

Fig. 1 Images were scored on a 4-point scale for image quality and diagnostic utility. **(a)** SSFP imaging in short-axis in a 26 year-old patient with tetralogy of Fallot and complete atrioventricular septal defect status post repair: No artifacts and good endocardial definition, scored 4 for both quality and diagnostic utility. **(b)** SSFP imaging in the four-chamber plane in a 32 year-old patient with dextrocardia and congenitally corrected transposition of the great arteries, who previously failed CMR on a 1.5 Tesla scanner: Flow-related artifact (arrows), which did not affect interpretation of ventricular size or function, scored 3 for quality, but 4 for diagnostic utility. **(c)** Volume-rendered reconstruction of gadolinium-enhanced MRA in a 57 year-old patient with pulmonary hypertension and reported history of atrial septal defect repair in a foreign country. The left upper pulmonary vein (white arrowhead) drains into the left innominate vein; the right upper and middle veins drain into a baffle within the superior vena cava (black arrowhead) to the left atrium. Scored 4 for both quality and diagnostic utility. **(d)** SSFP imaging in short axis in a 16 year-old patient with unbalanced atrioventricular septal defect status post Fontan: Significant coil artifact, obscuring portions of the heart, scored 2 for both quality and diagnostic utility (for right ventricular size and function)

size/function was scored on the ability to define and contour the endocardial border. Anatomy of the pulmonary arteries, coronary arteries, aortic arch, and pulmonary veins was scored on definition of the respective structures, course, and presence/absence of stenosis as appropriate. Flow measurements were scored by internal consistency of data. LGE images were scored by ability to determine presence or absence of LGE, and extent if present.

Due to the qualitative nature of grading image quality and diagnostic utility, a 20% subset of the cohort was randomly selected to evaluate reproducibility. A second reader, blinded to the scores of the first reader, re-evaluated the images to evaluate interobserver agreement. The initial reader, blinded to initial scores, also re-evaluated the images to evaluate intraobserver agreement.

SNR and CNR were calculated for cine SSFP, black blood, MRA, 3-dimensional SSFP, and LGE images. A region of interest (ROI) of approximately 1.0 cm^2 was drawn in two locations (Fig. 2). For cine SSFP and LGE images, a midventricular short-axis slice was used, and ROIs were drawn in the blood pool and in the interventricular septum. For black blood and 3-dimensional SSFP images, ROIs were drawn in the blood pool and in any adjacent myocardium. For the MRA, the first post-contrast dynamic was used, and ROIs were drawn in the aorta or main pulmonary artery (depending on timing of the contrast) and in the lung field. SNR was defined as the mean signal intensity in the blood pool (for cine SSFP, MRA, 3-dimensional SSFP and LGE images) or myocardium (for black blood images) divided by the standard deviation of signal intensity in that ROI [9]. CNR was defined as the difference in signal intensities of the two ROIs, divided by the average of the standard deviations of the two ROIs [9].

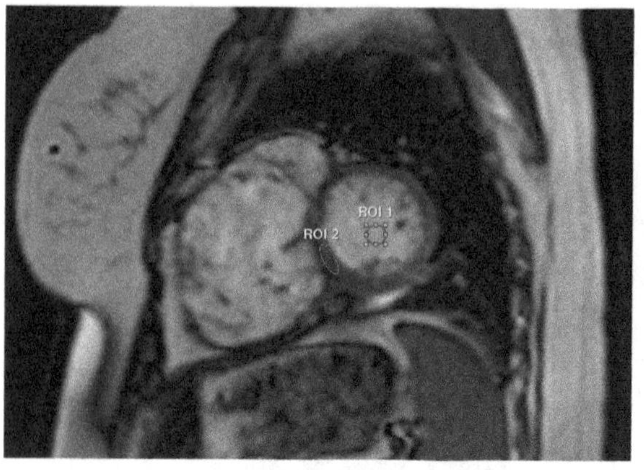

Fig. 2 Regions of interest for contrast to noise measurement. For cine images, an ROI of ~1.0 cm^2 was drawn in the blood pool and in the septum. Only ROI1 (the blood pool) was used for signal to noise ratio measurement

Table 2 Demographic data (N = 65)

Age (years)	17.3 (14.7-20.9)
Male gender	39 (60%)
Height (cm)	166 (154–175)
Weight (kg)	71.0 (60.5-87.7)
Body surface area (m^2)	1.83 (1.67-2.04)
Diagnosis of congenital heart disease	33 (51%)
Tetralogy of Fallot s/p repair	8
Bicuspid aortic valve	6
Aortic stenosis	4
Coarctation s/p repair	2
Ebstein anomaly	2
Partial anomalous pulmonary venous connections	2
Pulmonary stenosis	2
Other	7
Indications for CMR	
Left ventricular size/function	53 (82%)
Right ventricular size/function	26 (40%)
Regurgitant fraction	23 (35%)
Pulmonary artery anatomy	16 (25%)
Aortic root dimensions	15 (23%)
Late gadolinium enhancement	15 (23%)
Coronary artery anatomy	12 (18%)
Aortic arch anatomy	10 (15%)
Qp:Qs ratio	7 (11%)
Pulmonary venous anatomy	4 (6%)
Reason for open scanner	
Scheduling/equipment issue	52 (80%)
Claustrophobia	7 (11%)
Patient size	3 (5%)
Unspecified	3 (5%)

Data given as median (IQR) or number (percent). Qp:Qs, ratio of pulmonary to systemic blood flow

Statistical analysis

Data are presented as median (interquartile range [IQR]), mean ± standard deviation, or number (percent), as appropriate. SNR, CNR, and scan time on 1.0 Tesla and 1.5 Tesla studies were compared for each sequence using t-test. Age and body surface area among patients on 1.0 Tesla and 1.5 Tesla patients were not normally distributed, and were compared using Wilcoxon matched-pairs signed rank test. A p-value < 0.05 was considered statistically significant. Intraobserver and interobserver agreement was calculated using weighted kappa, to take into consideration closeness of agreement.

Results

A total of 65 patients were included, with demographic data presented in Table 2. The majority of the patients were adolescents and adults, with 6 patients under the age of 10, and the youngest 3.5 years old. Patients were referred to the open scanner primarily due to scheduling reasons, although 10 (15%) were referred for claustrophobia or patient size. Among patients referred for claustrophobia or body size, 4 had failed a previous attempt on a 1.5 Tesla scanner; all 4 patients successfully completed the study on the open scanner, without sedation. Of the remaining 6 patients, 4 were referred for first CMR on the open scanner; 2 had previously had a successful scan on a standard scanner. Only 2 patients in this cohort required sedation, due to age or developmental delay. Apart from sternal wires (20/65 patients, 31%), implanted metal objects were rare (1 with an embolization coil, 1 with a pulmonary artery stent, 1 with Harrington rods). Mean scan time was 54.1 ± 22.4 minutes. In the matched cohort of 1.0 Tesla and 1.5 Tesla patients, there was no significant difference in scan time (58.9 ± 20.9 vs. 51.7 ± 12.7 min, p = 0.15).

Image quality

All patients had good or excellent image quality on black blood, phase contrast, MRA, and LGE imaging (Fig. 3). There was below average image quality in 3/63 (5%) patients with cine images, and 4/15 (27%) patients with coronary artery imaging; all other sequences had at least good image quality in all patients. No sequences were rated as poor/nondiagnostic. Intraobserver agreement for grading image quality was good, with weighted kappa of 0.73. Interobserver agreement was fair, with weighted kappa of 0.32. The majority of disagreement was in differentiating between good and excellent image quality; the raters had 85% agreement in differentiating image quality 2 from values of 3–4.

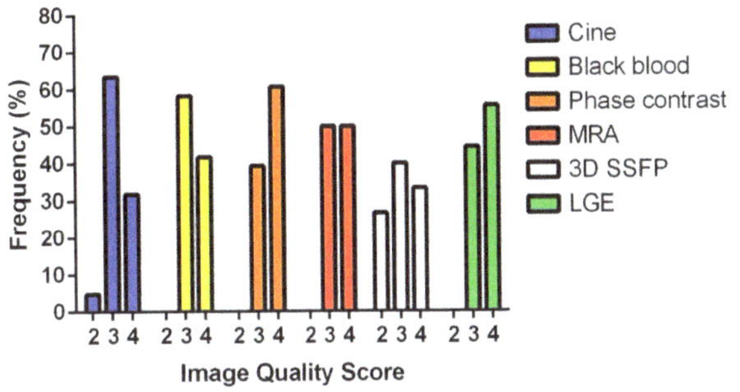

Fig. 3 Histogram of image quality score, by imaging sequence. MRA, magnetic resonance angiogram. 3D SSFP, three-dimensional steady state free precession. LGE, late gadolinium enhancement

In the subset of 25 patients for SNR and CNR analysis, there was no difference between patients on the 1.0 Tesla and 1.5 Tesla scanners in age (median 20.6, IQR 15.4-34.9, vs. 22.4, IQR 16.0-22.2, $p = 0.60$) or body surface area (1.83, IQR 1.62-2.09, vs. 1.84, IQR 1.66-2.07, $p = 0.62$). Both SNR (Fig. 4) and CNR (Fig. 5) were decreased on the open scanner for cine SSFP and MRA images, but similar to the 1.5 Tesla scanner for black blood, 3-dimensional SSFP, and LGE images. Use of 3-dimensional LGE imaging markedly increased SNR (26.5 ± 12.3 vs. 9.0 ± 0.8, $p = 0.004$) and CNR (19.2 ± 5.9 vs. 7.0 ± 1.4, $p = 0.0003$) compared to 2-dimensional LGE imaging at 1.0 Tesla.

Diagnostic utility

The clinical question was answered adequately (score 3+) in all but 2 patients (Fig. 6). In 1 patient status post Fontan procedure, susceptibility artifact due to an embolization coil limited evaluation of right ventricular volume. In 1 patient, the right coronary artery course appeared normal,

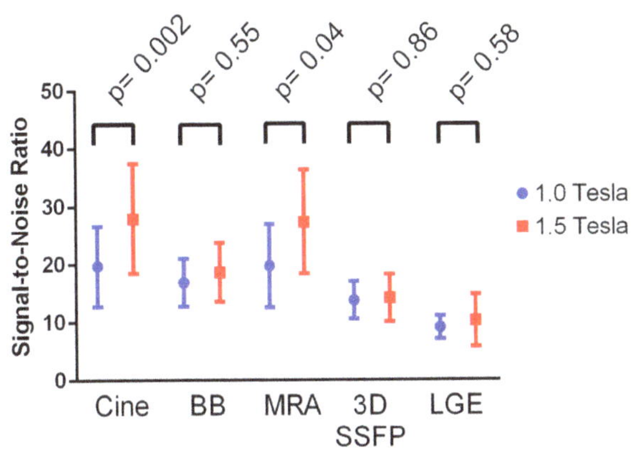

Fig. 4 Signal-to-noise ratio by sequence on 1.0 Tesla open or standard 1.5 Tesla scanner. BB, black blood; MRA, magnetic resonance angiogram; 3D SSFP, 3-dimensional steady state free precession; LGE, late gadolinium enhancement

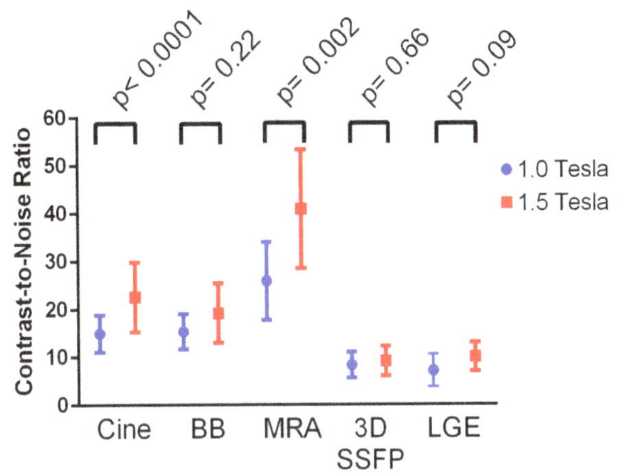

Fig. 5 Contrast-to-noise ratio by sequence on 1.0 Tesla open or standard 1.5 Tesla scanner. BB, black blood; MRA, magnetic resonance angiogram; 3D SSFP, 3-dimensional steady state free precession; LGE, late gadolinium enhancement

although the origin was suboptimally visualized; the left coronary artery was normal. No studies were scored as nondiagnostic, and no patients required callback for re-evaluation on a different scanner. Intraobserver and interobserver agreement for grading diagnostic utility was good, with weighted kappa 0.85 and 0.61, respectively. Again, the vast majority of disagreement was differentiating whether the clinical question was answered adequately or confidently; there was 97% agreement in differentiating score 2 from score 3–4.

Discussion

Open 1.0 Tesla scanners can be effective for evaluation of selected groups of patients with pediatric and congenital heart disease. Despite minor artifacts and decreased SNR and CNR, the majority of clinical questions can be answered adequately. To our knowledge, this is the first systematic report of CMR at 1.0 Tesla in the pediatric and congenital heart disease population.

The primary advantage of open scanners is the ability to increase the population eligible for CMR, including patients with larger body size or claustrophobia. A prior study demonstrated decreased anxiety in claustrophobic patients undergoing open CMR [5], although a randomized controlled trial demonstrated a significant persistent rate of claustrophobic events in the open scanner [10]. These studies included primarily patients with magnetic resonance imaging of other body parts; patients undergoing CMR, who must have the torso within the bore, could potentially be at higher risk for failure of CMR in a closed bore scanner. Although limited to a small subset of this cohort, the current results are promising, as all 4 patients who had failed a prior scan on a closed bore scanner completed the study on the open

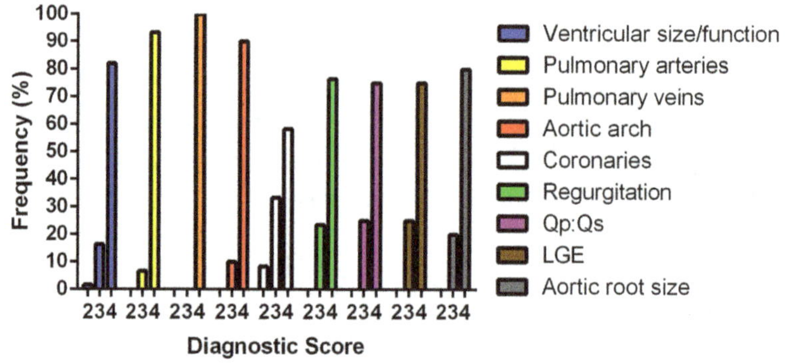

Fig. 6 Histogram of diagnostic utility, by clinical question. Qp:Qs, ratio of pulmonary to systemic blood flow. LGE, late gadolinium enhancement

scanner without sedation. Prospective identification of patients who may benefit from the open scanner could prevent lost scanner time or need to reschedule.

In this cohort, the majority of patients were referred to the open scanner due to scheduling or equipment issues, suggesting the primary practical advantage may be availability of scanner time. However, the diagnostic success of open CMR studies in this cohort confirms that selected patients in this population can appropriately take advantage of this scanner. Further work is needed to identify additional populations that can appropriately take advantage of open scanner availability.

Due to the lower magnetic field, signal to noise ratio suffers, and modifications to existing protocols are necessary to optimize image quality. De Bucourt and colleagues reported decreased SNR and CNR in extremely obese patients with an open 1.0 Tesla scanner [11]. However, this study used the integrated body coil, rather than the standard body coil, which was used for regular weight control patients. All patients in the current study used the standard body coil, which may partially explain more similar SNR and CNR in some sequences to studies at 1.5 Tesla. Furthermore, techniques to maximize signal, such as increased voxel size, avoidance of parallel imaging [12], and multiple signal averaging may partially offset differences due to magnetic field strength, at the cost of scan time and spatial resolution. In this cohort, studies on the 1.0 Tesla scanner had lower spatial resolution with more frequent usage of multiple signal averaging, without parallel imaging. By adjusting these parameters, SNR and CNR were actually similar among 1.0 Tesla and 1.5 Tesla scanners for black blood, 3-dimensional SSFP, and LGE imaging, but remained decreased for cine SSFP images and MRA. SNR and CNR could be further improved for LGE imaging with a 3-dimensional sequence, which is consistent with prior data at 1.5 Tesla [13]. Further evaluation is necessary for optimization of image quality, to minimize potential for diagnostic error. Furthermore, more technical and quantitative analysis may be necessary particularly for phase contrast data. Longer echo time has been shown to increase risk for error in flow measurements, due to intravoxel dephasing, particularly with stenotic jets [14-16]. This retrospective study did not allow for direct comparison of flow measurements in the same patients at 1.0 Tesla and 1.5 Tesla.

Despite some differences in image quality, the diagnostic score best reflects the clinical potential of the open scanner. Pertinent clinical findings were still detectable, particularly when the focus was ventricular size and systolic function. However, further optimization remains necessary, particularly for coronary artery imaging, which was the most limited of the indications in this study, or when evaluating small vessels. This cohort included few small children; further study is necessary, but patient selection based on clinical indication may be necessary.

This study has several limitations. Retrospective chart review is limited by documentation for determining reasons for the study or reasons for using the open scanner. However, only 3 patients did not have an identified reason for the open scanner. The retrospective nature of this study also prevented standardization of the imaging protocols, particularly between centers; further prospective study is necessary to optimize imaging parameters at 1.0 Tesla. This cohort consisted primarily of adolescents and adults, which may reflect selection bias. Although extrapolation to younger patients may not be appropriate, this does highlight that this population may benefit from use of the open scanner. This cohort cannot address whether need for sedation in smaller children can be lessened with the open scanner. The small sample size limits power to detect small differences in SNR and CNR, and verification in a larger cohort is necessary.

Conclusions

Open 1.0 Tesla scanners can successfully evaluate pediatric and congenital heart disease in selected patients. Despite some differences in image quality, SNR and CNR, the vast majority of studies were adequate to answer the clinical questions. Further work is necessary to optimize protocols for these indications, and to better define patient characteristics appropriate to this scanner. Use of the open scanner in this population could increase the potential cohort who can tolerate CMR without sedation or discomfort.

Competing interests

The authors declare that they have no competing interests.

Authors' contributions

JCL conceived of the study, participated in its design and coordination, analyzed the images, performed the statistical analysis, and helped to draft the manuscript. JCN participated in study design and coordination. LM and MM extracted demographic data and clinical indications. MGM and PPA assisted with study design and data collection. El-SHI assisted in interpretation of the data. ALD conceived of the study, participated in its design, and helped to draft the manuscript. All authors critically reviewed and approved the final manuscript.

Acknowledgements

This work had no external funding.

Author details

[1]Department of Pediatrics and Communicable Diseases, Division of Pediatric Cardiology, University of Michigan, Ann Arbor, MI, USA. [2]Department of Radiology, Section of Pediatric Radiology, University of Michigan, Ann Arbor, MI, USA. [3]Departments of Pediatrics and Radiology, Stony Brook University, Stony Brook, NY, USA. [4]Department of Medicine, Division of Cardiology, Stony Brook University, Stony Brook, NY, USA. [5]Department of Radiology, Division of Cardiothoracic Radiology, University of Michigan, Ann Arbor, MI, USA.

References

1. Valente AM, Cook S, Festa P, Ko HH, Krishnamurthy R, Taylor AM, et al. Multimodality imaging guidelines for patients with repaired tetralogy of fallot: a report from the American society of echocardiography: developed in collaboration with the society for cardiovascular magnetic resonance and the society for pediatric radiology. J Am Soc Echocardiogr. 2014;27:111–41.
2. Warnes CA, Williams RG, Bashore TM, Child JS, Connolly HM, Dearani JA, et al. ACC/AHA 2008 guidelines for the management of adults with congenital heart disease: a report of the American college of cardiology/ American heart association task force on practice guidelines (writing committee to develop guidelines on the management of adults with congenital heart disease). Circulation. 2008;118:e714–833.
3. Pemberton VL, McCrindle BW, Barkin S, Daniels SR, Barlow SE, Binns HJ, et al. Report of the national heart, lung, and blood Institute's working group on obesity and other cardiovascular risk factors in congenital heart disease. Circulation. 2010;121:1153–9.
4. Smith-Parrish M, Yu S, Rocchini A. Obesity and elevated blood pressure following repair of coarctation of the aorta. J Pediatr. 2014;164:1074–8.
5. Bangard C, Paszek J, Berg F, Eyl G, Kessler J, Lackner K, et al. MR imaging of claustrophobic patients in an open 1.0T scanner: motion artifacts and patient acceptability compared with closed bore magnets. Eur J Radiol. 2007;64:152–7.
6. Rupprecht T, Nitz W, Wagner M, Kreissler P, Rascher W, Hofbeck M. Determination of the pressure gradient in children with coarctation of the aorta by low-field magnetic resonance imaging. Pediatr Cardiol. 2002;23:127–31.
7. Tzifa A, Komnou A, Loggitsi D. Cardiac magnetic resonance imaging in a premature baby with interrupted aortic arch and aortopulmonary window. Cardiol Young. 2013;23:742–5.
8. Naehle CP, Kreuz J, Strach K, Schwab JO, Pingel S, Luechinger R, et al. Safety, feasibility, and diagnostic value of cardiac magnetic resonance imaging in patients with cardiac pacemakers and implantable cardioverters/defibrillators at 1.5 T. Am Heart J. 2011;161:1096–105.
9. Groarke JD, Waller AH, Vita TS, Michaud GF, Di Carli MF, Blankstein R, et al. Feasibility study of electrocardiographic and respiratory gated, gadolinium enhanced magnetic resonance angiography of pulmonary veins and the impact of heart rate and rhythm on study quality. J Cardiovasc Magn Reson. 2014;16:43.
10. Enders J, Zimmermann E, Rief M, Martus P, Klingebiel R, Asbach P, et al. Reduction of claustrophobia with short-bore versus open magnetic resonance imaging: a randomized controlled trial. PLoS One. 2011;6:e23494.
11. De Bucourt M, Streitparth F, Wonneberger U, Rump J, Teichgraber U. Obese patients in an open MRI at 1.0 Tesla: image quality, diagnostic impact and feasibility. Eur Radiol. 2011;21:1004–15.
12. Biglands JD, Radjenovic A, Ridgway JP. Cardiovascular magnetic resonance physics for clinicians: Part II. J Cardiovasc Magn Reson. 2012;14:66.
13. Peters DC, Appelbaum EA, Nezafat R, Dokhan B, Han Y, Kissinger KV, et al. Left ventricular infarct size, peri-infarct zone, and papillary scar measurements: A comparison of high-resolution 3D and conventional 2D late gadolinium enhancement cardiac MR. J Magn Reson Imaging. 2009;30:794–800.
14. O'Brien KR, Gabriel RS, Greiser A, Cowan BR, Young AA, Kerr AJ. Aortic valve stenotic area calculation from phase contrast cardiovascular magnetic resonance: the importance of short echo time. J Cardiovasc Magn Reson. 2009;11:49.
15. O'Brien KR, Cowan BR, Jain M, Stewart RA, Kerr AJ, Young AA. MRI phase contrast velocity and flow errors in turbulent stenotic jets. J Magn Reson Imaging. 2008;28:210–8.
16. Stahlberg F, Sondergaard L, Thomsen C, Henriksen O. Quantification of complex flow using MR phase imaging–a study of parameters influencing the phase/velocity relation. Magn Reson Imaging. 1992;10:13–23.

19

Measurement of myocardial blood flow by cardiovascular magnetic resonance perfusion: comparison of distributed parameter and Fermi models with single and dual bolus

Giorgos Papanastasiou[1,2*], Michelle C Williams[2], Lucy E Kershaw[3], Marc R Dweck[2], Shirjel Alam[2], Saeed Mirsadraee[1], Martin Connell[1], Calum Gray[1], Tom MacGillivray[1], David E Newby[1,2] and Scott IK Semple[1,2]

Abstract

Background: Mathematical modeling of cardiovascular magnetic resonance perfusion data allows absolute quantification of myocardial blood flow. Saturation of left ventricle signal during standard contrast administration can compromise the input function used when applying these models. This saturation effect is evident during application of standard Fermi models in single bolus perfusion data. Dual bolus injection protocols have been suggested to eliminate saturation but are much less practical in the clinical setting. The distributed parameter model can also be used for absolute quantification but has not been applied in patients with coronary artery disease. We assessed whether distributed parameter modeling might be less dependent on arterial input function saturation than Fermi modeling in healthy volunteers. We validated the accuracy of each model in detecting reduced myocardial blood flow in stenotic vessels versus gold-standard invasive methods.

Methods: Eight healthy subjects were scanned using a dual bolus cardiac perfusion protocol at 3T. We performed both single and dual bolus analysis of these data using the distributed parameter and Fermi models. For the dual bolus analysis, a scaled pre-bolus arterial input function was used. In single bolus analysis, the arterial input function was extracted from the main bolus. We also performed analysis using both models of single bolus data obtained from five patients with coronary artery disease and findings were compared against independent invasive coronary angiography and fractional flow reserve. Statistical significance was defined as two-sided P value < 0.05.

Results: Fermi models overestimated myocardial blood flow in healthy volunteers due to arterial input function saturation in single bolus analysis compared to dual bolus analysis (P < 0.05). No difference was observed in these volunteers when applying distributed parameter-myocardial blood flow between single and dual bolus analysis. In patients, distributed parameter modeling was able to detect reduced myocardial blood flow at stress (<2.5 mL/min/mL of tissue) in all 12 stenotic vessels compared to only 9 for Fermi modeling.

Conclusions: Comparison of single bolus versus dual bolus values suggests that distributed parameter modeling is less dependent on arterial input function saturation than Fermi modeling. Distributed parameter modeling showed excellent accuracy in detecting reduced myocardial blood flow in all stenotic vessels.

Keywords: Cardiovascular magnetic resonance, Myocardial blood flow, Fermi modeling, Distributed parameter modeling, Fractional flow reserve, Invasive coronary angiography

* Correspondence: G.Papanastasiou@ed.ac.uk
[1]Clinical Research Imaging Centre, University of Edinburgh,, Edinburgh, UK
[2]Centre for Cardiovascular Science, University of Edinburgh, Edinburgh, UK
Full list of author information is available at the end of the article

Background

Mathematical modeling of cardiovascular magnetic resonance perfusion (CMR) has the potential to allow quantitative assessment of myocardial blood flow [1,2]. Establishing absolute quantification of blood flow could have clinical benefits since it may lead to an improvement in the diagnosis and prognostication of patients with coronary artery disease [3-6].

Myocardial blood flow quantification using model-dependent analysis is based on fitting the convolution of a model with the arterial input function to the tissue contrast agent concentration-time curve. The model describes the passage of a contrast agent through the myocardium whilst the arterial input function is the observed contrast agent concentration-time curve derived from the blood pool [3]. Fermi deconvolution modeling is a popular approach used to estimate myocardial blood flow during the first-pass of gadolinium-based extracellular contrast agents (CA) [3,7,8]. It is an empirical-mathematical model, which is convolved with the first-pass of the arterial input function [3]. The distributed parameter model assumes that the extravascular-extracellular space exchanges CA with nearby regions in the intravascular space, restricting axial transport of CA inside the extravascular-extracellular space [4]. In addition to myocardial blood flow, this model can also be used to calculate other microvascular characteristics including intravascular space, extravascular-extracellular space, permeability surface area product, extraction fraction and volume of distribution [9].

The high concentration of CA during bolus passage leads to signal saturation and causes concentration underestimation in the left ventricular cavity [10] (which is used to generate an arterial input function for model deconvolution analysis). This can degrade the accuracy and reproducibility of myocardial blood flow quantification using Fermi modeling, leading to systematic myocardial blood flow overestimation [3]. The dual bolus acquisition technique can eliminate signal saturation allowing more reliable quantification of myocardial blood flow in first-pass magnetic resonance perfusion imaging. In the dual bolus technique, an initial injection of dilute CA is used to acquire a non-saturated arterial input function before the main CA bolus. This is commonly referred to as the "pre-bolus" [11,12]. However, compared to single bolus protocols [1-3,7-9], dual bolus imaging protocols are characterized by increased complexity both in image acquisition and data analysis [3,10-12].

In the present study, we compared single and dual bolus estimates of myocardial blood flow in healthy volunteers using both distributed parameter and Fermi models. We also assessed whether these models can reliably detect areas with reduced myocardial blood flow compared to a clinical gold standard of invasive coronary angiography and fractional flow reserve in patients with coronary artery disease.

Methods

Study population

Eight healthy volunteers with no previous history of cardiovascular or renal disease, diabetes mellitus, asthma or any other clinically significant illness and five patients with suspected coronary artery disease were recruited into the study. Exclusion criteria included severely compromised renal function (estimated glomerular filtration rate <30 mL/min) and contraindications to magnetic resonance imaging. The study was performed with the approval of the local research ethics committee, in accordance with the Declaration of Helsinki and with the written informed consent of all subjects. Prior to CMR perfusion, all subjects were asked to refrain from caffeine for 12 hours.

Image acquisition

All data were acquired using a 3T Verio system (Siemens AG, Healthcare Sector, Erlangen, Germany). Standard cardiac imaging planes and a short axis stack of left ventricular cine data were acquired using routine steady state free precession (TrueFISP) acquisitions. Native T_1 relaxation rates (i.e. in the absence of CA) were calculated using the modified Look-Locker inversion (MOLLI) recovery technique [13]. Stress imaging was performed by intravenous infusion of 140 μg/kg/min of adenosine (Adenoscan, Sanofi Aventis). Fifty dynamic perfusion images were obtained at diastole across three short-axis view slices: basal, mid-ventricular and apical slices according to the standard 16-segment heart model [14]. Perfusion images were acquired using a turbo-fast low angle shot (FLASH) saturation recovery prepared single-shot gradient echo pulse sequence (repetition time/ echo time 2.20 ms/1.07 ms, flip angle 12°, slice thickness 8 mm, preparation pulse delay (PD) to central line of k-space 100 ms, matrix size 192 × 108 and FoV 330 mm × 440 mm). With the application of GRAPPA (accelerator factor of 3) and partial Fourier acquisition of 0.75, each dynamic frame consisted of 48-phase encoded lines. All CMR perfusion data were acquired using electrocardiogram-gating.

Contrast agent bolus administration

In single bolus imaging, 0.05 mmol/kg of CA (Gadovist, Bayer Healthcare) was injected intravenously after 4 min of adenosine infusion, followed by 20 mL of 0.9% saline (Medrad Spectris Solaris, Medrad, USA) at 4 mL/s [3]. All patients with coronary artery disease were imaged using the single bolus protocol.

In the healthy volunteer cohort, an additional pre-bolus infusion was administered to allow dual bolus modeling to be applied without the risk of signal saturation in the arterial input function. In this dual bolus protocol, the two boluses were injected in a predetermined concentration ratio (pre-bolus:main bolus, 1:5) with the pre-bolus diluted using 0.9% saline. After 3.5 min of adenosine infusion, the pre-bolus of 0.006 mmol/kg CA was injected and adenosine was continued until the main bolus of 0.03 mmol/kg had also been administered. The pre-bolus allows determination of the arterial input function whilst the main bolus allows measurement of myocardial CA concentration curves [15]. To allow clearance of residual CA, the rest perfusion imaging was performed 15 min after the adenosine-stress scan with the same acquisition protocol in all subjects [3,7,8,15].

Invasive coronary angiography and fractional flow reserve

All five patients underwent invasive coronary angiography at the Royal Infirmary of Edinburgh. Fractional flow reserve was assessed for major epicardial vessels and defined as the ratio between distal coronary pressure and aortic pressure measured simultaneously at maximal adenosine-induced (intravenous 140μg/kg/min) hyperaemia [16,17]. Haemodynamically significant coronary artery disease was defined as luminal stenosis ≥70% on invasive coronary angiography, or fractional flow reserve < 0.80 and luminal stenosis ≥50 %. Outcomes from the three main coronary vessels were classified into 3 groups: Group 1, no or minor coronary artery disease with luminal stenosis <50%; Group 2, non-obstructive coronary artery disease with luminal stenosis ≥50% and fractional flow reserve > 0.80; and Group 3, obstructive coronary artery disease with luminal stenosis of ≥70% alone, or luminal stenosis ≥50% and fractional flow reserve ≤ 0.80 [16,17].

Cardiac contouring

Endocardial and epicardial contours were manually defined on the short axis magnetic resonance perfusion imaging data using dedicated cardiac image analysis software (QMass, Medis, The Netherlands) to generate a standardised 16-segment model of the heart [14]. Myocardial blood flow analysis was performed per myocardial segment. The signal intensity of the arterial input function was extracted from the left ventricular cavity excluding papillary muscles using customised in-house software created in Matlab (MathWorks Inc., Natick, MA) [18].

All arterial input function curves were extracted from the basal slice [3,7]. In single bolus analysis, the arterial input function was extracted from the standard (main bolus) CA dose component. For the dual bolus analysis in healthy subjects, the pre-bolus arterial input function was scaled and used for deconvolution analysis [3,11,15].

Image processing

To correct for signal saturation, myocardial and arterial input function signal intensity-time curves were converted to CA concentration-time curves using the method of Larsson *et al* [19], as described previously [3,7-9,11,12,19,20]. This method is based on the assumption that in a region of interest, the longitudinal relaxation rate R_1 $(1/T_1)$ changes linearly as a function of contrast agent concentration influx c(t) at time t multiplied by its relaxivity r_1 according to the following equation:

$$\frac{1}{T_1(t)} - \frac{1}{T_1(0)} = r1 \cdot c(t), \tag{1}$$

where $T_1(0)$ is the native longitudinal relaxation rate and $T_1(t)$ is the longitudinal relaxation rate at time t of contrast enhancement. By substituting $\Delta R_1 \frac{1}{T_1(t)} - \frac{1}{T_1(0)}$, equation (1) can be re-written as:

$$c(t) = \frac{\Delta R_1}{r_1} \tag{2}$$

In the above set of equations, $T_1(t)$ is unknown and can be calculated by adapting the MR signal equation for the saturation recovery prepared single-shot FLASH sequence as follows [3,7,19]:

$$SI = \psi \cdot \left[\left(1 - e^{-PD \cdot R_1}\right) \cdot a^{n-1} + b \cdot \frac{1-a}{1-a} \right] \tag{3}$$

where SI is the signal intensity, Ψ is a calibration constant dependent on receiver gain, instrumental conditions, proton density and α. PD is the pre-pulse delay which is the time between saturation pulse and the central line of k-space, $a = \cos(\alpha) \cdot e^{-TR \cdot R_1}$ and $b = 1 - e^{-TR \cdot R_1}$. TR is the time interval between repetitive α-radiofrequency pulses. Ψ is assumed to be constant throughout the dynamic perfusion image acquisition [19] and was initially calculated from equation (3) by using native T_1 and signal intensities derived from a region of interest (i.e. myocardial segment, arterial input function) in the absence of CA. $T_1(t)$ at time t of contrast enhancement was then calculated from equation (3) using Ψ and signal intensity values extracted from the same region of interest in each of the dynamic perfusion images. CA concentration-time curves were then calculated using equation (2).

Model equations

The model equations used for data fitting are summarized in Table 1. These equations represent the tissue impulse response R(t) the shape of which is determined by the fitted parameters [3]. To quantify myocardial blood flow and other parameters generated by the Fermi and distributed parameter models, we used model-constrained deconvolution [3,7,9]. The Fermi model was fitted in the time domain whilst the distributed parameter model was fitted in the Laplace domain in order to avoid discontinuities of the time step-function that can be present when fitting the distributed parameter model in the time domain [9,21]. We fitted the convolution of the Fermi function with the first-pass of the arterial input function, setting the end-point at the CA concentration minimum before the recirculation component begins (this range varies from patient to patient but is commonly in the range between 20-35 dynamic frames). We also fitted the convolution of the distributed parameter function with the entire CA concentration time course of the arterial input function (i.e. 50 dynamic frames per slice). To further investigate the behaviour of distributed parameter modeling in single and dual bolus analysis, we also fitted the convolution of the distributed parameter model with the first-pass of the arterial input function using the same number of time points as in Fermi modeling. All additional microvascular parameters were calculated using the relationships described in Table 2 [4,9].

A haematocrit value of 0.45 was assumed in order to convert myocardial blood flow into plasma flow which was used to calculate permeability surface area product, extraction fraction, extravascular-extracellular space and volume of distribution. Both models were fitted using a constrained nonlinear optimization (fmincon) in Matlab [22]. Myocardial perfusion reserve (myocardial blood flow at stress/ myocardial blood flow at rest) was calculated for all healthy volunteer data. Consistent with previous cardiac perfusion studies, vessel territories in patients with hyperaemic myocardial blood flow values less than 2.5 mL/min/mL of tissue were considered as regions with reduced myocardial blood flow [5,6].

Statistical analysis

The R software was used for statistical analysis (R Foundation for statistical computing, Vienna, Austria). Identification of any systematic bias between dual bolus and single bolus modeling estimates was performed using Bland Altman plots for both models. Statistical differences were investigated between Fermi and distributed parameter modeling, between distributed parameter and first-pass distributed parameter modeling, between stress and rest modeling values as well as between dual and single bolus analysis by implementing a paired *t*-test. A Welch two sample *t*-test was used to investigate statistical differences in myocardial blood flow values between the different groups (Groups 1-3) classified at the time of invasive coronary angiography.

Homogeneity of variances was verified using a Fisher's F-test. Comparison of mean myocardial blood flow and physiological parameters estimates in vessel territories of patients versus overall mean values in healthy volunteers was investigated using one sample *t*-test. Statistical significance was defined as two-sided P value < 0.05.

Results

The distributed parameter model was fitted in 8 healthy volunteers and 5 patients with coronary artery disease. Example images are shown in Figure 1. We generated 416 CA concentration-time curves in 13 subjects (16 myocardial segments per subject both at stress and rest). Distributed parameter model fits were successful in 398 CA concentration-time curves and non-convergent in 7 myocardial segments of one volunteer at stress, in 5 myocardial segments of one volunteer at rest and in 6 segments of one patient at stress. The Fermi model successfully fitted all CA concentration-time courses.

Comparison of Fermi and distributed parameter models in healthy volunteers

We initially fitted the Fermi and distributed parameter models to CA concentration-time curves for our healthy volunteer population using arterial input functions derived from the main bolus data. Examples of Fermi and distributed parameter model fits at rest and stress are presented in Figure 2. Examples of pre-bolus and main bolus arterial input functions are shown in Figure 3. Fermi-derived myocardial blood flow values were higher than distributed parameter-derived myocardial blood flow values for both stress and rest ($P = 0.0005$ and $P = 0.007$ respectively, Table 3).

Table 1 Model equations

Model	Fitted parameters	Fitting domain	Tissue impulse response R
Distributed parameter	Myocardial blood flow, T, T_c, T_e	Laplace	$R(s) = \frac{1 - \exp[-s \cdot (T + s \cdot T_c \cdot T_e)/(1 + s \cdot T_e)]}{s}$
Fermi	Myocardial blood flow, τ_0, k	Time	$R(t) = \frac{1}{\exp[(t - \tau_0) \cdot k] + 1}$

Fitted parameters for distributed parameter: myocardial blood flow, T is mean overall transit time, T_c is mean capillary transit time, T_e is mean interstitial (i.e. extravascular-extracellular) transit time. Where $s = i \cdot 2 \cdot \pi \cdot f$ and f is the frequency variable in the Fourier transformed data. Fitted parameters for Fermi: myocardial blood flow, τ_0 characterized the width of the shoulder of the Fermi function and k determined the decay rate of R(t) due to contrast agent wash-out. t is the time variable.

Table 2 Microvascular characteristics

Microvascular characteristics	Equation
v_b	$v_b = MBF \cdot T_c$
v_e	$v_e = MBF \cdot (T - T_c)$
v_d	$v_d = MBF \cdot T$
PS	$PS = \frac{MBF \cdot (T - T_c)}{Te}$
E	$E = 1 - \exp(-\frac{PS}{MPF})$
MPF	$MPF = MBF \cdot (1 - hct)$

Microvascular characteristics were calculated by incorporating the fitted parameters of the distributed parameter model into the following relationships (see reference [4]). Myocardial plasma flow (MPF) was used to calculate extravascular-extracellular space (v_e), distribution volume (v_d), permeability surface area product (PS) and extraction fraction (E) and myocardial blood flow (MBF) to calculate intravascular space (v_b). Hematocrit: hct.

We subsequently fitted the Fermi and distributed parameter models for our healthy volunteer population, using scaled arterial input functions from their prebolus data. Fermi-derived myocardial blood flow values were again higher than distributed parameter-derived myocardial blood flow values for both stress and rest ($P = 0.03$ and $P = 0.003$ respectively, Table 3).

Mean distributed parameter model-derived myocardial blood flow at stress was not different in dual bolus compared to single bolus analysis ($P = 0.22$) whilst mean Fermi model-derived myocardial blood flow at stress was higher in single bolus versus dual bolus analysis ($P = 0.00003$, Table 3).

Systematic bias of the above comparisons was investigated using Bland Altman method. The average bias was computed as the blood flow values at stress determined in dual bolus minus the relative values determined in the single bolus analysis. For the Fermi model, the average bias was -1.00 with 95% confidence intervals [-1.58, -0.42] and for the distributed parameter model, the average bias value was -0.30 with 95% confidence intervals [-1.61, 0.94].

Mean Fermi and distributed parameter-derived myocardial blood flow at rest did not significantly change between single and dual bolus analysis ($P = 0.07$ for both). The additional distributed parameter estimates were not significantly different in single bolus compared to dual bolus analysis (see values in Additional file 1).

Mean myocardial blood flow was higher during hyperaemia in all healthy volunteers for distributed parameter-dual bolus ($P = 0.00001$), Fermi-dual bolus ($P = 0.0000001$), distributed parameter-single bolus ($P = 0.0000005$), and Fermi-single bolus analysis ($P < 0.0000001$). Mean (SD) myocardial perfusion reserve values were: 2.59 (0.37) for distributed parameter-dual bolus, 2.42 (0.30) for distributed parameter-single bolus, 2.51 (0.48) for Fermi-dual bolus and 2.96 (0.34) for Fermi-single bolus analysis.

To investigate the lack of dependence of the distributed parameter model to arterial input function saturation observed in single bolus data, we also performed first-pass distributed parameter modeling. There was no difference between distributed parameter and first pass distributed parameter myocardial blood flow values ($P = 0.17$ in dual bolus, $P = 0.79$ in single bolus analysis, Table 3). No difference was observed in first-pass distributed parameter-derived myocardial blood flow values between single and dual bolus analysis, for both stress ($P = 0.31$) and rest ($P = 0.16$) (Table 3).

Distributed parameter and Fermi analysis in patients with coronary artery disease

Invasive coronary angiography and fractional flow reserve identified 7 vessels with obstructive lesions (Group 3), 5 vessels with non-obstructive lesions (Group 2) and 3 vessels with no or minor coronary artery disease (Group 1).

Mean myocardial blood flow values were calculated in vessel territories of the three main coronary arteries for each patient using both models (Table 4, Figure 2e and f).

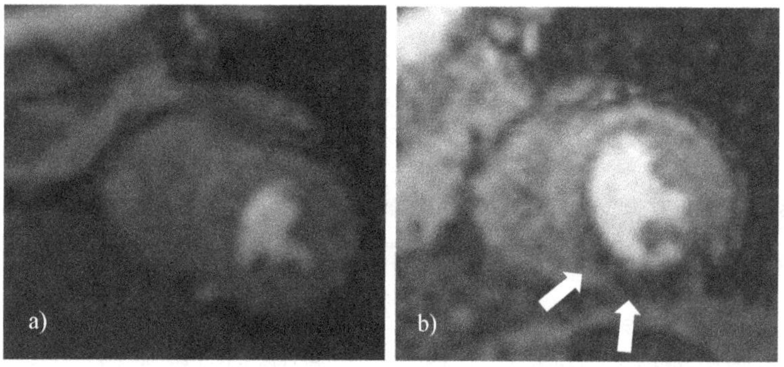

Figure 1 Mid-ventricular dynamic CMR perfusion images are shown. CMR perfusion image from **a)** a healthy volunteer and **b)** a patient with a perfusion abnormality in the infero-septal and inferior myocardial regions (white arrows).

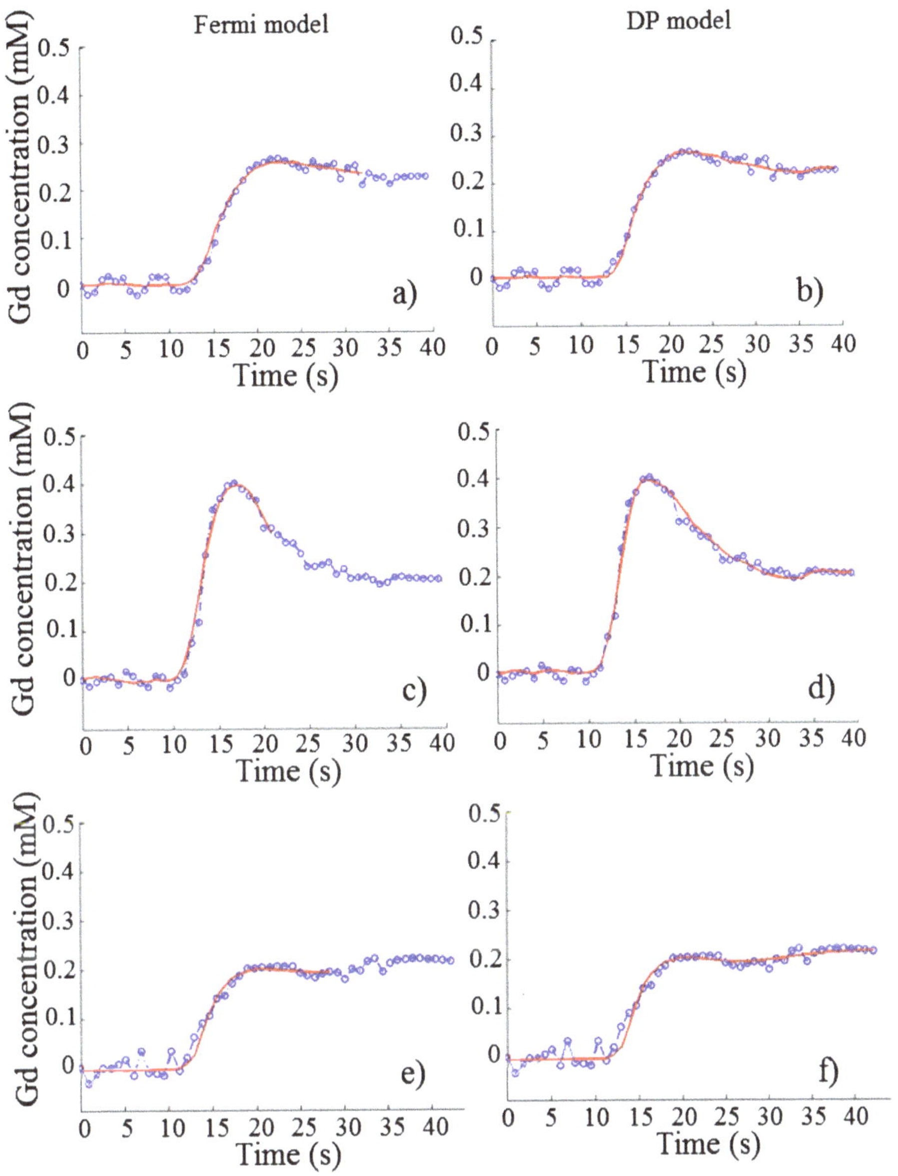

Figure 2 Examples of Fermi and distributed parameter model fits. Examples of model fits at rest **(a, b)** and at stress **(c, d)** from the same volunteer (dual bolus analysis). Fermi **(e)** and distributed parameter **(f)** model fits during hyperemia of a pathological myocardial segment (single bolus analysis). DP:distributed parameter model, Gd: gadolinium.

The Fermi and distributed parameter models correctly identified reduced myocardial blood flow in 6 and 7 of the 7 vessels in Group 3 respectively. In addition, the Fermi and distributed parameter models correctly identified reduced myocardial blood flow in 3 and 5 of the 5 vessels in Group 2 respectively. Both models estimated myocardial blood flow within normal range in Group 1. A difference was observed in myocardial blood flow at stress and in myocardial perfusion reserve between Group 1 versus Groups 2 and 3 for both models (Figure 4, Table 4).

Mean physiological parameter values were also calculated using distributed parameter modeling in all vessel territories for all patients (see Additional file 1).

Discussion

We have compared single and dual bolus estimates of myocardial perfusion in healthy volunteers using both Fermi and 2-region 1-barrier distributed parameter models. We demonstrate no difference in myocardial blood flow estimates using the distributed parameter model between single and dual bolus analysis. In

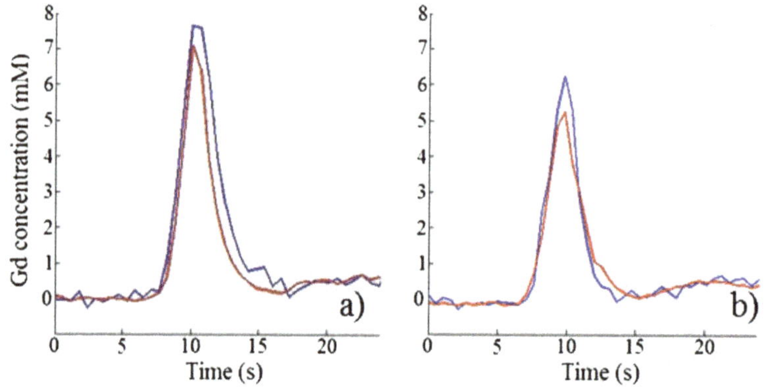

Figure 3 Scaled pre-bolus arterial input function versus standard arterial input function from the same examination. In volunteer 1 **(a)** and volunteer 2 **(b)** scaled pre-bolus (blue) arterial input function and main bolus arterial input function (red) are shown. Gd: gadolinium.

agreement with previous work, we demonstrate an increase in stress myocardial blood flow estimates with application of Fermi modeling using single bolus data analysis compared to dual bolus data analysis. For the first time, we have also successfully fitted the distributed parameter model in patients with coronary artery disease.

Model comparison in healthy volunteers

Using the distributed parameter model, we successfully fitted 96% of our data (398 in 416 CA concentration-time courses). Model comparison in 8 healthy volunteers suggested that single bolus analysis of the distributed parameter model shows no statistically significant difference compared to dual bolus analysis, indicating that this model may be less dependent on arterial input function saturation than the Fermi model. Furthermore, distributed parameter modeling using the first pass only, showed no statistically significant difference between single bolus and dual bolus analysis. This shows that the lack of dependence on single or dual bolus in the distributed parameter model using the full curve is not due to the increased number of time points used for fitting, compared to the first pass Fermi model. Dual bolus [11,12,15,23] and dual sequence [10,24] (which includes a low resolution dynamic acquisition of the left ventricle to eliminate arterial input function saturation), are the most widely suggested techniques to solve the issue of arterial input function saturation. However, both of these techniques involve increased complexity in image acquisition and data analysis that have led to ongoing debate regarding whether either method might replace standard single bolus protocols for CMR perfusion and myocardial blood flow quantification. Whilst single bolus protocols are prone to arterial input function saturation, they are still widely used in clinical imaging and are suitable for qualitative assessment of myocardial perfusion. Our analysis suggests that peak arterial input function saturation may not be such a dominant factor when quantifying myocardial blood flow in distributed parameter modeling compared with Fermi modeling.

Our calculated myocardial blood flow and microvascular characteristic parameter values generally agree with a previous study that was the first to introduce the two-region, one-barrier distributed parameter model in cardiac data [9]. Broadbent *et al* fitted a distributed parameter model in data acquired using a different protocol: short-axis view of the entire myocardial area across one mid-ventricular slice acquired in systole at 1.5 T. We applied the distributed parameter model using a 16-segment heart model across three mid-ventricular slices acquired in diastole at 3T.

The impact of contrast agent dose

We validated the dependence of Fermi and distributed parameter modeling in the presence of arterial input function saturation in single bolus data, using a relatively low CA dose (0.03 mmol/kg) in our healthy volunteer cohort. The administration of the specific CA dose has

Table 3 Healthy volunteer mean (SD) myocardial blood flow values calculated using dual and single bolus analysis

Modeling values/Method	Fermi	Fermi	DP	DP	DP-First pass	DP-First pass
	Dual bolus	Single bolus	Dual bolus	Single bolus	Dual bolus	Single bolus
Myocardial blood flow-Stress (mL/min/mL)	3.57 (0.59)*	4.57 (0.62)*	3.16 (0.71)	3.45 (0.48)	3.39 (0.56)	3.47 (0.50)
Myocardial blood flow-Rest (mL/min/mL)	1.48 (0.40)	1.57 (0.33)	1.23 (0.26)	1.46 (0.29)	1.18 (0.26)	1.34 (0.31)

Statistical differences between single and dual bolus analysis are indicated with *.

Table 4 Invasive coronary angiography/fractional flow reserve classification and mean myocardial blood flow (SD) at stress measured in mL/min/mL per vessel territories of the three main coronary arteries

		Invasive coronary angiography/Fractional flow reserve	Distributed parameter-Myocardial blood flow	Fermi-Myocardial blood flow	Distributed parameter-Myocardial perfusion reserve	Fermi-Myocardial perfusion reserve
Patient 1	LAD	3	0.82 (0.28)*	1.68 (0.60)*	0.88 (0.29)	1.54 (0.47)
	LCX	3	0.94 (0.20)*	1.99 (0.41)*	0.91 (0.16)	1.73 (0.44)
	RCA	2	0.84 (0.17)*	1.77 (0.79)*	0.91 (0.24)	1.77 (0.44)
Patient 2	LAD	2	1.99 (0.30)*	3.37 (0.49)	1.68 (0.37)	2.15 (0.49)
	LCX	2	1.98 (0.27)*	2.61 (0.41)	1.26 (0.30)	1.87 (0.80)
	RCA	3	1.27 (0.27)*	1.80 (0.81)*	0.86 (0.30)	1.08 (0.33)
Patient 3	LAD	2	1.20 (0.10)*	1.19 (0.34)*	0.71 (0.11)	0.78 (0.44)
	LCX	3	1.34 (0.13)*	1.84 (1.11)*	0.65 (0.30)	0.96 (0.26)
	RCA	2	1.58 (0.31)*	1.18 (0.16)*	0.81 (0.20)	0.70 (0.12)
Patient 4	LAD	3	1.99 (0.31)*	3.02 (0.64)	1.21 (0.31)	1.22 (0.23)
	LCX	3	1.61 (0.73)*	1.98 (0.58)*	0.90 (0.35)	1.05 (0.34)
	RCA	3	0.75 (0.29)*	1.00 (0.44)*	0.58 (0.23)	0.65 (0.24)
Patient 5	LAD	1	2.86 (0.59)	3.26 (0.88)	3.26 (0.40)	3.37 (0.50)
	LCX	1	2.54 (0.24)	2.79 (0.30)	3.01 (0.60)	2.91 (0.34)
	RCA	1	2.60 (0.36)	2.88 (0.33)	2.68 (0.35)	3.04 (0.85)

LAD, LCX and RCA: left anterior descending, left circumflex and right coronary artery respectively. Vessels with reduced myocardial blood flow are indicated with *.

possibly caused limited arterial input function saturation at the peak of contrast enhancement [3,10] (as shown in Figure 3), compared to higher CA doses. Our study demonstrates that Fermi modeling is still sensitive to any arterial input function saturation present in our single bolus data. In contrast, distributed parameter modeling is less dependent on any arterial input function saturation present in our data. Any increases in CA dose (at 3T), can increase the degree of arterial input function saturation in single bolus data of healthy volunteers, which would necessitate a de novo validation of distributed parameter modeling in single against dual bolus analysis.

Distributed parameter and Fermi analysis in patients

The distributed parameter model was capable of detecting reduced myocardial blood flow in patients with non-obstructive and obstructive coronary artery disease (Groups 2 and 3 respectively). Distributed parameter modeling correctly identified all 7 obstructive lesions and all 5 non-obstructive lesions. Fermi modeling correctly identified 6 out of 7 obstructive lesions and 3 out of 5 non-obstructive lesions. Both models showed decreased myocardial blood flow values as a function of luminal stenosis severity against invasive coronary angiography and fractional flow reserve classification (Figure 4).

Study limitations

The number of subjects included in this study is small. However, this is the first study demonstrating that a 1-barrier 2-region distributed parameter model approach may be less dependent on arterial input function saturation than Fermi modeling. Distributed parameter modeling needs to be applied in larger patient cohorts to further validate its diagnostic accuracy. We have not validated the behaviour of distributed parameter modeling in higher CA doses. To reduce patient discomfort during administration of adenosine, we did not implement a dual bolus stress-rest protocol in our patient cohort. As such, it was impossible to validate any systematic errors that may have contaminated our patient myocardial blood flow quantifications due to arterial input function saturation. To overcome this limitation and to complement our model comparison, we further assessed the ability of both models in detecting reduced myocardial blood flow in stenotic vessels versus current invasive gold standard methods. The CA dose used in patients was higher than in healthy volunteers to increase the signal-to-noise ratio due to an assumed reduction in blood flow in our patient cohort as compared to our healthy volunteer cohort. Although this higher dose in patients has possibly caused some myocardial blood flow overestimations in Fermi modeling (Table 4, in two epicardial vessels in patient 2, and one epicardial vessel in patient 4), the distributed parameter modeling showed excellent accuracy in detecting reduced haemodynamics at stress in all stenotic vessels compared to our invasive gold standard. The vessels with non-obstructive disease (Group 2) were all from patients who also had one or two other vessels with obstructive disease (Group 3).

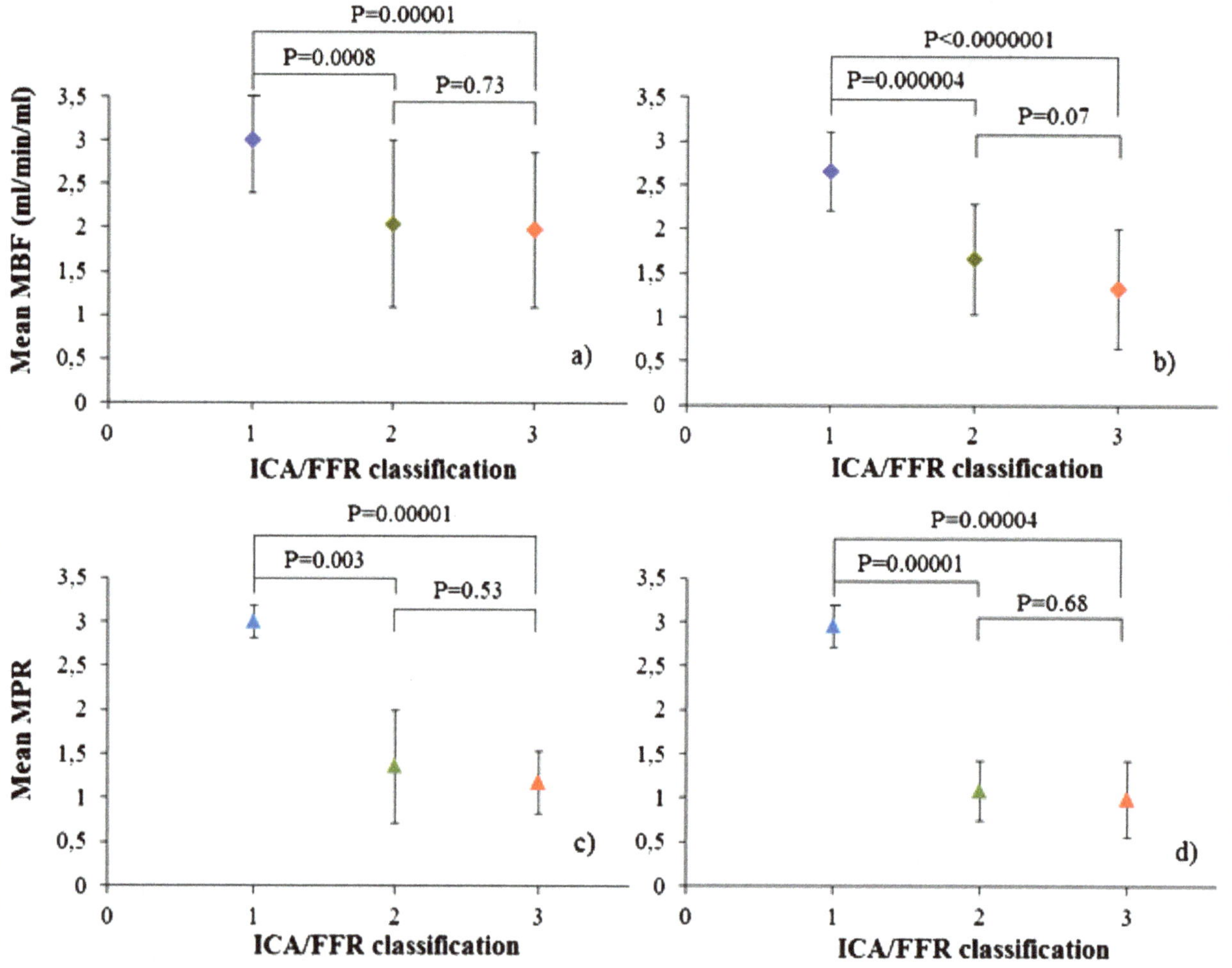

Figure 4 Mean Fermi-MBF (a), distributed parameter-MBF (b), Fermi-MPR (c), distributed parameter MPR (d) versus ICA/FFR classification. MBF: myocardial blood flow, MPR: myocardial perfusion reserve, ICA: invasive coronary angiography, FFR: fractional flow reserve.

The coincidental effect of microvascular dysfunction could therefore explain the low myocardial blood flow measurements in Group 2.

Conclusions

We implemented a two-region, one-barrier distributed parameter model in healthy volunteers and patients with coronary artery disease. Distributed parameter-derived myocardial blood flow did not significantly change when a single bolus arterial input function was used compared to the dual bolus case. Fermi modelling of the same data demonstrated significant overestimations in myocardial blood flow in single bolus compared to dual bolus analysis. This suggests that the distributed parameter model might be less dependent on arterial input function saturation than Fermi modeling.

The distributed parameter model detected reduced myocardial blood flow in all 7 vessels with obstructive lesions and in all 5 vessels with non-obstructive lesions as determined by invasive coronary angiography and fractional flow reserve classification in a pilot cohort of 5 patients with coronary artery disease.

Competing interests

The authors declare that they have no competing interests.

Authors' contributions

GP: Author of the manuscript. Developed the hypothesis and conceptualized the objectives of the manuscript. Participated in the design of the single and dual bolus acquisition protocols, prepared the data analysis software and performed quantitative and statistical analysis. MW: Recruited all patients, participated in the preparation of healthy volunteers and patients before the magnetic resonance (MR) imaging and supervised the scans. LK: Supported the design of the image analysis software and helped in the design of the dual bolus protocol. SA: Prepared the healthy volunteers before the MR scanning and supervised the scans. MD: Prepared the healthy volunteers before the MR scanning and supervised the scans. SM: Performed qualitative assessment of the MR images and reported incidental findings and/or myocardial infarction. MC: Supported the design of the image analysis software. CG: Supported the design of the image analysis software3. TM: Supported the design of the image analysis software. DN: Revised the manuscript. Gave final approval to be published and approved the validity of the research questions and scientific approaches. Planned the study, obtained funding. SS: Revised the manuscript. Gave final approval to be published and approved the validity of the research questions, methodology and scientific approaches. Planned the study, obtained funding. All authors read and approved the final manuscript.

Acknowledgements
This work was made possible through funding and continued support from the British Heart Foundation. We would also like to thank the radiographers of the Clinical Research Imaging Centre for their help in image acquisition and input to the protocol.

Funding
British Heart Foundation (RE/08/001/23904).

Author details
[1]Clinical Research Imaging Centre, University of Edinburgh,, Edinburgh, UK. [2]Centre for Cardiovascular Science, University of Edinburgh, Edinburgh, UK. [3]Christie Medical Physics and Engineering, The Christie NHS FT, Manchester, UK.

References

1. Hendel RC, Patel MR, Kramer CM, Poon M, Carr JC, Gerstad NA, et al. ACCF/ACR/SCCT/SCMR/ASNC/NASCI/SCAI/SIR 2006 appropriateness criteria for cardiac computed tomography and cardiac magnetic resonance imaging. J Am Coll Cardiol. 2006;48:1475–97.
2. Jaarsma C, Leiner T, Bekkers SC, Crijns HJ, Wildberger JE, Nagel E, et al. Diagnostic performance of noninvasive myocardial perfusion imaging using single-photon emission computed tomography, cardiac magnetic resonance, and positron emission tomography imaging for the detection of obstructive coronary artery disease. J Am Coll Cardiol. 2012;59:1719–28.
3. Jerosch-Herold M. Quantification of myocardial perfusion by cardiovascular magnetic resonance. J Cardiov Magn Reson. 2010;12:57.
4. Sourbron SP, Buckley DL. Tracer kinetic modelling in MRI: estimating perfusion and capillary permeability. Phys in Med Biol. 2012;57:R1–33.
5. Nesterov SV, Han C, Mäki M, Kajander S, Naum AG, Helenius H, et al. Myocardial perfusion quantitation with 15O-labelled water PET: high reproducibility of the new cardiac analysis software (Carimas). Eur J Nucl Med Mol Imaging. 2009;36:1594–602.
6. Kaufmann PA, Camici PG. Myocardial blood flow measurement by PET: technical aspects and clinical applications. J Nucl Med. 2005;46:75–88.
7. Biglands J, Magee D, Boyle R, Larghat A, Plein S, Radjenović A. Evaluation of the effect of myocardial segmentation errors on myocardial blood flow estimates from DCE-MRI. Phys in Med Biol. 2011;56(8):2423–43.
8. Jerosch-Herold M, Wilke N, Stillman AE. Magnetic resonance quantification of the myocardial perfusion reserve with a Fermi function model for constrained deconvolution. Med Phys. 1998;25:73–84.
9. Broadbent DA, Biglands JD, Larghat A, Sourbron SP, Radjenovic A, Greenwood JP, et al. Myocardial blood flow at rest and stress measured with dynamic contrast-enhanced MRI: Comparison of a distributed parameter model with a Fermi function model. Magn Reson Med. 2013;70:1591–7.
10. Gatehouse PD, Elkington AG, Ablitt NA, Yang G, Pennell DJ, Firmin DN. Accurate assessment of the arterial input function during high-dose myocardial perfusion cardiovascular magnetic resonance. J Magn Reson Im. 2004;20:39–45.
11. Christian TF, Rettmann DW, Aletras AH, Liao SL, Taylor JL, Balaban RS, et al. Absolute myocardial perfusion in canines measured by using dual-bolus first-pass MR imaging. Radiology. 2004;232:677–84.
12. Utz W, Greiser A, Niendorf T, Diet R, Schulz-Menger J. Single- or dual-bolus approach for the assessment of myocardial perfusion reserve in quantitative MR perfusion imaging. Magn Reson Med. 2008;59:1373–7.
13. Messroghli DR, Greiser A, Fröhlich M, Dietz R, Schulz-Menger J. Optimization and validation of a fully-integrated pulse sequence for modified look-locker inversion-recovery (MOLLI) T1 mapping of the heart. J Magn Reson Im. 2007;26:1081–6.
14. Cerqueira MD. Standardized myocardial segmentation and nomenclature for tomographic imaging of the heart: a statement for healthcare professionals from the cardiac imaging committee of the council on clinical cardiology of the american heart association. Circulation. 2002;105:539–42.
15. Ishida M, Schuster A, Morton G, Chiribiri A, Hussain S, Paul M, et al. Development of a universal dual-bolus injection scheme for the quantitative assessment of myocardial perfusion cardiovascular magnetic resonance. J Cardiov Magn Reson. 2011;13:28.
16. Tonino PAL, Fearon WF, De Bruyne B, Oldroyd KG, Leesar MA, Ver Lee PN, et al. Angiographic versus functional severity of coronary artery stenoses in the FAME study. J Am Coll Cardiol. 2010;55:2816–21.
17. Tonino PAL, De Bruyne B, Pijls NHJ, Siebert U, Ikeno F, van't Veer M, et al. Fractional flow reserve versus angiography for guiding Percutaneous Coronary Intervention. N Engl J Med. 2009;360:213–24.
18. Kershaw LE, Hutchinson CE, Buckley DL. Benign prostatic hyperplasia: evaluation of T1, T2, and microvascular characteristics with T1-weighted dynamic contrast-enhanced MRI. J Magn Reson Im. 2009;29:641–8.
19. Larsson HBW, Fritz-Hansen T, Rostrup E, Søndergaard L, Ring P, Henriksen O. Myocardial perfusion modeling using MRI. Magn Reson Med. 1996;35:716–26.
20. Fritz-Hansen T, Rostrup E, Ring PB, Larsson HB. Quantification of gadolinium-DTPA concentrations for different inversion times using an IR-turbo flash pulse sequence: a study on optimizing multislice perfusion imaging. Magn Reson Med. 1998;16:893–9.
21. Garpebring A, Ostlund N, Karlsson M. A novel estimation method for physiological parameters in dynamic contrast-enhanced MRI: application of a distributed parameter model using Fourier-domain calculations. IEEE Trans Med Imaging. 2009;28:1375–83.
22. Byrd RH, Gilbert JC, Nocedal J. A trust region method based on interior point techniques for nonlinear programming. Math Program. 2000;89:149–85.
23. Hsu L-Y, Rhoads KL, Holly JE, Kellman P, Aletras AH, Arai AE. Quantitative myocardial perfusion analysis with a dual-bolus contrast-enhanced first-pass MRI technique in humans. Journal of magnetic resonance imaging. J Magn Reson Im. 2006;23:315–22.
24. Cernicanu A, Axel L. Theory-based signal calibration with single-point T1 measurements for first-pass quantitative perfusion MRI studies. Acad Radiol. 2006;13:686–93.

20

The distribution and prognosis of anomalous coronary arteries identified by cardiovascular magnetic resonance: 15 year experience from two tertiary centres

David P Ripley[1,2], Ansuman Saha[2], Albert Teis[3], Akhlaque Uddin[1,2], Petra Bijsterveld[1], Ananth Kidambi[1,2], Adam K McDiarmid[1,2], Mohan Sivananthan[2], Sven Plein[1,2], Dudley J Pennell[3] and John P Greenwood[1,2*]

Abstract

Background: Aberrant coronary arteries represent a diverse group of congenital disorders. Post-mortem studies reveal a high risk of exercise-related sudden cardiac death in those with an anomalous coronary artery originating from the opposite sinus of Valsalva (ACAOS) with an inter-arterial course. There is little documentation of lifetime history and long-term follow-up of patients with coronary artery anomalies.

Methods: Patients with anomalous coronary arteries undergoing cardiovascular magnetic resonance over a 15-year period were identified and classified by anatomy and course. Medical records were reviewed for major adverse cardiovascular events (MACE). Revascularisation or myocardial infarction counted only if occurring in the distribution of the anomalous artery.

Results: Consecutive patients with coronary artery anomalies were retrospectively identified (n = 172). Median follow-up time was 4.3 years (IQR 2.5–7.8, maximum 15.6). 116 patients had ACAOS of which 64 (55%) had an inter-arterial course (IAC) and 52 (45%) did not. During follow up 110 ACAOS patients were alive, 5 died and 1 lost to follow-up. ACAOS patients experienced 58 MACE events (5 cardiovascular deaths, 5 PCI, 24 CABG and 24 had myocardial infarction). 47 MACE events occurred in ACAOS with IAC and 11 in those without ($p < 0.0001$), the statistical difference driven by surgical revascularisation and myocardial infarction.

Conclusions: In life, patients with an anomalous coronary artery originating from the opposite sinus of Valsalva taking an IAC have higher rates of both myocardial infarction and surgical revascularisation during long-term follow up, compared to those without IAC.

Keywords: Coronary vessel anomalies, Cardiovascular magnetic resonance, Prognosis

Background

Aberrant coronary arteries represent a diverse group of congenital disorders which affect between 0.3 to 1.3% of the unselected general population undergoing cardiac catheterisation [1,2]. They are increasingly recognised due to the expansion of advanced non-invasive cardiovascular imaging techniques including computed tomography (CT) imaging and cardiovascular magnetic resonance (CMR).

The majority of coronary anomalies go unrecognised and have no clinical significance, although a minority have been documented to have increased risk of myocardial infarction and ischaemia, congestive heart failure and sudden cardiac death (SCD). Congenital coronary abnormalities are the second leading cause of SCD in the young exceeded only by hypertrophic cardiomyopathy (HCM) [3]. Those with the highest risk include individuals with an anomalous coronary artery originating from the opposite sinus of Valsalva (ACAOS) with this

* Correspondence: j.greenwood@leeds.ac.uk
[1]Multidisciplinary Cardiovascular Research Centre (MCRC) & Leeds Institute of Genetics, Health and Therapeutics, University of Leeds, Leeds, UK
[2]Leeds Teaching Hospitals NHS Trust, Leeds General Infirmary, Leeds, UK
Full list of author information is available at the end of the article

risk higher in athletes than non-athletic persons [4]. Furthermore post mortem studies suggest this risk is limited to those ACAOS which take an inter-arterial course (IAC) between the aorta and pulmonary artery (PA), and this has been documented in both anomalous origins of the right coronary artery from the left coronary sinus (right-ACAOS) and in anomalous origins of the left coronary artery from the right coronary sinus (left-ACAOS); the latter appears to carry a higher risk of SCD [5-7]. Other anatomical features which are associated with high risk include intra-mural course, slit-like orifice and angulated take-off which are all thought to contribute to myocardial ischaemia [8].

Surgical intervention in patients with ACAOS, such as re-implantation of the anomalous vessel into the correct coronary sinus, unroofing of the intra-mural course or coronary artery bypass grafting may be performed which in theory prevents ischaemia and/or SCD. There are favourable early outcome data from surgical intervention [9,10] although little data regarding long term follow-up for late complications and outcomes. Although Krasuski et al. demonstrated contrasting results showing similar mortality rates between medically and surgically treated groups with ACAOS [10].

There is little published evidence describing the long term history and long-term follow-up of anomalous coronary arteries in life. The aim of this study was to demonstrate the distribution of anomalous coronary arteries referred for CMR and to document their long-term clinical outcome with respect to major adverse cardiovascular event (MACE) rates. A secondary aim was to confirm whether or not the anatomical course of anomalous coronary arteries conferred differential risk.

Table 1 Classification of anomalous coronary arteries*

1. Origin of both RCA and LMS (separate origins) from the right aortic sinus
   - 1a. Course of anomalous LMS between aorta and pulmonary artery (PA)
   - 1b. Course of anomalous LMS *not* between aorta and PA
2. Origin of both coronary arteries (separate origins) from the left aortic sinus
   - 2a. Course of anomalous RCA between aorta and PA
   - 2b. Course of anomalous RCA *not* between aorta and PA
3. Anomalous origin of the circumflex coronary artery from the right aortic sinus
   - 3a. Course of anomalous LCx between aorta and PA
   - 3b. Course of anomalous LCx *not* between aorta and PA
4. Anomalous origin of the left anterior descending artery from the right aortic sinus
   - 4a. Course of anomalous LAD between aorta and PA
   - 4b. Course of anomalous LAD *not* between aorta and PA
5. Single coronary artery (common origin)
   - 5a. Course of anomalous coronary artery between aorta and PA
   - 5b. Course of anomalous coronary artery *not* between aorta and PA
6. Anomalous origin or communication of a coronary artery with a cardiac chamber or major thoracic vessel
   - 6a. Abnormal origin from the pulmonary artery or one of its major arterial branches
   - 6b. Abnormal origin from the aorta or one of its major arterial branches
   - 6c. Abnormal communication of a coronary artery with a cardiac chamber or major thoracic vessel (fistula).
7. Miscellaneous/unclassified

*Adapted from Angelini Circulation 2002 [11] and Wilkins Texas Heart Institute Journal 1988 [12].

Methods

This study was approved by a regional research ethics committee and the National Information Governance Board for Health and Social Care (NIGB, section 251). Databases from two large UK cardiovascular MR centres were reviewed (Leeds General Infirmary and the Royal Brompton Hospital, London). All patients who were referred for clinically indicated CMR over a 15 year period (1995 to 2010) with anomalous coronary arteries identified on those scans were recorded. All CMR scans were performed with a 1.5 Tesla Philips Intera CV scanner (Philips Healthcare, Best, The Netherlands) or a 1.5 Tesla Siemens Sonata or Avanto scanner (Siemens Healthcare, Erlangen, Germany).

All CMR images were recalled and independently retrospectively reviewed. The anomalous coronary arteries were classified according to their anatomy and course, following strict criteria (Table 1).

Both the electronic and paper records of all patients were reviewed for MACE. Confirmation of events was further clarified from the general practitioner records. Their vital status (dead or alive) was ascertained from National Health Service Spine electronic record and if the patient was dead, the cause of death retrieved from the Office of National Statistics. MACE was defined as cardiovascular death, myocardial infarction in the distribution of the anomalous coronary artery, revascularisation in the distribution of the anomalous coronary artery or aborted SCD. Definition and adjudication of MACE was performed blinded to the coronary anomaly classification.

CMR pulse sequences

CMR pulse sequences were performed using a protocol which included a contemporary (at the time of patient study) coronary magnetic resonance angiography pulse sequence. A low-resolution coronary survey scan was initially performed during free breathing, using a respiratory navigator. For a targeted approach CMR was performed as follows: for the right coronary artery (RCA) double-oblique three dimensional volume along the long-axis of the RCA; for the left coronary system a double-oblique transverse three dimensional volume centred on the left main stem through the proximal left anterior descending and left circumflex arteries. For anomalous coronaries separate targeted views were typically acquired using a 3 point planning technique. 3-Dimensional targeted volumes were acquired using a three-dimensional gradient-echo sequence. Typical pulse sequence parameters: TE 2.2 ms, TR 7.7 ms, flip angle 25°, T2 and fat saturation pre-pulses, matrix 512 × 360, field of view 360 mm, 20 slices with slice thickness of 1.5 mm, acquired voxel size of 0.7 × 1.0 mm (reconstructed to 0.7 × 0.7 mm). Full details previously reported [13].

More recent techniques included a three dimensional whole heart acquisition. For this, timing of the diastolic coronary rest period was estimated from a high temporal resolution four-chamber free breathing cine scan. Three dimensional whole heart coronary MR angiography was acquired using a balanced SSFP sequence and a respiratory navigator to compensate for respiratory motion during free breathing. Typical pulse sequence parameters: TE 2.3 ms, TR 4.6 ms, flip angle 100°, T2 and fat saturation pre-pulses, duration of acquisition up to 120 ms per R-R interval (determined by length of diastolic rest period), matrix 304 × 304, field of view 320–460 mm, slice thickness 0.9 mm, 100–120 slices as required, acquired in-plane voxel size of 1.0 × 1.0 mm (reconstructed to 0.5 × 0.5 mm) [14].

Statistics

Data analysis was performed using SSPS 17.0 for Windows (SPSS, Chicago, Illinois, USA). Data are presented as mean ± SD or median (IQR) as appropriate. Ordinal data were compared using the Mann–Whitney U and χ^2 tests. Two-tailed testing with a probability value of ≤0.05 was considered statistically significant. Kaplan-Meier curves were used to estimate the distribution of time to first cardiac event and differences between time to first event curves compared with the log-rank test.

Results

In total, 59,844 CMR scans were performed between March 1995 and April 2010 at the two CMR institutions. 172 consecutive patients (0.3%) with coronary artery anomalies were retrospectively identified (90 and 82 from each centre) with a median age of 54 years (range 1–85; IQR 40–64). The median follow-up time was 4.3 years (IQR 2.5–7.8) with a maximum of 15.6 years. At the time of follow-up, 160 patients were alive (93%), 10 deceased (6%) and 2 lost to follow-up. The distribution of classified coronary anomalies are detailed in Table 2 and a selection of coronary anomalies imaged by CMR are shown in Figure 1. There were no cases where the anatomy could not be determined.

Of the 172 patients, 116 had ACAOS (61 and 55 from each centre) with a median follow-up of 4.6 years. Of these, 110 were alive (95%), 5 deceased (4.3%) and 1 lost to follow-up (1%). 21 patients had a separate right coronary artery (RCA) and left main stem (LMS) from the right coronary sinus of which 13 had an IAC of the LMS between the aorta and PA. Separate origins of both coronary arteries from the left aortic sinus all of which took an IAC were present in 34 patients. An anomalous circumflex from the opposite sinus occurred in 33 patients none of which took an IAC. An anomalous left anterior descending artery from the opposite sinus was present in 10 patients, with 4 following an IAC route. Finally, 18 had a single coronary artery of which 13 passed inter-arterially. Therefore of the 116 patients with ACAOS, 64 patients (55%) had an inter-arterial course and 52 (45%) without an inter-arterial course (Table 3). There was no statistical difference in the age of the two ACAOS populations (with or without IAC) (P = 0.63).

Table 2 Distribution of the coronary anomalies in the joint CMR Databases (n = 172)

Classification	Number	Age (median, range)
1a	13	58, 8 – 73
1b	8	36, 1 – 73
2a	34	55, 13 – 78
2b	0	
3a	0	
3b	33	58, 25 – 78
4a	4	56, 30 – 70
4b	6	19, 15 – 41
5a	13	60, 29 – 85
5b	5	70, 34 – 80
6a	11	36, 15 – 64
6b	2	53, 47 – 59
6c	18	56, 18 – 76
7	25	46, 8 – 78

Of those patients with ACAOS there were in total 58 MACE (5 cardiovascular deaths, 5 percutaneous coronary interventions (PCI) to the anomalous artery, 24 underwent surgical revascularisation to the anomalous territory and 24 had a documented myocardial infarction in the anomalous coronary artery territory). All PCI was performed for coronary artery disease with coronary stenosis visually measuring > 70% luminal stenosis. All myocardial infarctions were spontaneous related to atherosclerotic plaque (type 1) [15]. The mortality rate from cardiovascular causes was 4.3% (5 cardiovascular deaths in 116 ACAOS patients) during the median follow up period of 4.6 years. Of the 5 deaths 4 were from a documented myocardial infarction (all with a rise of cardiac biomarkers and ECG changes) and one

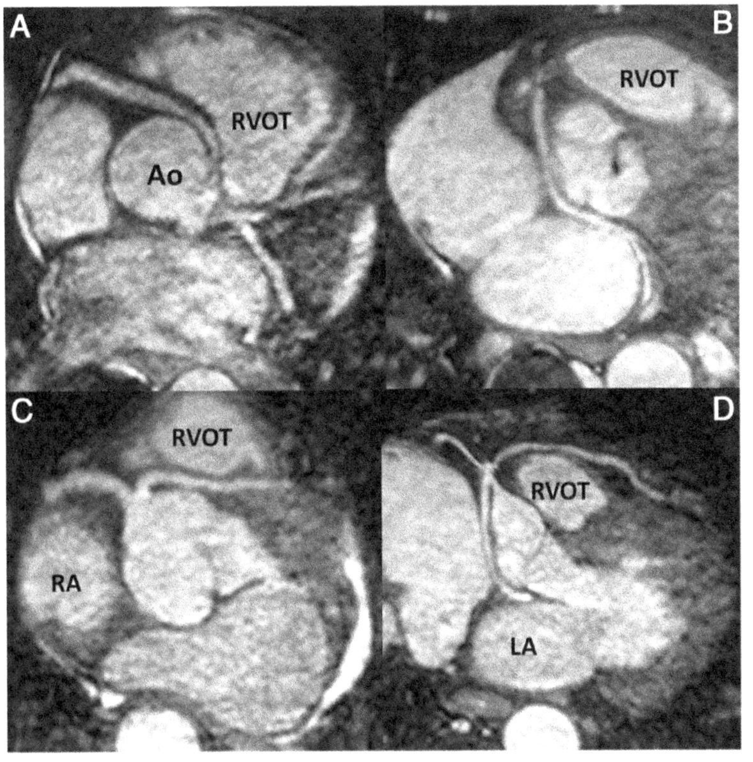

Figure 1 Examples of several different anomalous coronary arteries imaged by CMR: (A) Right coronary artery originating from the left coronary cusp passing anteriorly (class 2a), **(B)** Circumflex artery arising from the right coronary cusp (RCC) passing posteriorly (class 3b), **(C)** Left anterior descending (LAD) artery from the RCC anteriorly passing between the RVOT and aorta (class 4a) and **(D)** single ostium coronary system arising from the RCC with a retro-aortic circumflex artery and a pre-pulmonic LAD (class 5b). Images reconstructed using SoapBubble^{TM} software (Philips Medical Systems). Ao - Aorta; RVOT – Right Ventricular Outflow Tract; RA – Right Atrium; LA – Left Atrium.

death from chronic heart failure secondary to ischaemic heart disease.

47 MACE occurred in patients with ACAOS and an IAC and 11 in those without an IAC ($p < 0.0001$). There was significantly higher risk of both surgical revascularisation and myocardial infarction in the IAC group, with similar numbers of percutaneous revascularisation and cardiovascular deaths (Table 4). Age of first MACE was lower in those coronary abnormalities with an IAC ($p < 0.0001$) (Figure 2). The distribution of major cardiovascular events by coronary anomaly is presented in Table 5.

Table 3 Distribution of anomalous coronary arteries originating from the opposite sinus with and without inter arterial course

	Number	Age (median, range)
Total ACAOS	116	54, 1 – 85
- ACAOS with inter-arterial course	64	56, 8 – 85
- ACAOS without inter-arterial course	52	53, 1 – 80

ACAOS = anomalous coronary artery originating from the opposite sinus of Valsalva.

Discussion

This study has shown the distribution of coronary artery anomalies imaged by CMR in two large tertiary cardiac centres over the previous 15 years. Our study demonstrates the prognostic significance of an inter-arterial course for an anomalous coronary artery originating from the opposite sinus of Valsalva (ACAOS) passing between the aorta and pulmonary artery. We have also shown significantly higher myocardial infarction and surgical revascularisation rates for this group of anomalous arteries in those patients referred for CMR, over a median 4.6 year follow-up period.

Table 4 Major Adverse Cardiovascular Events in patients with an anomalous coronary artery originating from the opposite sinus of Valsalva (ACAOS) (n = 116)

	ACAOS with IAC (n = 64)	ACAOS without IAC (n = 52)	P value
Cardiovascular Deaths, n	3	2	NS
PCI, n	3	2	NS
Surgical revascularisation, n	23	1	P < 0.0001
Myocardial Infarction, n	18	6	P < 0.05

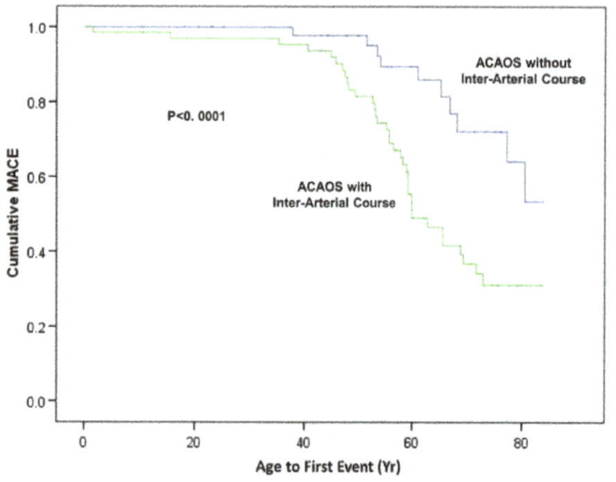

Figure 2 Kaplan-Meier curves showing the age at which the first major adverse cardiovascular event occurred, demonstrating a significant difference (log rank test, $p < 0.0001$) between those anomalous coronary arteries from the opposite sinus (ACAOS) with an inter-arterial course (IAC) and those without IAC.

Invasive X-ray angiography has traditionally been the diagnostic imaging test to identify coronary anomalies however the presence of an anomalous vessel may only be suspected after the procedure (e.g. after unsuccessful catheterisation). CMR has a number of advantages for diagnosing coronary artery anomalies. The non-invasive technique does not require contrast agents or ionising radiation, which is an important consideration particularly in children and young adults. The dose and stochastic effects of X-ray radiation are frequently misjudged [16] and the risk of developing a solid tumour is estimated at 1:2500

Table 5 Major Adverse Cardiovascular Events in patients by coronary anomaly in those patients with anomalous coronary artery originating from the opposite sinus of Valsalva (ACAOS)

Classification	Number	Major Adverse Cardiovascular Event				Total MACE
		CV Death	PCI	Surgical revascularisation	MI	
1a	13	0	1	7	5	13
1b	8	0	1	0	2	3
2a	34	1	1	12	6	20
2b	0	0	0	0	0	0
3a	0	0	0	0	0	0
3b	33	1	1	1	4	7
4a	4	0	0	0	2	2
4b	6	0	0	0	0	0
5a	13	2	1	4	5	12
5b	5	1	0	0	0	1

CV death – Cardiovascular death; PCI – Percutaneous coronary intervention; MI – myocardial infarction.

diagnostic coronary angiographic procedures [17,18]. Furthermore CMR clarifies the spatial relationship of these arteries with respect to the aorta and the pulmonary artery, which we and others have demonstrated confers differential risk; this is also important in surgical planning. The application of CMR for the detection and documentation of the origin and course of coronary anomalies is well established [19-22] and as such CMR is a recognised class I indication in international guidelines [23,24].

Anomalous coronary arteries cover a wide range of conditions the majority of which have no clinical significance [25]. Post mortem studies from both the military and in young athletes have shown that ACAOS is associated with a higher risk of SCD. The risk is higher in athletes with ACAOS, representing a 79 times higher relative risk than in non-athletic individuals [4] which is limited to those ACAOS taking an inter-arterial course between the aorta and main pulmonary artery. In one 25 year review of 126 non-traumatic military deaths, a high proportion of deaths (33%) were attributable to ACAOS and it was a more common cause of death than both myocarditis and hypertrophic cardiomyopathy [26]. In this review, the risk was exclusively limited to only those with a left-ACAOS (anomalous origination of the left coronary artery from the right sinus of Valsalva [27]) passing inter-arterially. However, there is also evidence that right-ACAOS (anomalous origination of the right coronary artery from the left sinus of Valsalva) may cause SCD, with one registry in athletes attributing 27 deaths to ACAOS (4 of which were a right coronary artery from the left coronary sinus) [28]. This registry also confirmed the relationship with exertion, detailing that all deaths occurred either during or shortly after exercise [28]. The prognostic risk of right-ACAOS was further corroborated by a contemporary review of consecutive patients referred for CT coronary angiography over a 4 year period, demonstrating malignant features which interestingly in this series were exclusive to right-ACAOS [29]. Those high risk features of an intramural inter-arterial course and severe lateral compression of the proximal vessel have been shown to have a clear relationship with ventricular fibrillation [30].

Whilst there is evidence that ACAOS is associated with SCD, there are little data regarding myocardial infarction and rates of revascularisation in the anomalous artery territory. Chaitman *et al.* [31] demonstrated the existence of coronary atheroma in 6 out of 17 patients (35%) with ACAOS, significantly higher than the 8% documented in a normal population [32]. Furthermore a history of MI and in patients with ACAOS with IAC and non-atherosclerotic arteries has been documented [31]. Although one long term follow-up of 87 patients with right-ACAOS and an inter-arterial course showed only 3 myocardial infarctions (3.4%) over a 2.5 year follow-up

[33] significantly lower than 15% we observe over 4.3 years in this sub-group (and 28% overall in our cohort). There are only a few published cases showing myocardial infarction in the anomalous territory.

The mechanism of myocardial infarction and SCD in ACAOS is not clear. The risk from ACAOS has been traditionally thought to be related directly to the haemodynamic significance of the inter-arterial course of the anomalous vessel, with SCD and myocardial infarction related to rising pressure in both aorta and pulmonary artery during exercise causing a scissoring or kinking of the vessel [34]. Angelini, however, has since developed a theory of intussusception, eloquently demonstrating with intravascular ultrasound (IVUS) that the main mechanism of ischaemia originates with hypoplasia and lateral luminal compression in the proximal vessel, which runs intramurally at the aortic root whilst crossing the aorto-pulmonary septum and demonstrated worsening of the proximal narrowing during physiological stress testing [35,36]. An extramural course has never been observed in those ACAOS with an inter-arterial course [25] however an intramural course has been demonstrated in some ACAOS without an inter-arterial course [25,27].

The location of the anomalous vessel in relation to the pulmonary trunk is therefore important and one long term follow up of right-ACAOS with inter-arterial course diagnosed by CT demonstrated higher MACE in those with a high inter-arterial course (RCA ostium located above the pulmonary valve) as opposed to low inter-arterial course (RCA ostium below pulmonary valve) and therefore hypothesised that the high inter-arterial course is more susceptible to compression between the aortic root and main pulmonary artery during systole [33]. The difference in MACE in this study was driven by unstable angina admissions and there was no statistical difference between myocardial infarction and cardiovascular death in both groups [33].

Krasuski *et al.* [10]. followed-up 301 patients with ACAOS (54 with an IAC) and demonstrated that ACAOS with an inter-arterial course were almost twice as likely to undergo surgical intervention and showed a higher rate of significant coronary artery disease in the distribution of the anomalous vessel (50% vs. 25%, $p = 0.02$) in those undergoing surgical intervention. Those undergoing surgery were also more likely to have had a myocardial infarction and an abnormal cardiac stress test [10]. They did not however, show any difference in the incidence of myocardial infarction between those with or without IAC, which is contrary to our data. Our study demonstrates a significantly higher rate of myocardial infarction in the territory of the anomalous coronary artery with 18 events in 64 ACAOS with IAC and only 6 in 52 ACAOS without IAC ($p < 0.05$). The lack of significance in myocardial infarction rates in the study by Krasuski may be due to the preference for early surgical intervention with 52% of patients with an inter-arterial course undergoing cardiac surgery, and after the year 2000, a 4:1 ratio of surgical versus medical management.

Krasuski also demonstrated a substantially higher mortality rate of 44% over a mean 9.2 year follow-up which is in contrast to the 4.3% mortality rate over 4.6 years in our study. Despite the high mortality rate they showed no difference in long term survival between those with or without IAC, which accords with our results, although contradicts the data from post-mortem studies. This lack of significance is unlikely to be due to the size of our cohort ($n = 116$) as this is higher than the population in many autopsy studies which reveal a statistical difference between the ACAOS with or without IAC. This may, however, reflect the limited number of young patients in our cohort with only 11% under the age of 30 years and a median age of 54 years. The under 30 age group in particular have been shown to have a significantly higher risk of SCD and exercise related death [8,37].

Limitations

This is a retrospective review of a selected population of patients referred to tertiary CMR centres for documentation of their coronary anatomy and therefore subject to referral bias. It is recognised that all cardiovascular MR scans performed showing coronary artery abnormalities may not have been identified, for example some those with complex adult congenital heart disease and incidental coronary anomalies could have been missed; we were careful to include all those with anomalous coronaries as the primary referral indication for CMR. The mean age of the patients was 54 years and therefore does not include many of the younger high risk patients who may have already died from SCD. We were unable to fully document referral indication, cardiovascular risk profile, co-morbidities and medication which may have influenced patient outcomes. Also, invasive angiography was not mandated in all to confirm the presence or absence of epicardial coronary artery disease. However we were careful to focus on hard cardiovascular events that could easily be validated. We were also meticulous in determining that myocardial infarction and revascularisation had to be related to the aberrant vessel in order to count as MACE for the purpose of our study. Whilst it is recognised that surgical revascularisation may have been performed for primary prevention on knowledge of the coronary anatomy in selected cases, we note the very large difference in surgical revascularisation between ACAOS with IAC (23, 36%) and those without (1, 2%). Furthermore there remained a significant difference in the number of myocardial infarctions (18 vs. 6) between the ACAOS with and without IAC.

Conclusion

In conclusion, we have shown distribution of anomalous coronary arteries imaged by CMR over a 15 year period from two large tertiary cardiac centres. This represents one of the largest series of anomalous coronary arteries, demonstrating that in life, patients with an anomalous coronary artery originating from the opposite sinus of Valsalva taking an inter-arterial course have higher rates of both myocardial infarction and surgical revascularisation during long-term follow up, compared to those without IAC.

Consent

Written informed consent was obtained from the patient for the publication of this report and any accompanying images.

Abbreviations

ACAOS: Anomalous coronary artery originating from the opposite sinus of Valsalva; CMR: Cardiovascular magnetic resonance; CT: Computed tomography; HCM: Hypertrophic cardiomyopathy; IAC: Inter-arterial course; IVUS: Intravascular ultrasound; LMS: Left main stem; MACE: Major adverse cardiovascular events; PA: Pulmonary artery; RCA: Right coronary artery; RVOT: Right ventricular outflow tract; SCD: Sudden cardiac death.

Competing interest

The authors declare that they have no competing interest.

Authors' contributions

DPR: Design, analysis and interpretation of data, drafting of the manuscript; AS: Analysis and interpretation of data; AT: Analysis and interpretation of data; AU: Interpretation of data, critical and intellectual revision of manuscript; PB: Analysis and interpretation of data; AK: Critical and intellectual revision of manuscript; AKM: Critical and intellectual revision of manuscript; MS: Critical and intellectual revision of manuscript; SP: Critical and intellectual revision of manuscript; DJP: Conception and design, critical and intellectual revision of manuscript. JPG: Conception and design, interpretation of data, drafting of manuscript. All authors have given approval of this manuscript for publication.

Funding

JPG and SP receive a research grant from Philips Healthcare. SP is funded by British Heart Foundation fellowship (FS/10/62/28409). DJP was supported from the NIHR Cardiovascular Biomedical Research Unit of Royal Brompton and Harefield NHS Foundation Trust and Imperial College London.

Author details

[1]Multidisciplinary Cardiovascular Research Centre (MCRC) & Leeds Institute of Genetics, Health and Therapeutics, University of Leeds, Leeds, UK. [2]Leeds Teaching Hospitals NHS Trust, Leeds General Infirmary, Leeds, UK. [3]NIHR Cardiovascular Biomedical Research Unit Royal Brompton Hospital, London, UK.

References

1. Click RL, Holmes DR Jr, Vlietstra RE, Kosinski AS, Kronmal RA. **Anomalous coronary arteries: location, degree of atherosclerosis and effect on survival–a report from the coronary artery surgery study.** *J Am Coll Cardiol.* 1989; **13**:531–7.
2. Yamanaka O, Hobbs RE. **Coronary artery anomalies in 126,595 patients undergoing coronary arteriography.** *Cathet Cardiovasc Diagn.* 1990; **21**:28–40.
3. Maron BJ, Shirani J, Poliac LC, Mathenge R, Roberts WC, Mueller FO. **Sudden death in young competitive athletes. Clinical, demographic, and pathological profiles.** *JAMA.* 1996; **276**:199–204.
4. Corrado D, Basso C, Rizzoli G, Schiavon M, Thiene G. **Does sports activity enhance the risk of sudden death in adolescents and young adults?** *J Am Coll Cardiol.* 2003; **42**:1959–63.
5. Roberts WC, Siegel RJ, Zipes DP. **Origin of the right coronary artery from the left sinus of valsalva and its functional consequences: analysis of 10 necropsy patients.** *Am J Cardiol.* 1982; **49**:863–8.
6. Cheitlin MD, De Castro CM, McAllister HA. **Sudden death as a complication of anomalous left coronary origin from the anterior sinus of valsalva, a not-so-minor congenital anomaly.** *Circulation.* 1974; **50**:780–7.
7. Kragel AH, Roberts WC. **Anomalous origin of either the right or left main coronary artery from the aorta with subsequent coursing between aorta and pulmonary trunk: analysis of 32 necropsy cases.** *Am J Cardiol.* 1988; **62**:771–7.
8. Taylor AJ, Byers JP, Cheitlin MD, Virmani R. **Anomalous right or left coronary artery from the contralateral coronary sinus: "High-risk" abnormalities in the initial coronary artery course and heterogeneous clinical outcomes.** *Am Heart J.* 1997; **133**:428–35.
9. Frommelt PC, Sheridan DC, Berger S, Frommelt MA, Tweddell JS. **Ten-year experience with surgical unroofing of anomalous aortic origin of a coronary artery from the opposite sinus with an interarterial course.** *J Thorac Cardiovasc Surg.* 2011; **142**:1046–51.
10. Krasuski RA, Magyar D, Hart S, Kalahasti V, Lorber R, Hobbs R, Pettersson G, Blackstone E. **Long-term outcome and impact of surgery on adults with coronary arteries originating from the opposite coronary cusp.** *Circulation.* 2011; **123**:154–62.
11. Angelini P, Velasco JA, Flamm S. **Coronary anomalies: incidence, pathophysiology, and clinical relevance.** *Circulation.* 2002; **105**:2449–54.
12. Wilkins CE, Betancourt B, Mathur VS, Massumi A, De Castro CM, Garcia E, Hall RJ. **Coronary artery anomalies: a review of more than 10,000 patients from the clayton cardiovascular laboratories.** *Tex Heart Inst J.* 1988; **15**:166–73.
13. Kim WY, Danias PG, Stuber M, Flamm SD, Plein S, Nagel E, Langerak SE, Weber OM, Pedersen EM, Schmidt M, Botnar RM, Manning WJ. **Coronary magnetic resonance angiography for the detection of coronary stenoses.** *N Engl J Med.* 2001; **345**:1863–9.
14. Greenwood JP, Maredia N, Radjenovic A, Brown JM, Nixon J, Farrin AJ, Dickinson C, Younger JF, Ridgway JP, Sculpher M, Ball SG, Plein S. **Clinical evaluation of magnetic resonance imaging in coronary heart disease: the ce-marc study.** *Trials.* 2009; **10**:62.
15. Thygesen K, Alpert JS, Jaffe AS, Simoons ML, Chaitman BR, White HD. **Third universal definition of myocardial infarction.** *Nat Rev Cardiol.* 2012; **9**:620–33.
16. Shiralkar S, Rennie A, Snow M, Galland RB, Lewis MH, Gower-Thomas K. **Doctors' knowledge of radiation exposure: questionnaire study.** *BMJ.* 2003; **327**:371–2.
17. Razavi R, Hill DL, Keevil SF, Miquel ME, Muthurangu V, Hegde S, Rhode K, Barnett M, Van Vaals J, Hawkes DJ, Baker E. **Cardiac catheterisation guided by mri in children and adults with congenital heart disease.** *Lancet.* 2003; **362**:1877–82.
18. NRPB. *Guidelines on Patient Dose to Promote the Optimisation of Protection for Diagnostic Medical Exposures. Vol 10: No. 1 Radiological Protection Board, Chilton.* : ; 1999.
19. McConnell MV, Ganz P, Selwyn AP, Li W, Edelman RR, Manning WJ. **Identification of anomalous coronary arteries and their anatomic course by magnetic resonance coronary angiography.** *Circulation.* 1995; **92**:3158–62.
20. Post JC, Van Rossum AC, Bronzwaer JG, De Cock CC, Hofman MB, Valk J, Visser CA. **Magnetic resonance angiography of anomalous coronary arteries. A new gold standard for delineating the proximal course?** *Circulation.* 1995; **92**:3163–71.
21. Taylor AM, Thorne SA, Rubens MB, Jhooti P, Keegan J, Gatehouse PD, Wiesmann F, Grothues F, Somerville J, Pennell DJ. **Coronary artery imaging in grown up congenital heart disease: complementary role of magnetic resonance and x-ray coronary angiography.** *Circulation.* 2000; **101**:1670–8.
22. Bunce NH, Lorenz CH, Keegan J, Lesser J, Reyes EM, Firmin DN, Pennell DJ. **Coronary artery anomalies: assessment with free-breathing three-dimensional coronary mr angiography.** *Radiology.* 2003; **227**:201–8.
23. Pennell DJ, Sechtem UP, Higgins CB, Manning WJ, Pohost GM, Rademakers FE, Rossum AC, Shaw LJ, Yucel EK. **Clinical indications for cardiovascular magnetic resonance (cmr): consensus panel report.** *Eur Heart J.* 2004; **25**:1940–65.

24. Hundley WG, Bluemke DA, Finn JP, Flamm SD, Fogel MA, Friedrich MG, Ho VB, Jerosch-Herold M, Kramer CM, Manning WJ, Patel M, Pohost GM, Stillman AE, White RD, Woodard PK. **Accf/acr/aha/nasci/scmr 2010 expert consensus document on cardiovascular magnetic resonance: a report of the american college of cardiology foundation task force on expert consensus documents.** *Circulation.* 2010; **121:**2462–508.
25. Angelini P. **Coronary artery anomalies: an entity in search of an identity.** *Circulation.* 2007; **115:**1296–305.
26. Eckart RE, Scoville SL, Campbell CL, Shry EA, Stajduhar KC, Potter RN, Pearse LA, Virmani R. **Sudden death in young adults: a 25-year review of autopsies in military recruits.** *Ann Intern Med.* 2004; **141:**829–34.
27. Angelini P, Walmsley RP, Libreros A, Ott DA. **Symptomatic anomalous origination of the left coronary artery from the opposite sinus of valsalva. Clinical presentations, diagnosis, and surgical repair.** *Tex Heart Inst J.* 2006; **33:**171–9.
28. Basso C, Maron BJ, Corrado D, Thiene G. **Clinical profile of congenital coronary artery anomalies with origin from the wrong aortic sinus leading to sudden death in young competitive athletes.** *J Am Coll Cardiol.* 2000; **35:**1493–501.
29. Opolski MP, Pregowski J, Kruk M, Witkowski A, Kwiecinska S, Lubienska E, Demkow M, Hryniewiecki T, Michalek P, Ruzyllo W, Kepka C. **Prevalence and characteristics of coronary anomalies originating from the opposite sinus of valsalva in 8,522 patients referred for coronary computed tomography angiography.** *Am J Cardiol.* 2013; **111:**1361–7.
30. Jo Y, Uranaka Y, Iwaki H, Matsumoto J, Koura T, Negishi K. **Sudden cardiac arrest: associated with anomalous origin of the right coronary artery from the left main coronary artery.** *Tex Heart Inst J.* 2011; **38:**539–43.
31. Chaitman BR, Lesperance J, Saltiel J, Bourassa MG. **Clinical, angiographic, and hemodynamic findings in patients with anomalous origin of the coronary arteries.** *Circulation.* 1976; **53:**122–31.
32. Tuzcu EM, Kapadia SR, Tutar E, Ziada KM, Hobbs RE, McCarthy PM, Young JB, Nissen SE. **High prevalence of coronary atherosclerosis in asymptomatic teenagers and young adults: evidence from intravascular ultrasound.** *Circulation.* 2001; **103:**2705–10.
33. Lee HJ, Hong YJ, Kim HY, Lee J, Hur J, Choi BW, Chang HJ, Nam JE, Choe KO, Kim YJ. **Anomalous origin of the right coronary artery from the left coronary sinus with an interarterial course: subtypes and clinical importance.** *Radiology.* 2012; **262:**101–8.
34. Grollman JH Jr, Mao SS, Weinstein SR. **Arteriographic demonstration of both kinking at the origin and compression between the great vessels of an anomalous right coronary artery arising in common with a left coronary artery from above the left sinus of valsalva.** *Cathet Cardiovasc Diagn.* 1992; **25:**46–51.
35. Hariharan R, Kacere RD, Angelini P. **Can stent-angioplasty be a valid alternative to surgery when revascularization is indicated for anomalous origination of a coronary artery from the opposite sinus?** *Tex Heart Inst J.* 2002; **29:**308–13.
36. Angelini P, Velasco JA, Ott D, Khoshnevis GR. **Anomalous coronary artery arising from the opposite sinus: descriptive features and pathophysiologic mechanisms, as documented by intravascular ultrasonography.** *J Invasive Cardiol.* 2003; **15:**507–14.
37. Taylor AJ, Rogan KM, Virmani R. **Sudden cardiac death associated with isolated congenital coronary artery anomalies.** *J Am Coll Cardiol.* 1992; **20:**640–7.

Permissions

All chapters in this book were first published in JCMR, by BioMed Central; hereby published with permission under the Creative Commons Attribution License or equivalent. Every chapter published in this book has been scrutinized by our experts. Their significance has been extensively debated. The topics covered herein carry significant findings which will fuel the growth of the discipline. They may even be implemented as practical applications or may be referred to as a beginning point for another development.

The contributors of this book come from diverse backgrounds, making this book a truly international effort. This book will bring forth new frontiers with its revolutionizing research information and detailed analysis of the nascent developments around the world.

We would like to thank all the contributing authors for lending their expertise to make the book truly unique. They have played a crucial role in the development of this book. Without their invaluable contributions this book wouldn't have been possible. They have made vital efforts to compile up to date information on the varied aspects of this subject to make this book a valuable addition to the collection of many professionals and students.

This book was conceptualized with the vision of imparting up-to-date information and advanced data in this field. To ensure the same, a matchless editorial board was set up. Every individual on the board went through rigorous rounds of assessment to prove their worth. After which they invested a large part of their time researching and compiling the most relevant data for our readers.

The editorial board has been involved in producing this book since its inception. They have spent rigorous hours researching and exploring the diverse topics which have resulted in the successful publishing of this book. They have passed on their knowledge of decades through this book. To expedite this challenging task, the publisher supported the team at every step. A small team of assistant editors was also appointed to further simplify the editing procedure and attain best results for the readers.

Apart from the editorial board, the designing team has also invested a significant amount of their time in understanding the subject and creating the most relevant covers. They scrutinized every image to scout for the most suitable representation of the subject and create an appropriate cover for the book.

The publishing team has been an ardent support to the editorial, designing and production team. Their endless efforts to recruit the best for this project, has resulted in the accomplishment of this book. They are a veteran in the field of academics and their pool of knowledge is as vast as their experience in printing. Their expertise and guidance has proved useful at every step. Their uncompromising quality standards have made this book an exceptional effort. Their encouragement from time to time has been an inspiration for everyone.

The publisher and the editorial board hope that this book will prove to be a valuable piece of knowledge for researchers, students, practitioners and scholars across the globe.

List of Contributors

Manish Motwani, Ananth Kidambi, Timothy A Fairbairn, Akhlaque Uddin, John P Greenwood and Sven Plein
Multidisciplinary Cardiovascular Research Centre & The Division of Cardiovascular and Diabetes Research, Leeds Institute of Genetics, Health & Therapeutics, University of Leeds, Leeds, UK

Steven Sourbron
Division of Medical Physics, University of Leeds, Leeds, UK

Sebastian Kozerke
Institute for Biomedical Engineering, University and ETH Zurich, Zurich, Switzerland

Andreas Schuster and Gerd Hasenfuß
University Medical Center Goettingen, Clinic of Cardiology and Pneumology, Goettingen, Germany

Verena Reupke
Department of Experimental Animal Medicine, Georg-August University, Goettingen, Germany

Andreas Schuster, Gerd Hasenfuß, Christian Oliver Ritter and Christina Unterberg-Buchwald
DZHK (German Centre for Cardiovascular Research), Partner Site Goettingen, Berlin, Germany

Christine Stadelmann
Department of Neuropathology, University Medical Center Goettingen, Goettingen, Germany

Michael Steinmetz
University Medical Center Goettingen, Clinic of Pediatric Cardiology and Intensive Care Medicine, Goettingen, Germany

Martin Uecker, Joachim Lotz and Robin Niklas Wilke
University Medical Center Goettingen, Institute for Diagnostic and Interventional Radiology, Goettingen, Germany

Reuben Thomas, Xiuling Qi, Jennifer Barry and Graham A. Wright
Physical Sciences Platform, Sunnybrook Research Institute, 2075 Bayview Avenue, Room M7-510, Toronto, ON M4N 3M5, Canada

Nilesh R. Ghugre
Department of Medical Biophysics, University of Toronto, Toronto, ON, Canada

Bradley H. Strauss and Mihaela Pop
Schulich Heart Research Program, Sunnybrook Health Sciences Centre, Toronto, ON, Canada

Susan Newbigging
The Toronto Centre for Phenogenomics, Mount Sinai Hospital, Toronto, ON, Canada

Susie Parnham, Suchi Grover, Craig Bradbrook, Carmine G. De Pasquale and Joseph B. Selvanayagam
Department of Cardiovascular Medicine, Flinders Medical Centre, Bedford Park, Adelaide, SA 5042, Australia

Jonathan M. Gleadle
Department of Renal Medicine, Bedford Park, Adelaide, SA, Australia

Darryl Leong, Joseph B. Selvanayagam, Carmine G. De Pasquale and Susie Parnham
School of Medicine, Flinders University, Bedford Park, Adelaide, SA, Australia

Richard J. Woodman
Flinders Centre for Epidemiology and Biostatistics, School of Medicine, Flinders University, Bedford Park, Adelaide, SA, Australia

Darryl Leong
Population Health Research Institute, Hamilton, ON, Canada

Per Hammar
Västmanland County Hospital Västerås, Department of Radiology, Västerås S-72189, Sweden

Anna M. Nordenskjöld
Department of Cardiology, Örebro University Hospital, S-70182 Örebro, Sweden

Nermin Hadziosmanovic and Bertil Lindahl
Uppsala Clinical Research Centre, S-75237 Uppsala, Sweden

Bertil Lindahl
Department of Medical Sciences, Cardiology, Uppsala University, Uppsala S-75105, Sweden

Tomas Bjerner, Olov Duvernoy and Håkan Ahlström
Department of Radiology, Oncology and Radiation Science, Uppsala University, S-75185 Uppsala, Sweden

Lars Johansson
Astra Zeneca, Molndal, Sweden

Florian von Knobelsdorff-Brenkenhoff and Jeanette Schulz-Menger
Working Group Cardiovascular Magnetic Resonance, Experimental and Clinical Research Center, a joint cooperation between the Charité Medical Faculty and the Max-Delbrueck Center for Molecular Medicine; and HELIOS Klinikum Berlin Buch, Department of Cardiology and Nephrology, Berlin, Germany

Jannike Nickander, Magnus Lundin, Goran Abdula, Andreas Sigfridsson and Martin Ugander
Department of Clinical Physiology, Karolinska Institutet and Karolinska University Hospital, Stockholm, Sweden

Peder Sörensson
Department of Medicine, Unit of Cardiology, Karolinska Institutet and Karolinska University Hospital, Stockholm, Sweden

Stefania Rosmini and James C. Moon
Institute of Cardiovascular Science, University College London, London, UK

Peter Kellman
National Heart, Lung, and Blood Institute, National Institutes of Health, Bethesda, MD, USA

Michael S. Hansen, Sonia Nielles-Vallespin and Hui Xue
National Heart, Lung, and Blood Institute, National Institutes of Health, DHHS, 10 Center Drive MSC-1061, Bethesda, MD 20892, USA

Martin Ugander and Raquel Themudo
Department of Clinical Physiology, Karolinska Institutet and Karolinska University Hospital, Stockholm, Sweden

Ashita Barthur, Anish Kirpalani, Joseph J. Barfett, Gauri R. Karur and Djeven P. Deva
Department of Medical Imaging, St. Michael's Hospital, University of Toronto, Toronto, ON, Canada

Jannike Nickander, Rashida Haq, Vinita Dhir and Christine Brezden-Masley
Division of Hematology/Oncology, St. Michael's Hospital, University of Toronto, Toronto, ON, Canada

Djeven P. Deva, Anish Kirpalani, Joseph J. Barfett and Christine Brezden-Masley
Keenan Research Centre, Li Ka Shing Knowledge Institute, St. Michael's Hospital, University of Toronto, Toronto, ON, Canada

Andrew T. Yan and Kim A. Connelly
Terrence Donnelly Heart Centre, St. Michael's Hospital, University of Toronto, Toronto, ON, Canada
Division of Cardiology, St. Michael's Hospital, University of Toronto, Toronto, ON, Canada

Kelvin K. W. Chan
Sunnybrook Health Sciences Centre, University of Toronto, Cancer Care Ontario, Canadian Center for Applied Research in Cancer Control, Toronto, ON, Canada

Laura Jimenez-Juan
Department of Medical Imaging, Sunnybrook Health Sciences Centre, University of Toronto, Toronto, ON, Canada

Linyuan Jing, Arichanah Pulenthiran, Christopher D. Nevius, Abba Mejia-Spiegeler, Jonathan D. Suever and Christopher M. Haggerty
Department of Imaging Science and Innovation, Geisinger Health System, 100 North Academy Avenue, Danville 17822-4400, PA, USA

H. Lester Kirchner, Linyuan Jing and Arichanah Pulenthiran
Biomedical and Translational Informatics Institute, Geisinger Health System, Danville, PA, USA

Gregory J. Wehner
Department of Biomedical Engineering, University of Kentucky, Lexington, KY, USA

Brandon K. Fornwalt
Department of Radiology, Geisinger Health System, Danville, PA, USA

Maximilian Fuetterer, Julia Busch, Sophie M. Peereboom, Constantin von Deuster, Lukas Wissmann, Christian T. Stoeck and Sebastian Kozerke
Institute for Biomedical Engineering, University and ETH Zurich, Gloriastrasse 35, 8092 Zurich, Switzerland

Thea Fleischmann, Nikola Cesarovic and Miriam Lipiski
Division of Surgical Research, University Hospital Zurich, Sternwartstrasse 14, 8091 Zurich, Switzerland

Kihei Yoneyama, Bharath A. Venkatesh and João A.C. Lima
Department of Cardiology, Johns Hopkins University, Baltimore, MD, USA

David A. Bluemke
Radiology and Imaging Sciences, National Institutes of Health Clinical Center, Bethesda, MD, USA

Robyn L. McClelland
Department of Biostatistics, University of Washington, Seattle, WA, USA

Kihei Yoneyama
St. Marianna University School of Medicine, Kawasaki, Japan

João A. C. Lima
Professor of Medicine, Radiology and Epidemiology, Johns Hopkins Hospital, Johns Hopkins University, Blalock 524D1, 600 North Wolfe Street, Baltimore, MD 21287, USA

Henrik Engblom, Shahnaz Akil, Marcus Carlsson, Fredrik Hedeer and Håkan Arheden
Department of Clinical Physiology, Clinical Sciences, Lund University and Lund University Hospital, Lund, Sweden

Peter Kellman, Michael S. Hansen and Hui Xue
National Heart, Lung, and Blood Institute, National Institutes of Health, DHHS, 10 Center Drive, Bethesda, MD 20892, USA

Cecilia Hindorf and Jenny Oddstig
Department of Radiation Physics, Lund University Hospital, Lund, Sweden

Anthony H. Aletras
Laboratory of Computing, Medical Informatics and Biomedical - Imaging Technologies, School of Medicine, Aristotle University of Thessaloniki, Thessaloniki, Greece

Toby Rogers, Jaffar M. Khan, Annette Stine, William H. Schenke, Laurie P. Grant, Jonathan R. Mazal, Adrienne Campbell-Washburn, Michael S. Hansen, Rajiv Ramasawmy, Daniel A. Herzka, Hui Xue, Peter Kellman and Anthony Z. Faranesh
Cardiovascular and Pulmonary Branch, Division of Intramural Research, National Heart Lung and Blood Institute, National Institutes of Health, Bethesda, MD, USA

Kanishka Ratnayaka
Department of Cardiology, Rady Children's Hospital, San Diego, CA, USA

Elena K. Grant
Department of Cardiology, Children's National Medical Center, Washington, DC, USA

Robert J. Lederman
Division of Intramural Research, National Heart Lung and Blood Institute, National Institutes of Health, Building 10, Room 2c713, Bethesda, MD 20892-1538, USA

Benjamin Zorach, Pelbreton C. Balfour Jr, Yang Yang, Roshin Mathew, Jonathan Pan and Angela M. Taylor
Department of Medicine, Cardiology Division, University of Virginia Health System, Charlottesville, VA, USA

Peter W. Shaw
Berkshire Medical Center, Pittsfield, MA,USA

Jamieson Bourque
Department of Radiology, Cardiovascular Imaging Center, University of Virginia Health System, Charlottesville, VA, USA

Sujith Kuruvilla
Department of Medicine, Philadelphia VA Medical Center, University of Pennsylvania, Perelman School of Medicine, Philadelphia, PA, USA

Frederick H. Epstein, Christopher M. Kramer, Craig H. Meyer and Yang Yang
Department of Biomedical Engineering, University of Virginia Health System, Charlottesville, VA, USA

Jorge A. Gonzalez
Division of Cardiovascular Disease, Scripps Clinic, Division of Cardiology, Cardiovascular Imaging, Division of Radiology, La Jolla, San Diego, CA, USA

Stefan K. Piechnik, Alexander Liu, Rohan S. Wijesurendra, Masliza Mahmod, Rina Ariga, Jane M. Francis, Stefan Neubauer and Vanessa M. Ferreira
University of Oxford Centre for Clinical Magnetic Resonance Research, Division of Cardiovascular Medicine, Radcliffe Department of Medicine, University of Oxford, Oxford, UK

Eylem Levelt
Department of Cardiovascular Sciences, University of Leicester, Leicester, UK

Andreas Greiser
Siemens Healthcare GmbH, Erlangen, Germany

Kieran Clarke
Department of Physiology, Anatomy and Genetics, University of Oxford, Oxford, UK

Theodoros D. Karamitsos
1st Department of Cardiology, Aristotle University of Thessaloniki, AHEPA Hospital St. Kyriakidi 1, 54636 Thessaloniki, Greece

Harrie C M van den Bosch, Wikke Setz-Pels and John Wondergem
Department of Radiology, Catharina Hospital, Michelangelolaan 2, 5623EJ, Eindhoven, The Netherlands

Albert de Roos and Jos J M Westenberg
Department of Radiology, Leiden University Medical Center, Leiden, The Netherlands

Ron Wolterbeek
Department of Medical Statistics, Leiden University Medical Center, Leiden, The Netherlands

Lucien E M Duijm
Department of Radiology, Canisius-Wilhelmina Hospital, Nijmegen, The Netherlands

Joep A W Teijink
Department of Vascular Surgery, Catharina Hospital, Eindhoven, The Netherlands

Jimmy C Lu and Adam L. Dorfman
Department of Pediatrics and Communicable Diseases, Division of Pediatric Cardiology, University of Michigan, Ann Arbor, MI, USA

Maryam Ghadimi Mahani
Department of Radiology, Section of Pediatric Radiology, University of Michigan, Ann Arbor, MI, USA

James C Nielsen and Layne Morowitz
Departments of Pediatrics and Radiology, Stony Brook University, Stony Brook, NY, USA

Muzammil Musani
Department of Medicine, Division of Cardiology, Stony Brook University, Stony Brook, NY, USA

Prachi P. Agarwal and El-Sayed H. Ibrahim
Department of Radiology, Division of Cardiothoracic Radiology, University of Michigan, Ann Arbor, MI, USA

Saeed Mirsadraee Martin Connell, Calum Gray and Tom MacGillivray
Clinical Research Imaging Centre, University of Edinburgh, Edinburgh, UK

Marc R Dweck, Shirjel Alam, Michelle C Williams, David E Newby, Scott IK Semple and Giorgos Papanastasiou
Centre for Cardiovascular Science, University of Edinburgh, Edinburgh, UK

Lucy E Kershaw
Christie Medical Physics and Engineering, The Christie NHS FT, Manchester, UK

Akhlaque Uddin, Petra Bijsterveld, Ananth Kidambi, Adam K McDiarmid, Sven Plein and John P Greenwood
Multidisciplinary Cardiovascular Research Centre (MCRC) & Leeds Institute of Genetics, Health and Therapeutics, University of Leeds, Leeds, UK

Mohan Sivananthan, Ansuman Saha, David P Ripley, Akhlaque Uddin, Petra Bijsterveld and Ananth Kidambi
Leeds Teaching Hospitals NHS Trust, Leeds General Infirmary, Leeds, UK

Dudley J Pennell and Albert Teis
NIHR Cardiovascular Biomedical Research Unit Royal Brompton Hospital, London, UK

Index

A

Acute Myocardial Infarction (AMI), 23

Adenosine, 2, 36-37, 70, 80-82, 86, 91, 94, 115, 138-141, 144, 146, 160, 164-165, 167-169, 171-176, 195, 201

Analysis Of Variance, 3, 25, 32, 105, 108, 113

Aortic Arch, 63, 68, 189, 193

Arterial Input Function, 3, 82, 85, 89, 94-95, 125-126, 139-140, 146, 161, 165, 170, 194-195, 197-198, 200-203

Atherosclerosis, 43-45, 51, 69, 103, 127-128, 130, 135-137, 146, 159-160, 165, 176-177, 183-185, 210-211

B

Bicuspid Aortic Valve, 59, 63, 68, 186

C

Cardiovascular Magnetic Resonance, 1, 32-33, 35, 42-45, 51, 53, 68-69, 71-72, 80-83, 95-96, 102, 104-105, 114-115, 125-127, 135-136, 165-168, 171, 175-177, 186, 193-194, 203-204, 210-211

Cardiovascular Magnetic Resonance (LGE CMR), 44

Carotid Arteries, 181

Chronic Kidney Disease (CKD), 35

Cine Images, 161, 186, 190

Cmr Fluoroscopy, 147-149, 153, 158

Coefficient Of Variation, 108, 113, 184

Computed Tomography, 42-43, 59, 68, 125, 127, 135, 139-140, 145, 161, 165, 176, 203-204

Congenital Heart Disease, 53-54, 63-65, 70, 100, 150, 158, 186-187, 190-193, 209-210

Contrast-to-noise Ratio, 86, 94, 123, 125-126, 187, 191

Coronary Artery Bypass Graft (CABG), 45

Coronary Artery Disease (CAD), 1-2, 6-7, 9, 35-36, 138-139, 160, 167

Coronary Microvascular Dysfunction, 52, 146, 165-168, 173-176

Coronary Sinus, 205-206, 208, 210

D

Displacement Encoding With Stimulated Echoes (DENSE), 105

Distal Aorta, 177-179, 181-184

Distributed Parameter Modeling, 194, 197-201

E

Endomyocardial Biopsies (EMB), 12-13

Extracellular Volume Fraction (ECV), 78, 161

F

Fast Low Angle Shot (FLASH), 195

Fermi Modeling, 194-195, 200-202

First-pass Perfusion, 3-4, 115, 121, 125, 139, 143-144, 161, 164, 167, 169

Fractional Flow Reserve, 9-10, 40, 43, 51-52, 143, 145, 166, 174, 176, 194-195, 201-202

G

Gradient Recalled Echo (GRE), 85

H

Hyperpolarization, 115, 118

Hypertrophic Cardiomyopathy, 54, 58, 67, 69-70, 80, 208, 210

I

Interquartile Range (IQR), 47

Intima-media Thickness, 178, 184

Intravascular Ultrasound, 209-211

Invasive Coronary Angiography, 42, 174, 194, 197, 201-202

Ischemia-reperfusion Injury (IRI), 23

Ischemic Heart Disease, 47, 53, 59, 61, 139, 143, 145-146, 165

L

Late Gadolinium Enhancement, 12, 15, 20, 24, 32, 38, 44, 51, 68, 72, 79, 94, 136, 140-141, 145, 161, 167, 169, 171, 186, 191-192

Luminal Stenosis, 3, 167-169, 206

M

Major Adverse Cardiovascular Events, 28, 207-208

Metabolic Syndrome, 130, 136, 159-160, 165, 175

Microvascular Disease, 40, 43, 83, 142, 159-160, 163, 165

Microvascular Obstruction, 22-23, 25-26, 31-34, 168

Modified Look-locker Inversion Recovery (MOLLI), 80

Mr Coronary Angiography (MRCA), 35

Multi-ethnic Study Of Atherosclerosis, 103, 127, 135-137, 176

Myocardial Blood Flow (MBF), 1-2, 124, 163, 198

Myocardial Hemorrhage, 22-23, 28, 30-34

Myocardial Infarction, 2, 5, 22-23, 28, 31-34, 36, 44, 49, 51-52, 54, 62, 69, 72, 80, 95, 118, 130, 132, 136, 140, 145-146, 148, 161, 173, 176, 183-184, 204-207, 209-210

Myocardial Ischemia, 35-36, 42-43, 58, 139, 160, 174

Myocardial Perfusion, 1, 6-11, 35, 37-43, 62-63, 66-67, 82-84, 86, 91-95, 115-116, 123, 125-126, 130-131, 136, 138-146, 159-174, 176, 197-199, 201-203

Myocardial Perfusion Reserve (MPR), 1, 138, 159-160, 163

Myocardial Perfusion Reserve Index (MPRI), 37-38, 40, 167, 170

Myocarditis, 12-13, 20, 55, 57-58, 62-63, 65, 67, 70, 72, 80, 176, 208

N

Nonlinear Inverse Reconstruction (NLINV), 12

Normalized Wall Index, 177, 180-182

O

Opposite Sinus Of Valsalva, 204, 207

P

Parallel Acquisition Technique (PAT), 73

Percutaneous Coronary Intervention (PCI), 45, 139

Perfusion Quantification, 82-83, 125, 146, 161, 163

Peripheral Arterial Occlusive Disease, 177, 184-185

Positron Emission Tomography, 1, 11, 43, 62, 66, 138-139, 142-146, 165-166, 203

Principal Component Analysis (PCA), 2

Proximal Aorta, 134, 177-178, 182-184

Pulmonary Artery, 56, 103, 112, 114, 147-152, 156-157, 189-190, 205, 207-210

Pulmonary Hypertension (PH), 79

Pulmonary Venous Anatomy, 188

Pulse Wave Velocity, 134, 176-179, 182-185

R

Region Of Interest (ROI), 3

Renal Transplant (RT), 35-36

Right Coronary Artery (RCA), 37, 47, 205

Right Heart Catheterization, 147-150, 158

S

Saturation Recovery (SR) Sequence, 83

Shortened Modified Look-locker Inversion Recovery (SHMOLLI), 81, 176

Signal-to-noise Ratio, 82, 85, 116, 119, 125-126, 187, 191

Specific Absorption Rate (SAR), 83, 187

T

Targeted Biopsy, 12-13, 17

Thoracic Aorta, 179

Type 2 Diabetes Mellitus, 167-168, 171-172, 175, 185

U

Unrecognized Myocardial Infarction (UMI), 44

www.ingramcontent.com/pod-product-compliance
Lightning Source LLC
LaVergne TN
LVHW080654210926
848485LV00003B/377